RADIOLOGIC AND OTHER BIOPHYSICAL METHODS IN TUMOR DIAGNOSIS

Proceedings of the Annual Clinical Conferences on Cancer
sponsored by The University of Texas System Cancer Center
M. D. Anderson Hospital and Tumor Institute,
and published by Year Book Medical Publishers, Inc.

TUMORS OF THE SKIN

TUMORS OF BONE AND SOFT TISSUE

RECENT ADVANCES IN THE DIAGNOSIS OF CANCER

CANCER OF THE GASTROINTESTINAL TRACT

CANCER OF THE UTERUS AND OVARY

NEOPLASIA IN CHILDHOOD

BREAST CANCER: EARLY AND LATE

LEUKEMIA-LYMPHOMA

REHABILITATION OF THE CANCER PATIENT

ENDOCRINE AND NONENDOCRINE
HORMONE-PRODUCING TUMORS

NEOPLASIA OF HEAD AND NECK

RADIOLOGIC AND OTHER BIOPHYSICAL
METHODS IN TUMOR DIAGNOSIS

RADIOLOGIC AND OTHER BIOPHYSICAL METHODS IN TUMOR DIAGNOSIS

A Collection of Papers Presented at the Eighteenth Annual Clinical Conference on Cancer, 1973, at The University of Texas System Cancer Center M. D. Anderson Hospital and Tumor Institute, Houston, Texas

YEAR BOOK MEDICAL PUBLISHERS, INC.
35 East Wacker Drive, Chicago

Library of Congress Catalog Card Number: 74-19963

International Standard Book Number: 0-8151-0211-9

Acknowledgments

FOR THEIR SUPPORT in making possible both the Eighteenth Annual Clinical Conference and the publication of this monograph, the staff of M. D. Anderson Hospital and Tumor Institute of The University of Texas System Cancer Center gratefully acknowledges the assistance of the Texas Division of the American Cancer Society, American Cancer Society, Inc., and the Division of Continuing Education of The University of Texas Health Science Center at Houston.

The program was arranged and organized by a committee composed of the following staff members of M. D. Anderson Hospital: Gerald D. Dodd, Jr., and Thomas P. Haynie, III, co-chairmen; and members H. Stephen Gallager, Howard J. Glenn, Arnold M. Goldman, James M. Hevezi, Monroe F. Jahns, William O. Russell, Robert J. Shalek, Sidney Wallace, and Alfonso Zermeno.

This volume was prepared for publication by the members of the M. D. Anderson Hospital Department of Publications, under the direction of Dr. Russell W. Cumley and the supervision of Joan E. McCay, as follows: Susan B. Freitag and Dorothy M. Beane, associate editors; and Larry W. Dybala, Carol A. Flynn, Walter J. Pagel, Jane E. Parker, and D. Ruth SoRelle, assistant editors. Secretarial assistance was provided by Connie C. Fox and Alice S. Rojas; and Joyce M. Johnston, (Dept. of Diagnostic Radiology).

Many of the illustrations in this volume were prepared by members of the M. D. Anderson Hospital Department of Medical Communications.

Contents

vii

Introduction

R. LEE CLARK, M.D., M.Sc., D.Sc. (Hon.)
President, The University of Texas System Cancer Center; and Professor of Surgery, The University of Texas M. D. Anderson Hospital and Tumor Institute, Houston, Texas

THE ANNUAL CLINICAL CONFERENCES of The University of Texas M. D. Anderson Hospital and Tumor Institute began in 1956 for the purposes of exchanging and discussing the newest applicable and reliable methods for the diagnosis and treatment of cancer, and to learn about the development of more refined or totally new devices and techniques for the discovery of human physiological messages awaiting interpretation.

During these 18 years, M. D. Anderson Hospital and the Division of Continuing Education of the Graduate School of Biomedical Sciences, now within The University of Texas Health Science Center at Houston, have had the unstinting encouragement and support of The University of Texas Board of Regents, represented today by Dr. Joe Nelson, and of the American Cancer Society, both the Texas and the national divisions, for these conferences.

Nine years ago, in 1964, our ninth clinical conference was entitled "Recent Advances in the Diagnosis of Cancer." Some of the techniques discussed as possibly useful for the future are standard diagnostic procedures today. Yet, some that were available as long as 2 decades before that conference, as was Dr. George Papanicolaou's exfoliative cytologic technique for the detection of early carcinoma of the uterine cervix, are still not adequately and routinely used for the significant reduction of the incidence and mortality of cancer that they are capable of achieving.

The ideal of all oncologists is not only the cure or control of cancer

1

but the prevention of as many cancers as possible. We should all feel the urgency of the responsibility to devise sensitive techniques to detect precancerous states, and to incorporate these techniques in our routine medical examinations. One promising possibility for the achievement of the ideal of cancer prevention lies in investigations in the field of immunodiagnosis. There is evidence that tumor antigens are present in premalignant as well as malignant lesions. Detection of these precancerous tumor antigens in serum by immunodiagnostic techniques might lead to massive screening programs, if not of the entire population at least of those individuals deemed to be at higher risk for the development of cancer because of hereditary, environmental, or genetic factors.

For those lesions not detected prior to malignant cell transformation, equally sensitive techniques for the detection of tumor antigens and cancer cells in their earliest phases of growth, and prior to the opportunity for spread to other areas, are urgently needed.

During the ninth clinical conference, Dr. Douglas H. Sprunt of the Department of Pathology of the University of Tennessee, said in his address:

"If a method of curing cancer in its early stages were discovered tomorrow, we would not be able to use it effectively, as we have no means for detecting many early cancers. We cannot even use effectively the methods we now have for curing cancer, as we have no test that can be applied on a large scale to healthy individuals for the detection of cancer in its early and asymptomatic stage."

Although that was true nine years ago, this statement is fortunately becoming less and less in accord with the facts. Diagnostic tools that have been available for many years have undergone progressive refinement and modification, and our understanding of molecular mechanisms, microanatomical structures, cell kinetics, biochemical, immunological, pharmacological, and radiophysical interrelationships has been expanding rapidly. Unfortunately, many of the techniques capable of detecting and diagnosing cancer during its early development are performed with expensive and specialized equipment and by highly trained personnel working in teams. These techniques are of little value to the individual who does not have access to assistance from these teams and their equipment. The government, however, through the National Cancer Institute, is attempting to make such services more accessible to practicing physicians and their patients by constructing and helping to develop geographically distributed major comprehensive clinical cancer research and demonstration centers.

With such modifications of traditional approaches to medical services as a greater emphasis on outpatient rather than inpatient care of many cancer patients, automation and computerization of many previously time-consuming laboratory evaluation procedures, and eventual widespread activation of routine screening procedures to detect early cancers through the Cancer Control Program in communities throughout the nation, more patients will be diagnosed before their cancers have reached advanced stages.

We have very effective methods of cancer treatment and cure now for some types of cancer, but they are curative primarily for cancers treated in the early phases of growth. We still have very limited skills in controlling and curing widespread and systemic disease.

During this meeting, some of the highly reliable and accurate diagnostic procedures which are available were described. Few of them are so highly accurate that they can stand alone. Most are used in conjunction with one or several other diagnostic procedures for confirmation.

William Cowper, English surgeon of the 18th century, might have been describing the defeatist attitudes of most physicians of the past toward the chances for cancer cure when he wrote:

> " . . . . .from the toil of dropping
> buckets into empty wells,
> and growing old in drawing nothing up."

Our foe, the malignant process, constantly challenges our imaginations, flexibility, resourcefulness, and ingenuity. The present generation of physicians considers cancer an intellectual challenge and wishes only to find the proper tools to reverse its implacable course toward death. Their "buckets" of curiosity are eagerly lowered into wells of investigation with every expectation, frequently fulfilled, of drawing forth new facts to add to the increasing sea of knowledge about the process of life and of its alterations.

Introduction of Heath Memorial Award Recipient

ROBERT C. HICKEY, M.D.

Director, The University of Texas System Cancer Center M. D. Anderson Hospital and Tumor Institute, Houston, Texas

THE HEATH MEMORIAL LECTURE for this year will be delivered by Leo G. Rigler, M.D., Professor of Radiology and Chief, Resident Training at the University of California, Los Angeles.

Our awardee and lecturer is well known in the field of diagnostic radiology. He has had many honors and accomplishments—the teaching and leadership skills which have produced so many prominent students, now themselves professors in leading institutions, are perhaps his greatest. He was born the same year, 1896, that Professor Wilhelm Roentgen discovered X rays.

I knew of Dr. Rigler, a pioneer in roentgenology and now a recognized leader, especially in cancer diagnosis, from the late Dr. Dabney Kerr. This was during the time Dr. Rigler was at Minneapolis General Hospital. A native of Minnesota, he began his career there after graduating from the University of Minnesota. He became Chief of Radiology at Minneapolis General Hospital in 1927, then Professor and Chairman of the Department of Radiology at the University of Minnesota for 20 years. He did much of his fruitful work there, as an educator, clinical observer, and interpreter of radiologic techniques as they relate to cancer and neoplastic diseases.

Our distinguished guest has been an editor and a leader of radiological societies, as for example, Chancellor of the American College

5

of Radiology, President of the Radiological Society of America, and Trustee of the American Board of Radiology.

Among others, his awards include: Gold Medal, American College of Radiology; Gold Medal, Radiological Society of America; Caldwell Medal, American Roentgen Ray Society; and Bronze Medal, American Medical Association.

We are honored to present the eighth annual Heath Memorial Award to Dr. Leo G. Rigler.

THE HEATH MEMORIAL LECTURE:

Peripheral Carcinoma of the Lung: Incidence, Possibilities for Survival, Methods of Detection, Identification

LEO G. RIGLER, M.D.

Department of Radiology, University of California at Los Angeles, Los Angeles, California

PRIMARY CARCINOMA of the lung has been investigated so intensively for so many years that it is difficult to add anything to our present store of knowledge. There are extensive efforts at prevention, but so far they have not been highly successful. The prevalence of carcinoma of the lung in males is continuing upward at a somewhat slower rate, but the incidence in females is increasing rapidly. There is, of course, only one effective therapy, surgical extirpation. This is an extraordinarily crude method when one considers the sophisticated and subtle procedures which science has produced in other areas, but it is the only one available with any prospect of producing a cure. Unfortunately, the present 5-year survival of all patients seen throughout the country is a dreadful 8 to 10 per cent.

Peripheral carcinoma of the lung may be defined as a lesion arising in a bronchus of the third order or smaller, as contrasted to a central tumor which arises in a major, lobar, or primary segmental bronchus. This selection is made deliberately because it is this cancer which can be found most readily on X-ray examination and in the management of which the greatest therapeutic success has been attained. In a previous publication, I have delineated the first visible X-ray signs of various types of this tumor (Rigler, 1966). I have also selected peripheral carcinoma because it is my contention that the majority of

7

primary carcinomas of the lung arise in the periphery, although at operation, and especially at autopsy, they are largely found to be central. In extensive, retrospective studies of the past roentgen history of carcinoma of the lung, we have found that at least 60 per cent of all the cases were either in the periphery or had arisen in the periphery and extended centrally by the time of diagnosis (Rigler, 1957, 1964). Many therefore appeared to be of central origin but, in fact, had been peripheral at the outset (Fig. 1). These observations have since been borne out by many others (Garland *et al.*, 1962; Liebow, 1955; Tala, 1967; Veeze, 1968) and particularly by the rather remarkable studies of the pathology of lung cancer by Raeburn (1951) and Raeburn and Spencer (1953). In 750 autopsies done in the conventional manner, on individuals not suspected of having cancer, these pathologists found only one occult cancer. Raeburn (1951), however, in a study of 400 autopsies, cut the lungs in .5 mm. slices and found 4 more occult carcinomas measuring from 1 to 12 mm. in diameter, all of which would have been missed in a conventional autopsy study. Raeburn and Spencer (1953) gathered together 15 such small lesions from various autopsies and surgical specimens. Only 4 of these were found to be central in origin, while 11 were peripheral. Spencer has demonstrated by detailed pathological sections the spread from the periphery to the major bronchi by lymphatics (Spencer, personal communication). Walter and Pryce (1955), studying surgical cases, came to somewhat the same conclusion. Garland and his associates (1962), using the same method of retrospective study, concluded that 60 per cent of all primary carcinomas arose in the periphery. Tala, in Finland (1967), has presented the data on a series of 168 cases in which he was able to trace the roentgen signs of the development of the tumor back to the time when the roentgenogram was still negative. Of the total group, 38.1 per cent were located in a peripheral or intermediate area at the time of diagnosis. But when he went back to the beginnings of the process, using the method we had originally described (Rigler, O'Loughlin, and Tucker, 1953), 21 per cent more were found to have originated far away from the major bronchi so that the total noncentral lesions were about 60 per cent. Veeze (1968), in Holland, has also come to the same conclusion. It would appear, therefore, that if we could recognize carcinoma of the lung at a stage before lymphatic extension had occurred, the majority would, in fact, be in the periphery of the lung.

Carcinoma arising in a small bronchus is likely to remain asymptomatic until it has grown to a large size. It can, therefore, only be discovered when small by some form of routine examination. Once it

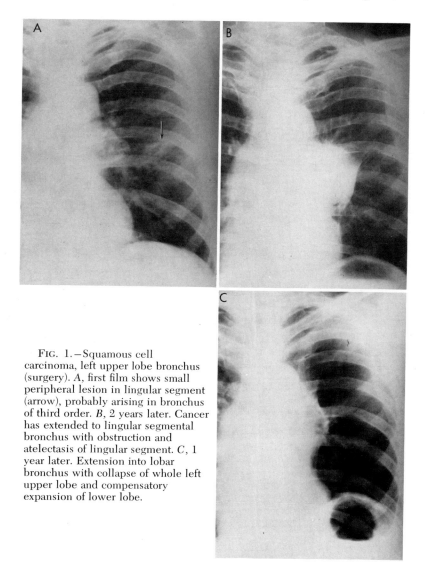

FIG. 1.—Squamous cell carcinoma, left upper lobe bronchus (surgery). *A*, first film shows small peripheral lesion in lingular segment (arrow), probably arising in bronchus of third order. *B*, 2 years later. Cancer has extended to lingular segmental bronchus with obstruction and atelectasis of lingular segment. *C*, 1 year later. Extension into lobar bronchus with collapse of whole left upper lobe and compensatory expansion of lower lobe.

extends to a large bronchus, symptoms appear rapidly and this will lead to further examination. However, if the tumor can be detected and identified in the asymptomatic phase and then resected, the outlook for survival is fairly good—far better than for the carcinomas which have either arisen centrally or have extended to a major bronchus.

Many studies in the past 10 years concern the survival of patients with peripheral carcinoma of the lung after surgical treatment. These cases are generally asymptomatic, usually found on routine X-ray examination, and show no evidence of obvious metastasis. From these surgical observations it is clear that the survival rates are far better than those obtained for all carcinomas of the lung. In addition, they indicate that the chances of survival depend largely upon the size of the lesion rather than upon its histologic type.

The reports of Steele and his associates (Steele, Kleitsch, Dunn, and Buell, 1966), who studied 392 patients from Veterans and Army Hospitals in whom a peripheral nodule in the lung was found on X-ray examination, submitted to surgery, proved histologically to be primary carcinoma, and extirpated by lobectomy or pneumonectomy, are most significant. None of the cases showed obvious clinical or roentgen evidence of regional distant metastasis. All were 6 cm. or less in diameter. Some of this group have been followed as long as 8 years. The most recent data (Steele and Buell, 1970) present the following significant figures. The 8-year relative survival of all curative resections was 40 per cent. When one divides these cases along histological lines the survival at 6 years, with a reasonable number exposed to risk, showed relatively small differences between the various cell types—not more than 9 per cent. But a substantial difference occurs when the nodules are classified as to size. At the 6-year period, for example, the survival of patients with tumors 2 cm. or less in diameter was 51 per cent, of those 2.5 to 4 cm. 41 per cent, and in those of 4.5 to 6 cm. 26 per cent. Further confirmation of these data comes from the study of Jackman, Good, Clagett, and Woolner (1969), who reported 195 cases in which malignant nodules were found on X-ray examination in asymptomatic individuals. They used an upper limit of 4 cm. in diameter; all tumors were resectable. At the end of 5 years the survival of all patients was approximately 47 per cent. Here again, the results based on histology showed relatively small differences except for a group of 17 patients with bronchioloalveolar carcinoma in whom the 3-year survival was over 90 per cent. However, in all cases there was a 5-year survival of almost 70 per cent for those lesions 2 cm. and less, 48 per cent for those 3 cm. and less, and about 40 per cent for those 4 cm. and less. Buell (1971), following patients from California hospitals for as long as 10 years, showed similar results. He was so impressed with the importance of size that he predicted that if we could reduce the minimal detectable size on X-ray examination to 5 mm. instead of the 1 to 2 cm. presently possible, a cure index of 80 per cent could be achieved in all cases less than 2 cm.

If we accept the thesis that at least 60 per cent of all cases of carcinoma of the lung begin as peripheral lesions, and that a survival of 70 per cent could possibly be achieved if the lesions could all be found when they were 2 cm. or less in size, there would, of course, be a remarkable improvement in the mortality from carcinoma of the lung.

Even if such survival rates could not be achieved, I emphatically reject the proposition that it is useless to undertake widespread efforts for the discovery of cancer of the lung in asymptomatic individuals. We should carry this on for other reasons than immediate curability, for only in this way can we discover the true prevalence of the disease, its morbidity, and its relationship to environment and to other disease processes. We need to know where carcinoma of the lung is located and in what individuals, so that if a more effective means of therapy were introduced tomorrow, one which would necessitate the finding of small or early lesions, we would be prepared for it. Persistence in such efforts at mass detection may be the only means by which we will learn to increase our ability, to improve our technical processes for detecting small tumors, and to identify them when detected.

Various methods have been used in the effort to detect carcinoma of the lung in its asymptomatic phase. One method, the obtaining of bronchial secretions and their cytological examination, which has had some trials, seems to me to be impractical for mass survey use. The difficulties attending the procedure are obvious and have been demonstrated in many trials.

In fact, the only available procedure which is presently universally applicable, reasonably cheap, produces no distress on the part of the individual examined, and which has a reasonable probability for the detection of small carcinomas of the lung in their asymptomatic phase is routine X-ray examination of the lungs in apparently well individuals. Yet presently we find relatively few such small tumors, and the reasons are many. The first, of course, is that we are not doing semiannual or even annual examinations of the vulnerable population. Some efforts have been made in this direction, but mostly these have been examinations on one occasion or occasional examinations of special individuals.

The second difficulty is that even when survey examinations are made, the X-ray techniques have often been deficient; the importance of an exacting technique cannot be overemphasized. This is well illustrated in Figure 2, in which a very large carcinoma might easily be missed if the posteroanterior view alone (Fig. 2A) had been made. The exposure was insufficient to penetrate the heart to show

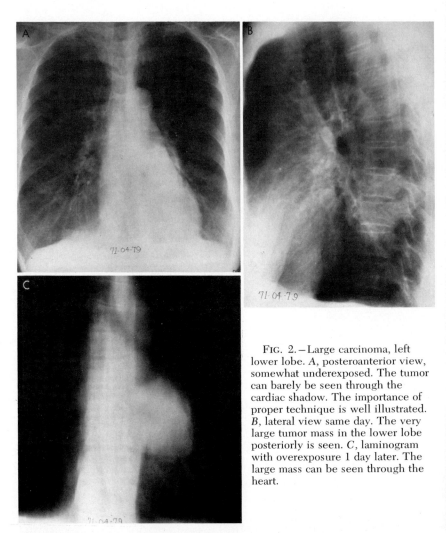

FIG. 2.—Large carcinoma, left lower lobe. *A*, posteroanterior view, somewhat underexposed. The tumor can barely be seen through the cardiac shadow. The importance of proper technique is well illustrated. *B*, lateral view same day. The very large tumor mass in the lower lobe posteriorly is seen. *C*, laminogram with overexposure 1 day later. The large mass can be seen through the heart.

the overlying mass. Furthermore, films have commonly been interpreted in a relatively rapid superficial fashion with insufficient attention to small densities. As a result, we are still seeing many cases in which a lesion, clearly present in the roentgenogram, has been overlooked or its significance underestimated. One example of the hundreds of this type which I have personally observed is illustrated in Figure 3. Here, a small nodule, overlooked on a routine examination when the patient was apparently well, has grown within 2 years into a very large mass, symptomatic, and showing extension into the

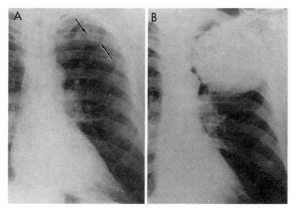

FIG. 3.—Undifferentiated carcinoma, left upper lobe. *A*, routine posteroanterior view in asymptomatic patient. Small round density, left (arrows) was not observed. Surgery at this time might have good prognosis. *B*, 2 years later. Symptomatic, rapid growth to a large mass, metastasis present, prognosis now hopeless.

regional nodes. The outlook, if it had been removed surgically on the first occasion, would have been good. When discovered because of symptoms, the prognosis was extremely poor.

The second case of this type is shown in Figure 4. Here a patient with scars of tuberculosis was being re-examined at various intervals, even though he was completely asymptomatic. A small lesion is seen in the left subclavicular region (Fig. 4A) which might well be interpreted as being a part of the tuberculous scar process. In Figure 4B, however, 1 year later, this lesion has enlarged, and this by itself should have aroused apprehension; 2 years later (Fig. 4C) the nodule measured about 2 cm. in diameter, was round and fairly demarcated, and proved at operation to be an adenocarcinoma. Thus 2 years had been allowed to elapse from the time the lesion might first have been discovered until definitive therapy was undertaken.

The third difficulty lies in the nature of the lesion itself and the corollary to that, the character of the roentgen image, which we must interpret. Goldmeier (1965) has called attention to the reasons why carcinomas less than 2 cm. in diameter are so seldom found on X-ray examination of the lungs, even with good techniques and skilled interpretation. He points out that primary carcinoma of the lung, in contrast to such tumors as hamartoma or metastasis, does not produce a solid mass. When a malignant tumor is small, areas of uninvolved lung tissue remain within the substance of the tumor itself and around its periphery. As a result, its total X-ray density is smaller

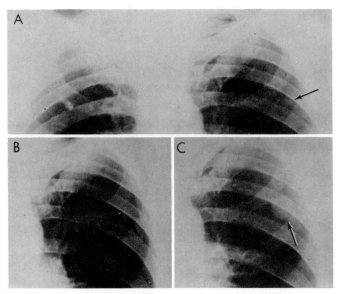

FIG. 4.—Adenocarcinoma in a patient with residual tuberculous scars. *A*, very small lesion left upper (arrow) thought to be extension of tuberculosis. *B*, 1 year later. Modest increase in size (arrow). Not recognized. *C*, 1 more year later. Nodule measures 2 cm. (arrow) and is readily recognized. Surgery.

than it should be considering its diameter, and therefore it is difficult to see. An illustration of this is shown in Figure 5, a posteroanterior roentgenogram of a patient being treated for coronary heart disease. There were no pulmonary symptoms, and the lesion shown here was overlooked. It measures 2½ cm. in diameter, but its density is low enough that a casual and somewhat unskilled interpretation of the film failed to detect the lesion. Several years later it had extended into the lower lobe bronchus and had involved the nodes, producing symptoms for the first time. The need for an exacting technique or a definite improvement in our methods, which will permit such faint shadows to become obvious, is clearly desirable. In studying large groups of cases in which films were made at a date long before diagnosis, we have found a great many failures to recognize lesions which were, in fact, present and visible although difficult to distinguish from their surroundings. Veeze (1968) reports on a series of cases in which he studied the roentgenograms made fortuitously years before the diagnosis was entertained. Six per cent of all cases of carcinoma of the lung were evident in the films made 3 years before a definitive diagnosis was established. In 14 per cent, the lesion

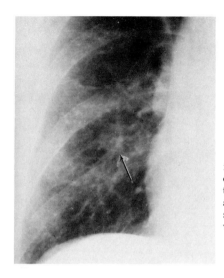

FIG. 5.—Squamous cell carcinoma right lower lobe. Although it measures 2.5 cm. (arrow), the density is very low and the lesion was not recognized. It was asymptomatic at this time; 2 years later symptoms developed but lymph nodes were already involved.

was obvious 2 years before, in 56 per cent, 1 year before, and in 87 per cent, 6 months before. He concludes from this that the X-ray examination should be made at semiannual intervals, but what we learn from these studies is that we are failing to find lesions even though they are visible in the roentgenogram, both prospectively and retrospectively.

That it is possible to detect small lesions, especially nodular ones, in the lungs is illustrated by a study which I once made on metastases. Patients with carcinoma of the breast or bone sarcoma were examined at monthly intervals using posteroanterior roentgenograms only. In a few cases, we were able to demonstrate that it was possible to determine the presence of metastases when they were even less than 3 mm. in size if they occurred in the periphery of the lung. We have, in addition, been able to demonstrate some primary carcinomas .5 cm. or less in size.

The lesion shown in Figure 6 is a primary carcinoma. It is extremely small, less than 1 cm., but clearly visible although it is much easier to detect when a few months have passed and the tumor has grown (Fig. 6B). It is notable, however, that in the cases reported by Steele, Kleitsch, Dunn, and Buell (1966), of almost 400 carcinomas, of which 87 were 2 cm. or less in size, there were none less than a centimeter in diameter and only 9 less than 1.5 cm. In the 195 cases presented by Jackman, Good, Clagett, and Woolner (1969), all measuring 4 cm. or less, there were only 2 which were a centimeter or

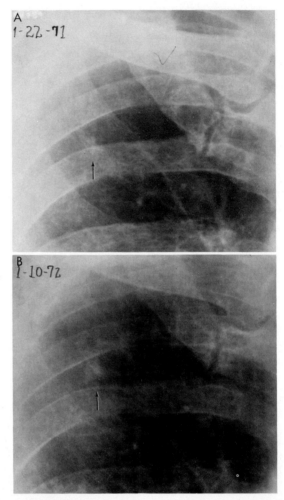

FIG. 6.—Carcinoma less than 1 cm. in diameter. *A*, small irregular nodule, left upper (arrow). This was not recognized partly because it was superimposed upon a rib. *B*, 3 months later. Still asymptomatic, lesion is somewhat larger (arrow), extends into the interspace and is readily detected.

less in diameter. Since all these cases were discovered because of routine X-ray examination, it is obvious that there is something wrong with our method or with our ability to utilize the method.

That the image of the lungs seen in the roentgenogram is far from satisfactory is known to all experienced radiologists. The complex anatomical structure of the lungs, the overlying bony structures, the blood vessels and supporting tissues, and the anatomical variations give shadows, some of which are indistinguishable from an abnormal process. Furthermore, the presence of diffuse interstitial lesions which are common in elderly individuals adds complications to the process. For these reasons, the minimum size of a lesion which can be distinguished is generally given as 3 mm. The fact is, however, that many carcinomas of the lung up to 2 cm. in diameter are difficult to visualize and are often overlooked. Figure 7A presents the posteroanterior view of a primary carcinoma measuring 2.5 cm. in diameter. Despite this, it was overlooked because its density is so low and it is not a solid shadow. The lateral view (Fig. 7B) exhibits a more solid density, projecting just beyond the spine.

We have used many conventional methods to improve this situation, bearing in mind that we are sharply limited as to the extent of the procedures which can be undertaken, since the vast majority of the patients on whom routine chest examination is made will present no disease process. Monetary costs, the practicalities of the situation from the point of view of radiation exposure, and time factors all limit our effort. The importance of such special positions is well illus-

FIG. 7.—Bronchioloalveolar carcinoma right upper lobe. *A*, tumor (arrows) measured more than 2 cm. in diameter but its total density is low. It was overlooked, although with magnification it is evident. *B*, lateral view shows a more solid mass (arrows) extending just anterior to the vertebral body. The difficulties in detection, even of tumors of this size, and the value of the lateral view are well shown.

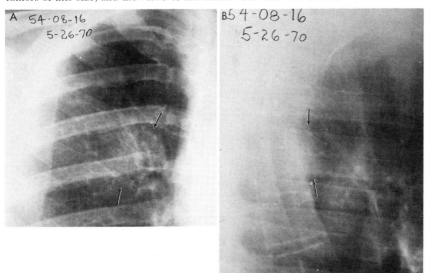

trated in Figure 8, in which a lesion is almost completely hidden because it is overlapped by the clavicle and the first rib. Clearly, the increased density of this area (Fig. 8A) should have called attention to the process, but it was not observed. About 7 months later, the carcinoma had grown and extended into the apex where it can be seen partially free of the bony structures (Fig. 8B). Presently, we are using stereoscopic and apical lordotic views to expose such lesions, but many other procedures, such as obliques, could be undertaken, and with all this, much more could be accomplished. The standard procedure is to make posteroanterior and lateral exposures, the latter may be of very great importance. This is well illustrated in Figure 9A which is the posteroanterior view of a female cigarette smoker, aged 48, who had a routine examination of the lungs. The film is somewhat overexposed but, even with a bright light, showed no evidence of a lesion whatever. The lateral view (Fig. 9B) does show a nodule measuring about 1.5 cm. in diameter, just behind the trachea at the aortic arch. This shadow was observed and, as a result, laminograms were made. The laminogram (Fig. 9C) exhibits the lesion just to the right of the spine in the medial portion of the posterior segment of the upper lobe. At operation, it proved to be a squamous cell carcinoma and a lobectomy was done. We have many other illustrations of the importance of the lateral view in demonstrating lesions, especially those that are medial and which may be invisible because they are

Fig. 8.—Carcinoma, right upper lobe. *A*, tumor (arrow) is partly concealed by the clavicle and the first rib. Stereoscopic or apical lordotic views would have made it visible and prevented this failure. *B*, 7 months later, still asymptomatic. The lesion is readily recognized as it now extends above the bony structures into the apex.

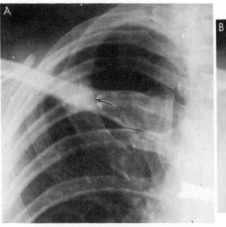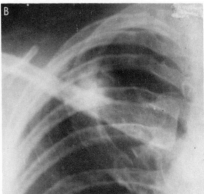

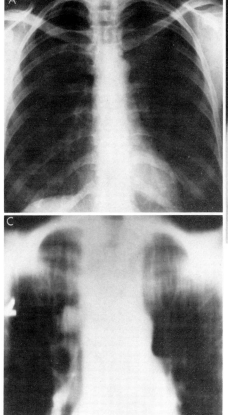

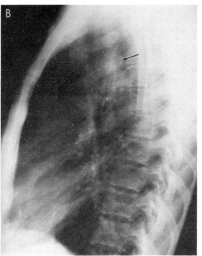

FIG. 9.—Squamous cell carcinoma, presymptomatic, found on routine examination. *A*, posteroanterior view, somewhat overexposed. No evidence of any tumor. *B*, lateral view, same time. A round nodule is seen (arrow) just behind the trachea and above the aorta. The tumor was recognized from this film although invisible in the posteroanterior view. *C*, laminogram, posteroanterior view. A nodule measuring 1.5 cm. is seen in the medial portion of the posterior segment of the right upper lobe. The difference between this and the conventional posteroanterior view is startling and illustrates how easily such cancers can be missed if the technique is faulty, but often even with good technique. Lobectomy. (Courtesy of Dr. Rolf Dieter Arndt, personal communication).

hidden within the shadows of the large vessels. Laminography would indeed assist greatly in this effort to find small lesions, as seen in this case, but it is obviously too expensive, too time-consuming, and too costly in radiation exposure to be used on a routine basis. It is effective when it is necessary to prove the presence of a lesion and it adds information as to the nature of a nodule. Practically, we must restrict ourselves, and mass surveys could scarcely be done using more than 2, or possibly 3, films, even if limited to the vulnerable population.

Many new methods to improve the roentgen image are presently being explored in this country. Such technical changes as using high kilovolt exposures, X-ray magnification, and photographic magnification have all been used to a limited extent but without as yet producing a large impact on the problem. The use of X-ray tubes with minimal-sized focal spots, even in the micron range, shows some promise, but there are practical problems which have not yet been solved.

For some years I have been investigating a method for conversion of the conventional roentgenogram to a television image in order to magnify the shadows, vary the amount of light transmission, change the contrast, increase the detail, enhance the edge of the shadows, change the gamma, and even reverse the image. Two examples are shown here (Figs. 10 and 11). The conventional posteroanterior view (Fig. 10A) barely exhibits a tiny nodule at the left base, but the same film converted into a TV-gram (Fig. 10B) shows the nodule effectively; this was a hamartoma. A patient with very small carcinomatous metastases was examined in the usual fashion (Fig. 11) and the nodular metastases were not found; the TV conversion of the same film (Fig. 11B) exhibits them (arrows) without difficulty. The results of this study are equivocal as yet and many other efforts in this direction are being carried on (Kundel, Revesz, and Shea, 1969; Kundel, 1969, 1972; Revesz and Haas, 1972). Certainly, by this method one can enhance the visibility of some nodules, but I am not yet certain as to its practical application.

Bedrossian and Martin (1973) have tried using xeroradiography, also an electronic process, but it is only effective in the excised lung. It may well be valuable to guide the pathologist so that he may find small lesions without the laborious slicing procedures practiced by Raeburn and Spencer, but it is not a method useful for the living individual. Another electronic method most recently developed and now being studied by Stanton and Brady (1973) in which greater detail and enhancement of the edge of shadows may be obtained with sufficient penetration to secure satisfactory films, is called electron radiography. Another method, being studied by Dr. Michael Stamm at UCLA (Stamm, personal communication), with which I have had some experience, is the conversion of a conventional roentgenogram by television into a color image using the Kolor-rad apparatus. Because of the increased perception of color by the eye, it may be possible that small lesions will be made to stand out more vividly in this way.

I have no doubt that methods will be devised in the near future which will improve the image sufficiently to permit more frequent detection of small lesions. But even if these efforts are unsuccessful,

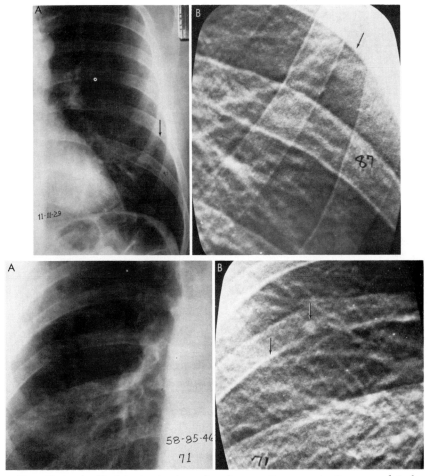

FIG. 10 *(top)*.—Nodule in the lung found on routine examination proved to be hamartoma. *A,* posteroanterior view shows small nodule in the left lower lobe (arrow), measuring 5 mm.; easily overlooked. *B,* television conversion by magnification and intensification shows the nodule (arrow) more definitively and makes its presence certain.

FIG. 11 *(bottom)*.—Metastases to right lung, conventional film and TV-gram. *A,* posteroanterior roentgenogram. A number of faint shadows slightly suspicious of metastases are seen, but clear-cut nodules are not exhibited. The patient does have some overexpansion in the upper lobes and some compression of the lower lobes from previous chronic pulmonary disease. *B,* 2 definite nodules overlying the rib can be clearly made out in the TV-gram (arrows). Several others are seen but these are in an area in which it is difficult to distinguish them from normal vessels. The effect of magnification and image improvement of the film shown in *A* is well exhibited here and no doubt indicates some potential in this television process.

there is still a great opportunity, using present methods, to improve the frequency with which we detect small cancers. I repeat, many small lesions which should be obvious in the roentgenogram are being overlooked even today, and the opportunity for a cure is lost because of our own carelessness, ineptitude, or indifference.

The criticisms of mass X-ray surveys have been extensive, many of them based upon the lack of results in the Philadelphia neoplasm project as reported in the many papers by Weiss, Cooper, and Boucot (1969); Weiss, Boucot, and Cooper, (1971); and Boucot and Weiss (1973). Many of us who have had experience in this field find their results difficult to understand, and the editorial by Fontana (1973) points up many of these doubts. Boucot and Weiss (1973) have answered this editorial, but the doubts remain. Gilbertsen (1964) likewise has expressed serious reservations as to the efficacy of X-ray examination in the detection of curable carcinoma, but the number of cases on which this is based is so small that I do not believe his criticisms are valid. Brett (1969), in England, had done semiannual X-ray examinations on a group of industrial workers. He used a control group who were examined at only 3-year intervals. The difference in 5-year survivial was substantial. He tells me (Brett, personal communication) that if errors in the management of the semiannual examined group were considered with a critical reanalysis of the control group, the semiannually examined group would have had a potential of 23 per cent 5-year survival, as compared to 6 per cent in the controls. These data include all carcinomas, not merely peripheral ones. There are numerous reports in the literature on the results of mass X-ray surveys, especially in Germany and in Russia. Most of these present data indicating that operable carcinoma of the lung is found by surveys 4 times as frequently as by all other methods (Cooley, 1969; Lindig, 1968). Göttsching has also demonstrated the effectiveness of mass surveys in carcinoma of the lung. I would quote only one specific series reported by Kirsch (1970), in which the 5-year survival was 6 per cent in cases discovered because of symptoms, 14 per cent in patients in whom the lesion was found by X-ray examination in the presence of minor symptoms, and 24 per cent in symptomless individuals whose cancer was detected in a mass survey. Cooley (1969) has considered the various results achieved by routine X-ray examination of the chest. Influenced by the results of the Philadelphia neoplasm project, he is somewhat pessimistic as to the outlook. Conversely, Veeze (1968), in a thorough review of mass surveys, presents a very different opinion, and from my experience I share his viewpoint. I am confident that an annual roentgen examination, properly done and properly interpreted, in smokers over the age of 40, would bring to light a much greater number of small, resectable carcinomas of the lung than is presently the case and would thus improve the salvage rate appreciably.

Programs of routine X-ray examination, however, should not be undertaken without due regard for the harmful effects which may ensue. The possibility that many benign nodules will be found which will make thoracotomy and lung resection more frequent, with the inevitable risks of morbidity and mortality which this entails, is one such deterrent. The second difficulty lies in the psychic trauma induced by repeated examinations which might well be imposed upon individuals with completely benign processes. I believe these can be effectively managed if sufficient effort is made and if there is a proper relationship between physician and patient. The third objection might be the cost of repeated annual or possibly semiannual examinations, even if only the vulnerable population were included. However, when one considers the enormous costs which we now undergo in the diagnosis, intensive investigation, and treatment of patients with completely hopeless cases of carcinoma of the lung, it seems to me that the cost of finding lesions in which there would be a reasonable chance for survival would be of small consequence.

What I have been discussing here is the detection of an abnormality in the lungs which might conceivably be a carcinoma. I should point out at once that this is not the end of the trail; once a lesion has been detected, numerous difficulties are encountered and efforts, often frustrating, must be made to determine whether the lesion is malignant and the patient should be subjected to an operation. In this kind of study, no doubt as many nonmalignant as malignant lesions will be found. In some instances, regardless of all the armamentaria of differential diagnosis available to us, a definite statement as to the malignancy cannot be made prior to microscopic examination. I would emphasize, however, that the most important problem for us is to find something on which to exercise our abilities in diffferential diagnosis. The latter is of no importance whatever if the lesion is not found. The indentification of the nature of the lesion may be difficult and at times impossible, but the failure to recognize the presence of an abnormality is an irretrievable error, possibly a failure to save a life.

To illustrate some of the difficulties in differential diagnosis, I would present some recent cases of small lesions. All of these patients were completely free of pulmonary symptoms; the nodules were found on routine X-ray examination. All of the patients were over 40 and cigarette smokers, that is, they were a part of the vulnerable population. In all but one, the lesion had been overlooked or at least not given any significance in earlier examinations, although it was definitely present.

CASE 1. A routine film of the chest in an asymptomatic individual (Fig. 12A) actually showed a nodule which was, however, not detected. One year later, the nodule had increased somewhat in size (Fig. 12B) and was more visible. The laminogram (Fig. 12C) demonstrates

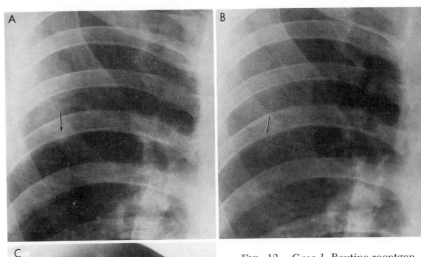

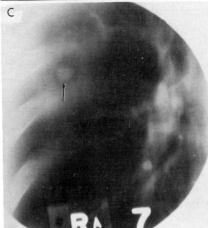

FIG. 12.—*Case 1*. Routine roentgen examination with nodule found in right upper lobe; asymptomatic. *A*, posteroanterior view shows a small nodule overlapping the posterior and anterior ribs (arrow), and not observed at the time of this examination. *B*, 2 years later the nodule has increased in size from about 5 mm. to 8 mm. and is seen impinging upon the interlobar fissure with its upper surface quite flat. This degree of density in a nodule of this size and the limitation by the fissure should suggest that it is benign. *C*, laminogram confirming the presence of the nodule. Note the halo around the rather solid density which likewise is usually suggestive of a benign lesion. Surgical excision showed a 7-mm. nodule which, on microscopic examination, proved to be an adenomatoid hamartoma with no cartilage in the lesion, but undoubtedly benign.

the lesion more effectively. Nodules as small as this, 7 mm. in diameter, and which are so dense are likely to be solid tumors such as as hamartomas; this indeed proved, on resection, to be an adenomatoid hamartoma. There was no cartilage in the lesion, but there was fairly typical adenomatoid tissue.

CASE 2. Routine examination of the chest on this patient (Fig. 13A) showed a small nodule measuring about 4 mm. In a film made one month later (Fig. 13B), it is most difficult to identify the same shadow. This illustrates again the problems involved in the detection of very small lesions. The laminogram of the same date (Fig. 13C) shows the nodule as a clearly visible density. Lobectomy was done because the first pathologist who saw the frozen sections considered it to be malignant. Later studies, however, indicated that it was an adenomatoid hamartoma of unusual cellularity simulating an oat cell carcinoma. Another interpretation of the same section is that this is a vascular malformation and no doubt it is benign.

CASE 3. This patient had multiple routine chest films, beginning in 1970, in all of which a lesion in the right upper lobe is seen in retrospect. Nevertheless, it was not recognized until the film made late in 1973 (Fig. 14A). Another film, (Fig. 14B) made just a few days later, shows the lesion hidden behind ribs and very easily overlooked. There was, in fact, little or no change in size over this interval of 3 years, which indicated the low growth potential of this tumor. A lobectomy was done and the tumor proved to be a mucin-secreting bronchiolar adenoma, considered by many pathologists to be at least a precancerous tumor, if not truly malignant from the beginning. The major shadow was produced by the mucin in the alveoli rather than by the tumor itself, which was almost microscopic in size. It is possible that the varying X-ray findings were the result of changes in the quantity of mucus in the alveoli.

CASE 4. This patient, also on routine examination of the chest, presented with a nodule in the lung. No previous films were available. The nodule was difficult to see and a number of films (Fig. 15A) were made, but it was finally brought out well in the TV-gram, the conversion film (Fig. 15B). Laminography (Fig. 15C) made it visible as well. It measured 4 mm. at operation and proved to be a papillary adenocarcinoma, probably the smallest carcinoma I have ever found prospectively.

It is clear that small lesions can be found. The probabilities are that in the majority of cases, lesions found in the roentgenogram which are well under 1 cm. in size will be benign rather than malig-

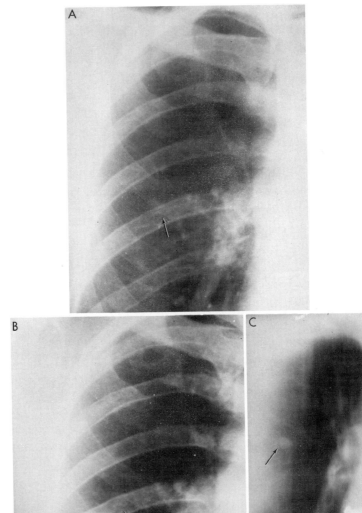

FIG. 13.—*Case 2.* Routine examination in an asymptomatic patient with a nodule in the lung. *A,* posteroanterior roentgenogram of the chest shows a nodule measuring about 5 mm. (arrow), fairly well demarcated and only moderately dense. *B,* film of same

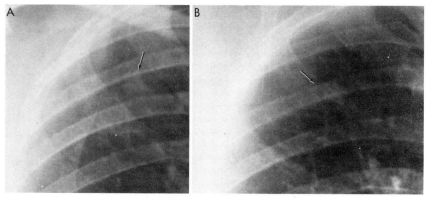

FIG. 14.—*Case 3.* Routine examination of the chest in an asymptomatic individual exhibiting a lesion in the right upper lobe. *A,* a somewhat irregular, not well-defined density is shown in the right first interspace (arrow). It measures about 1 cm. in diameter, and on this film is very readily seen. *B,* film of the same patient a few days later in which the lesion is superimposed upon the ribs and thereby almost undetectable (arrow). A surgical excision with microscopic examination revealed a mucin-secreting bronchiolar adenoma. Most of the shadow was caused by the mucin secretion in the alveoli rather than the tumor itself which was almost microscopic in size. It is probable that the differences seen in the many films were the result of the degree of mucin secretion at any one time. Most pathologists consider this a precursor of malignant disease, if not malignant disease itself.

nant. Nevertheless, malignant tumors less than 1 cm. can be detected in the roentgenogram, and of course the opportunity for cure here is far greater than when they are larger.

That roentgen examination can be negative, even in the presence of positive cytology or bronchoscopic observation of a cancer with positive biopsy, has been repeatedly observed as described by Marsh, Frost, Erozan, and Carter (1972). Most of these false-negatives occur in the lesions of the larger bronchi in which the tumor is mucosal, has not yet extended to the extrabronchial tissues to produce a mass, and has not produced any appreciable degree of obstruction. This failure of X-ray examination may also occur in peripheral lesions but it is rare, in our experience, to find positive cytology

---

patient taken 3 weeks later showing almost no evidence of the nodule in the area where it was previously seen (arrow). This illustrates how easily such small lesions of the lungs can merge into the normal pulmonary structures. *C,* laminogram of the same area shows the nodule (arrow), well outlined and fairly dense. Lobectomy revealed a rather unusual lesion, probably an adenoma, although an extremely cellular one, first thought to be an oat cell carcinoma; later sections proved it benign.

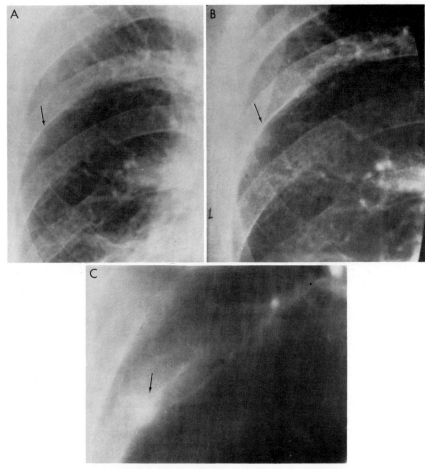

FIG. 15.—*Case 4*. Routine examination in an asymptomatic individual. *A*, numerous films revealed a very small (4 mm.) nodule in the right upper lobe (arrow). Several radiologists questioned whether there was any abnormality whatever. *B*, television conversion of the same film shows a lesion (arrow) just below the rib as a fairly well demarcated nodule of low density. There was no doubt with this TV-gram that the nodule was present. *C*, laminogram confirms the finding and the nodule can be made out in the periphery (arrow). Surgical excision and microscopic study showed papillary adenocarcinoma.

with a negative film in which the lesion is eventually demonstrated to be in the periphery.

There are many procedures for the identification of the nature of a nodule. Multiple X-ray examinations should be made when a nodule is suspected such as is indicated above. Laminography is of the greatest importance, first to make certain that a nodule is in fact present, and second, to get a clearer picture of the nature of the process. The presence or absence of calcification can be best determined in this way. Irregularities in the contour of the nodule, notches, streaked areas, etc. will also become visible in the laminogram when they may be doubtful in the conventional film. In any case suspected of a tumor, stereoscopic, oblique, and apical lordotic views all may be used for help in determining the presence of any definitive sign. Obviously, all clinical and laboratory evidence available must be used under these circumstances.

Such negative X-ray signs as the presence of gross amounts of calcium which almost rules out a primary malignancy, a marked density in a lesion less than 1 cm. in diameter which indicates a hamartoma, and failure to change in size over a 6-month period are all good negative signs. Such positive signs as fairly rapid growth as seen on a comparison of films from an earlier date; the notch sign (Rigler and Heitzman, 1955) which, while not pathognomonic, is highly suggestive; the linear crease sign in bronchioloalveolar carcinoma and occasionally in adenocarcinoma (Rigler, 1964); the Fleischner line (Baron, personal communication); the "rabbit ear" sign reported by Shapiro, Wilson, Yesner, and Shuman, 1972; spiculation around the margin of the nodule; cavitation with thick walls; and many other signs all may be helpful. I will not go into this in great detail at this time since it represents a subject of its own. It may be necessary in some cases to wait for 3 months to determine whether any change has occurred. This is only feasible when the lesion is well under 2 cm. in size, but it is in that group that the greatest difficulty will be encountered in trying to make a differential diagnosis. In other cases, needle biopsy, bronchial brushing, or local excision may be necessary to arrive at a final diagnosis. With the exception of the mucin-secreting adenomas, some hamartomas, and some atypical granulomas, as illustrated in the cases I have shown, the difficulties have not been overwhelming. Much more needs to be done, however, to permit a more accurate identification without resorting to surgery. Again, let me emphasize that improving the roentgen image may well make identification more certain. Numerous clinical and laboratory tests are available which, combined with the roentgen findings, are helpful in establishing the nature of the lesion. Present-day use of the fiberoptic bronchoscope and the securing of bronchial secretions for cytology are of great importance, but apply more especially to tumors of the larger bronchi. Cytology may be useful even in the small peripheral lesion, but it is not as effective. As in many other diagnostic situations, it is necessary to adopt a policy of attention to the individual situation. It is impossible to lay down rules which will fit all cases. With sufficient effort and avoidance of undue haste, unnecessary surgery may be precluded to a large extent.

Summary and Conclusions

Peripheral carcinoma of the lung, arising from a small bronchus, presents different clinical and roentgen findings than do tumors of larger bronchi.

Certain features are discussed:

1. The majority of cases of primary carcinoma arise in a small bronchus, but some extend centrally to simulate a major bronchial origin.

2. The peripheral lesion is asymptomatic until it becomes very large or extends into a larger bronchus.

3. Peripheral lesions must be found by routine examination of apparently well individuals.

4. The most effective method of discovery is by X-ray examination.

5. The surgical results in small, asymptomatic, peripheral carcinomas are of such an order, 50 to 70 per cent 5-year survival, that it is imperative to discover them.

6. Primary carcinomatous nodules in the periphery, less than 2 cm. in diameter, frequently are not found on X-ray examination, and those less than 1 cm. are rarely detected.

7. We should improve our present techniques of X-ray examination and our ability to interpret routine films in order to find such lesions.

8. Experiments to improve the image in the roentgenogram by a variety of means, largely electronic, are underway. Future improvements may make it possible to find many more small lesions and to identify their nature.

9. Great improvement could now be accomplished with conventional films if excellent technique and proper interpretation were more commonly accomplished.

10. Mass annual X-ray examinations of the vulnerable population are economically feasible and would result in a substantial increase in survival in primary carcinoma of the lung.

REFERENCES

Arndt, R. D.: Personal communication.
Baron, M.: Personal communication.
Bedrossian, C. M. W., and Martin, J. E.: Xeroradiography of the lung. *Radiology*, 107:217–218, April 1973.

Boucot, K. R., and Weiss, W.: Is curable lung cancer detected by semiannual screening? *The Journal of the American Medical Association*, 224:1361–1365, June 4, 1973.

_____: Letter: Screening for lung cancer. *The Journal of the American Medical Association*, 226:566–567, October 29, 1973.

Brett, G. Z.: Earlier diagnosis and survival in lung cancer. *British Medical Journal*, 4:260–262, November 1969.

_____: Personal communication.

Buell, P. E.: The importance of tumor size in prognosis for resected bronchogenic carcinoma. *Journal of Surgical Oncology*, 3:539–551, 1971.

Cooley, R. N.: Radiographic detection of preclinical and asymptomatic cancer of the lung. *The American Journal of Roentgenology, Radium Therapy and Nuclear Medicine*, 107:440–442, October 1969.

Fontana, R. S.: The Philadelphia Pulmonary Neoplasm Research Project. *The Journal of the American Medical Association*, 225:1372–1373, September 10, 1973.

Garland, L. H. Beier, R. L., Coulson, W., Heald, J. H., and Stein, R. L.: The apparent sites of origin of carcinomas of the lung. *Radiology*, 78:1–11, January 1962.

Gilbertsen, V. A.: X-ray examination of the chest. *The Journal of the American Medical Association*, 188:1082–1083, June 2, 1964.

Goldmeier, E.: Limits of visibility of bronchogenic carcinoma. *American Review of Respiratory Diseases*, 91:232–239, February 1965.

Göttsching, H.: Roentgen survey examinations and bronchial carcinoma. *Zeitschrift fur Allgemeinmedizin*, 47:1683–1685, November 20, 1971.

Jackman, R., Good, C. A., Clagett, O. T., and Woolner, L.: Survival rates in peripheral bronchogenic carcinomas up to four centimeters in diameter presenting as solitary pulmonary nodules. *Journal of Thoracic and Cardiovascular Surgery*, 57:1–8, January 1969.

Kirsch, M., Ansbett, F., and van de Kamp, W.: Concerning the influence of mass survey roentgen examinations on the late results in the surgery of bronchial carcinoma. *Zeitschrift fur Erkrankungen der Atmungsorgane mit Folia Bronchologica*, 133:177–184, December 1970.

Kundel, H., and LaFollette, P. S., Jr.; Visual search patterns and experience with radiological images. *Radiology*, 103:523–528, June 1972.

Kundel, H., Revesz, G., and Shea, F. J.: Display format and decision making in television processing of chest radiographs. *Investigative Radiology*, 4: 264–267, July–August 1969.

Kundel, H., Revesz, G., and Stauffer, H. M.: The electro-optical processing of radiographic images. *Radiologic Clinics of North America*, 7:447–460, December 1969.

Liebow, A.: Pathology of carcinoma of the lung as related to the roentgen shadow. *The American Journal of Roentgenology, Radium Therapy and Nuclear Medicine*, 74:383–401, September 1955.

Lindig, W.: Importance of mass x-ray screening for the diagnosis of lung cancer. *Zeitschrift fur Tuberkulose und Erkrankungen der Thorax Organe*, 129:237–244, December 1968.

Marsh, B., Frost, J., Erozan, Y. S., and Carter, D.: Occult bronchogenic carcinoma. *Cancer* 30:1348–1352, November 1972.

Raeburn, C.: Primary carcinoma of peripheral bronchi. *The Lancet*, 2:474–476, September 15, 1951.

Raeburn, C., and Spencer, H.: Study of origin and development of lung cancer. *Thorax.* 8:1–10, March 1953.

Rigler, L., and Heitzman, E.: Planigraphy in the differential diagnosis of the pulmonary nodule with particular reference to the notch sign of malignancy. *Radiology,* 65:692–702, 1955.

Rigler, L. G.: A roentgen study of the evolution of carcinoma of the lung. *Journal of Thoracic Surgery,* 34:283–297, 1957.

————: The natural history of untreated lung cancer. *Annals of the New York Academy of Sciences,* 114:755–766, April 2, 1964.

————: The earliest roentgenographic signs of carcinoma of the lung. *The Journal of the American Medical Association,* 195:655–657, February 1966.

Rigler, L. G., O'Loughlin, B. J., and Tucker, R. C.: The duration of carcinoma of the lung. *Diseases of the Chest,* 23:50–71, January 1953.

Shapiro, R., Wilson, G. L., Yesner, R., and Shuman, H. A.: Useful roentgen sign in the diagnosis of localized bronchioloalveolar carcinoma. *The Americal Journal of Roentgenology, Radium Therapy and Nuclear Medicine,* 114:516–524, March 1972.

Spencer, H.: Personal communication.

Stamm, M.: Personal communication.

Stanton, L., and Brady, L.: Electron radiography, a new x-ray imaging system. *Applied Radiology,* 2:53, 1973.

Steele, J. D., and Buell, P.: Survival in bronchogenic carcinomas resected as solitary pulmonary nodules. *Proceedings of the National Cancer Conference,* 6:835, 1970.

Steele, J. D., Kleitsch, W. P., Dunn, J. E., Jr., and Buell, P.: Survival in males with bronchogenic carcinoma resected as asymptomatic solitary pulmonary nodules. *Annals of Thoracic Surgery,* 2:368–376, May 1966.

Tala, E.: Carcinoma of the lung. A retrospective study with special reference to prediagnosis period and roentgenographic signs. *Acta Radiologica Supplement,* 268:1+, 1967.

Veeze, P.: *Rationale and Methods of Early Detection in Lung Cancer.* Groningen, Holland, Van Gorcum Co., 1968, 177 pp.

Walter, J. B., and Pryce, D. M.: The site of origin of lung cancer and its relation to histological type. *Thorax,* 10:117–126, June 1955.

Weiss, W., Boucot, K., and Cooper, D. A.: The Philadelphia Pulmonary Neoplasm Research Project. Survival factors in bronchogenic carcinoma. *The Journal of the American Medical Association,* 216:2119–2123, June 28, 1971.

Weiss, W., Cooper, D. A., and Boucot, K. R.: Operative mortality and 5-year survival rates in men with bronchogenic carcinoma. *Annals of Internal Medicine,* 71:59–65, July 1969.

Nuclear Techniques in Brain Tumor Detection

HENRY N. WAGNER, Jr., M.D.
Divisions of Nuclear Medicine and Radiation Health,
The Johns Hopkins Medical Institutions, Baltimore,
Maryland

THERE ARE TWO MAJOR REASONS why radioactive tracers have achieved widespread use in clinical medicine and biomedical research: first, they permit exquisitely sensitive and technically easy measurement of important chemical substances in body fluids; and second, they permit measurement of regional function. The latter is the basis of brain scanning.

The father of the technique of brain scanning is G. E. Moore, a Minneapolis surgeon who tried to visualize brain tumors better by injecting fluorescent dyes into his patients prior to surgical treatment. In 1948, he substituted a radioactive indicator, di-iodo-fluorescein, and used a single radiation detector to help locate the tumor containing the radioactive tracer. He began to use radioiodine (^{131}I) labeled albumin shortly thereafter, and this tracer remained the brain scanning agent used through most of the decade of the 1950's. The instrument used at the time was the rectilinear scanner equipped with a sodium iodide crystal 3 inches in diameter and based on the principles of the first rectilinear scanner invented by Cassen in 1951. Cassen's 2 innovations were to replace the gas-filled Geiger counter with a crystal scintillation detector and to attach motors so that it could be moved automatically back and forth over the patient's head. Initially, a stylus was used to portray on paper the spatial distribution of radioactivity, but in the commercial version this was changed to the photographic recording system invented by Kuhl.

A major advance in brain scanning was the development of sodium pertechnetate (^{99m}Tc). This agent was produced by Stang and Richards in 1960 as a by-product of their development of a chemical separation system (radionuclide generator) for production of iodine-132. The latter radionuclide was used extensively in the United Kingdom because its short (3-hour) half-life made it useful for daily studies in the same patient. The development of the molybdenum-99/technetium-99m generator system resulted from 2 considerations: first, tellurium-132, their source of iodine-132, was obtained from nuclear fission and the molybdenum-99 was a by-product of separation of fission fragments; second, the same type of generator developed for iodine-132 could be used for the molybdenum-99/technetium-99m system. This was commercially available for 3 years before Harper and Richards realized the great potential of this radionuclide for brain scanning. The introduction of ^{99m}Tc into nuclear medicine in 1963 marked the beginning of a steady increase in the number of brain scans performed in nuclear medicine departments. This increase came about because the information provided to neurologists, neurosurgeons, and internists increased greatly in value as a result of the better images. At the same time as technetium-99m was being introduced (1963), commercial versions of the Anger scintillation camera appeared, 5 years after Anger's first description of his initial camera which had only a 4-inch crystal. The commercial version, when it came into use, not only facilitated the performance of brain imaging, but also made possible studies of the cerebral circulation. The increasing use of the latter procedure is illustrated by the recent report of the Joint Committee for Stroke Facilities of the American Heart Association, which stated:

> "Scintigraphy utilizing a scintillation camera (gamma camera) and serial display of the image may provide the information necessary to determine whether a patient has an arteriovenous malformation, an ischemic cerebral infarct, or a cerebral neoplasm . . ."

Diagnostic tests usually fall by the wayside if they do not provide information useful in patient care. This is clear from the widespread popularity that brain scanning has achieved since technetium-99m became available. It is estimated that in 1972, nearly 3 million persons in the United States received a tracer study involving technetium-99m. Presumably, about half of these were brain scans.

Let us ask ourselves the following questions: (1) What are the most common indications for brain scanning? (2) What percentage of the studies reveal abnormalities? (3) What is the accuracy of the procedure? (4) In which patients have the results been most helpful?

While we do not have precise answers to all of these questions in adults, we have tried to answer them in children by analyzing the results of brain scanning in 556 children examined at our hospital between 1966 and 1971. Follow-up data were available in 409 children. We found that 37 per cent had brain scans because of seizures. Other frequent indications were motor abnormalities (7.4 per cent), headache (5.0 per cent), suspected optic neuritis (4.9 per cent), raised intracranial pressure (4.9 per cent), and trauma (4.7 per cent). Fifteen per cent of the scans were abnormal, most often because of tumors of the brain, pituitary fossa, brain stem, and cerebellum; subdural collections; cerebral abcess; and encephalitis. Three scans were false-positive and 12 patients with tumor had normal scans.

The finding that 15 per cent of our scans were abnormal is in keeping with the observations of others in children and the usual experience in adults. Scans gave misleading information, most often of the "false-negative type," in only 4 per cent (15) of the 409 patients. The scans were abnormal in all known cases of cerebral or cerebellar abcess, encephalitis, Schilder's disease, and cerebral contusion. Seventy-six per cent of all supratentorial and 60 per cent of all posterior fossa tumors were detected, as were 70 per cent of subdural collections. The over-all detection rate for scanning was 82 per cent (54 of 66 patients with confirmed lesions). This compares with figures of 80 per cent (7 of 9) and 62 per cent (13 of 21) for pneumoencephalography and arteriography, respectively. In earlier reports, the accuracy of scanning was also found to be similar to that of pneumoencephalography and arteriography in adults.

Which children should have brain scans? The categories in which scanning was most often "very helpful" or "helpful" were usually those in which the incidence of abnormal scans was highest. An exception was the group of patients with focal seizures—only 9 per cent of this group had abnormal scans; however, in many of the studies, these were valuable because they moved the patient into a "no evidence" category from a higher probability category, in addition to detecting lesions. Other instances in which scanning was found valuable involved focal neurological disease such as posterior fossa disease, trauma and metastases, and raised intracranial pressure. It has been suggested that scanning is never indicated in children with generalized seizures without focal signs; 5 of our 129 patients did have abnormal scans, however, and considering the harmless nature of the tests, we believe that there remains a place for scanning of selected children with generalized seizures.

The incidence of false results was low. Scans were most often abnormal in patients with localizing signs of recent onset and in those with symptoms of posterior fossa disease or raised intracranial pressure.

Another major conclusion of our study was that often we do not appreciate the value of a normal study. Perhaps the greatest usefulness of brain scanning is in eliminating the possibility of serious disease, usually cerebral neoplasm, in patients with clinical evidence that raises the possibility of cerebral neoplasm. An example is the child with the onset of seizures. The probability of the patient having a neurosurgical lesion is about 5 per cent, which is too high a risk to simply assume that the child has idiopathic epilepsy. Prior to the availability of brain scanning, it was necessary to hospitalize such a child to perform procedures, such as arteriography or pneumoencephalography, to be certain that there was no surgically correctable lesion. With a normal brain scan that can be performed without hospitalizing the patient, we lower the probability to about 1:200, which is low enough to permit the physician to proceed with drug therapy.

It is a tribute to the farsightedness of the pioneers of nuclear medicine that they were able to see that brain scanning would eventually become a widely accepted diagnostic tool. This is surprising when we look back at the brain scans performed with a rectilinear scanner with a crystal 3 inches in diameter and with radioiodinated human serum albumin as the tracer. It is difficult to see how we ever interpreted such images. Since then, important advances have been made in both instruments and radiopharmaceuticals.

Radiopharmaceuticals used for brain scanning fall into 2 major categories: high and low photon agents. The criterion that is used to judge radiopharmacueticals is the yield of photons/rad of radiation dose to the patient. The goal is to have this number as high as possible.

Figure 1 shows the progressive increase in photons/rad as each new radiopharmaceutical was introduced into nuclear medicine. When we compare technetium-99m pertechnetate and iodine-131 albumin we see that the ratio has increased nearly 200-fold.

Today, both rectilinear scanners and scintillation cameras are used for brain imaging; each has its strong and weak points. For brain scanning, the use of a dual detector with crystals 5 inches in diameter permits the anterior and posterior views or both lateral views to be obtained simultaneously. The crystal area of the 2 crystals com-

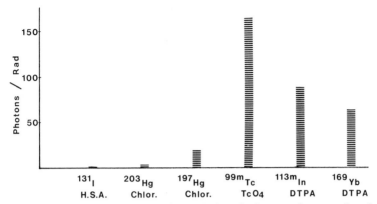

FIG. 1.—Progressive increase in photons/rad with the introduction of each new radiopharmaceutical into nuclear medicine.

bined is nearly equal to that of the scintillation camera; thus the sensitivity of the 2 instruments is comparable. The rectilinear scanners employ focused collimators and therefore the resolution is better for deep-seated lesions than it is with the camera. The camera has the advantage of being more flexible in the positions in which it can be placed relative to the patient's head. This can be an important advantage, for example, in looking at the posterior fossa with the pinhole collimator. The scintillation camera has permitted the development of nuclear cerebral angiography. This procedure consists of the intravenous injection of radionuclide and the obtaining of rapid-sequence scintigrams to visualize the major regions of cerebral blood supply.

The relationship between the circulation studies and the brain scan is important. Our experience has been that a finding of decreased blood flow in the distribution of a cerebral artery, coupled with a normal brain scan, greatly increases the probability of cerebral ischemic disease. In ischemic disease involving carotid artery distributions, the circulation study is twice as likely to be abnormal as in the conventional brain scan. Decreased circulation in the region of a lesion seen in the scan reduces the probability of tumor, which is more likely to show normal or increased flow in the region of the lesion. Occasionally, a neoplasm is observed which has a blood flow nearly equal to or greater than normal brain, but is within a cerebral hemisphere in which the total flow is reduced compared with the opposite site. In cerebral neoplasia, the circulation study helps evaluate the vascularity of the lesion. The greatly increased flow through arteriovenous malformations or aneurysms is easily identified. Meningioma and glioblastoma are characterized by increased activity in the lesion soon after the injection, but with a progressive increase of contrast between the lesion and surrounding tissues.

Acknowledgment

This study was supported by National Institutes of Health Grant No. GM-10548.

Gallium-67 Citrate for Tumor Scanning

C. LOWELL EDWARDS, M.D. and
RAYMOND L. HAYES, Ph. D.
*Medical Division, Oak Ridge Associated Universities,
Oak Ridge, Tennessee*

TUMOR SCANNING with ⁶⁷Ga citrate has evoked a great deal of interest among clinicians and investigators in nuclear medicine, and in a short period of time has been widely applied to many clinical problems. Numerous reports of clinical experience with this radionuclide have appeared in the literature. These range from reports of single cases to groups of more than 200 cases from multiple cooperating institutions (Table 1), and vary widely as to patient selection, scanning, and conditions. Occasionally, these publications have contained results or conclusions that seem contradictory in ways that are not easily explained by the known variables; however, in some areas a consensus seems to be emerging.

In this paper we will attempt to: (1) summarize the clinical experience in ⁶⁷Ga scanning, emphasizing points where there is agreement; (2) discuss specific clinical applications of ⁶⁷Ga scanning; and (3) point out significant problems involved in the use of ⁶⁷Ga as a general tumor-scanning agent.

The initial observation that ⁶⁷Ga localizes in neoplastic tissue was serendipitous in nature (Edwards and Hayes, 1969) and its clinical application continues to be empirical, despite extensive investigation in human beings and experimental animals. As yet, we have no satisfactory explanation of the basic mechanism responsible for the concentration of ⁶⁷Ga into tumors. However, there is substantial

Table 1
Summary of Results of [67]Ga Tumor Scans Obtained at
Various Institutions and Reported in the English Literature

Author	Lymphoma	Lung	Breast
Kay and McCready, 1972	76/96°	—	—
Turner et al., 1972	11/12	—	—
Higasi et al., 1972	2/2	25/35	8/16
Langhammer et al., 1972	22/35	64/72	3/9
Berelowitz and Blake, 1971	6/8	1/1	1/1
Fogh and Edeling, 1972	17/17	70/73	15/19
Lavender et al., 1971	1/2	—	5/13
Ito et al., 1971	7/7	21/21	4/4
Vaidya et al., 1970	2/3	0/2	3/4
Winchell et al., 1970	5/5	0/1	0/1
Edwards and Hayes, 1972	33/51	11/20	10/14
TOTALS	182/238	192/225	49/81
Per cent Positive	76%	85%	60%
CGSLR TOTALS†	270/319	146/172	—
Per cent Positive	84%	84%	—

°Positive scans/total number of scans.
†References: Greenlaw et al., in press; DeLand et al., in press; Johnston et al., in press.

evidence that ^{67}Ga is taken up by lysosomes within the cytoplasm of tumor cells and certain normal cells (Hayes and Edwards, 1973; Haubold and Aulbert, 1973). Electron microscopic autoradiograms have indicated that ^{67}Ga is associated with lysosomelike dense bodies (Swartzendruber, Nelson, and Hayes, 1971); enzymatic analysis of zonal centrifugation fractions has provided additional evidence of the association between the ^{67}Ga and lysosomes (Brown *et al.* 1973). Sephadex G-200 gel filtration of extracts of tissue has shown that the ^{67}Ga is mainly associated with 2 macromolecular components having molecular weights of $4-5 \times 10^4$ and $1.0 - 1.2 \times 10^5$, the former being quite prominent in tumor tissue (Hayes and Carlton, 1973).

The Normal Gallium-67 Scan

Autopsy studies have shown that after the intravenous injection of carrier-free ^{67}Ga as citrate, no tissue or organ is completely free of the isotope, although levels in the brain, cerebral-spinal fluid, fat, and skeletal muscle are quite low (Nelson *et al.*, 1972). Organs consistently showing the greatest concentrations of ^{67}Ga on scans include the liver, spleen, bone marrow, and central skeleton (Fig. 1). Other tissues or anatomical areas that may show increased activity on scans include the salivary glands (Fig. 2), the lacrimal glands (Fig. 3), the renal cortex, the external genitalia, and the ends of long bones of the

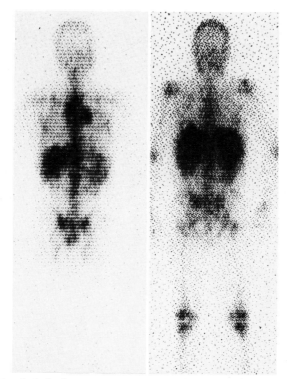

FIG. 1.—*Left*, whole body ⁶⁷Ga scan of a 21-year-old man with Hodgkin's disease of the mediastinum, showing radioactivity concentrated in tumors of the mediastinum. Normal concentration also is seen in the bone and bone marrow of the central skeleton, as well as in the liver, spleen, and skull. Note the ⁶⁷Ga activity at the tip of each scapula in the midthoracic region. *Right*, a whole body ⁶⁷Ga scan of a 19-year-old man with acute leukemia. Note the radioactivity in the enlarged spleen and liver and that at the ends of the long bones of the extremities.

extremities (Fig. 1 *right*) (Edwards, Hayes, and Nelson, 1972; Larson, Milder, and Johnston, 1973).

At times, ⁶⁷Ga will be concentrated in the normal adult breast and may pass into the human milk. This was first noted in postpartum and postabortal lactating and prelactating women with tumors (Larson and Schall, 1971; Fogh, 1971). An increased uptake of ⁶⁷Ga also has been noted in gynecomastia (Winchell *et al.*, 1970). We have also seen extensive uptake in the breasts of a nonlactating, nonpregnant, 15-year-old girl who had no evidence of tumor in her breasts (Fig. 4). Others have also noted variable uptake in breasts of women who were neither pregnant nor lactating.

Often, scans show an increased density in the center of the face

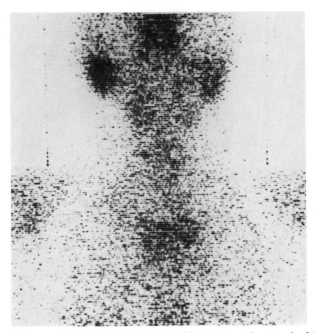

FIG. 2.—An anterior ^{67}Ga scan of a 76-year-old woman with a poorly differentiated thyroid carcinoma showing an accumulation of radioactivity in the tumor. Note also the activity in the salivary glands and in the center of the face. Neither of these latter areas contained tumor.

(Fig. 2), attributable to activity in the nasal pharynx; in the upper mediastinum, attributable to activity in the overlying sternal marrow and dorsal vertebrae; and in the posterior lateral aspects of the mid-thorax, attributable to activity in the inferior angle of the scapulae (Fig. 1 *left*). The uptake of ^{67}Ga in all these sites normally varies a great deal from patient to patient, often for no apparent reason. This variability accounts for much of the difficulty encountered in interpreting ^{67}Ga scans. Abdominal and pelvic ^{67}Ga scans are particularly difficult to interpret largely because of the variable amounts of isotope retained by the viscera, especially the bowel (Fig. 5).

LUNG CANCER

Cancer of the lung, whether primary or metastatic, can be detected by ^{67}Ga scanning in a high percentage of patients (Fig. 6). In the literature, we find reports varying from about 55 per cent to 100 per cent, with an average of about 85 per cent (Table 1). A similar per-

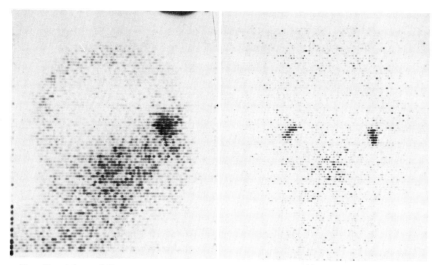

FIG. 3.—A lateral *(left)* and an anterior *(right)* [67]Ga scan of a 45-year-old woman with undifferentiated carcinoma of the lung showing concentration of the radioactivity in the lacrimal glands. The focus of activity appears larger on the lateral view because the lacrimal glands were not in the focal plane of the collimator. There is also a slight accumulation of activity in the nasopharynx showing in the center of the face.

centage was found by The Cooperative Group to Study Localization of Radiopharmaceuticals (CGSLR) for a large group of patients with untreated lung cancer (DeLand *et al.,* in press). There is no general agreement as to whether the morphologic features determining a tumor's histopathologic classification are important factors affecting its affinity for [67]Ga. The experience of the CGSLR suggests only a slightly greater frequency of positive scans in well-differentiated squamous cell carcinoma than in adenocarcinoma or small cell carcinoma (Table 2) (DeLand *et al.,* in press). Higasi and associates have reported that squamous cell carcinoma and adenocarcinoma take up ^{67}Ga less readily than the undifferentiated carcinomas (Higasi *et al.,* 1972), and Langhammer and co-workers found no dependence on the morphologic type of tumor (Langhammer *et al.,* 1972).

Unfortunately, the uptake of ^{67}Ga is not limited to malignant neoplastic lesions and a positive scan over a known lesion does not prove that it is malignant. Gallium's lack of specificity for malignancy has been repeatedly demonstrated with a variety of lesions, *e.g.,* sarcoidosis, acute tuberculosis, abscesses, and acute pneumonias, which are particularly likely to produce localized concentrations of ^{67}Ga resembling the scan findings of cancer (VanDer Schoot, Groen, and

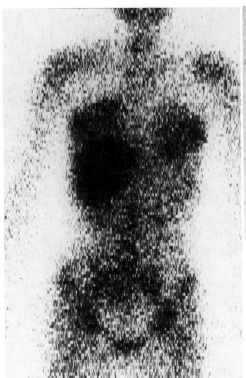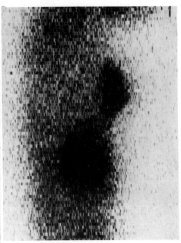

FIG. 4.—Anterior *(left)* and lateral *(right)* ⁶⁷Ga scans of a 15-year-old girl with Hodgkin's disease showing radioactivity concentrated in both breasts. The patient was neither pregnant nor lactating at the time of the scan.

DeJong, 1972; Dige-Petersen, Heckscher, and Hertz, 1972). Detecting these lesions on scans may be equally as important to the patient as finding a tumor, but in a specific search for cancer, ⁶⁷Ga concentrated in these benign lesions may lead to erroneous conclusions by the unwary.

Presently, the minimum tumor size necessary for detection limits the clinical application of ⁶⁷Ga scanning. In actual practice, the frequency of positive scans in patients with untreated lung cancer drops off sharply for lesions with diameters of less than 2 cm. (DeLand *et al.*, in press). It is quite probable that the critical size is somewhat smaller for superficial lesions, but even larger for deeper lesions or lesions adjacent to normal structures having a higher concentration of ⁶⁷Ga. From the standpoint of curative surgery, tumors 2 cm. in diameter usually are not early lesions. At the present it appears that ⁶⁷Ga scanning probably will not help the clinician in screening for early, unsuspected, curable, primary lung cancers.

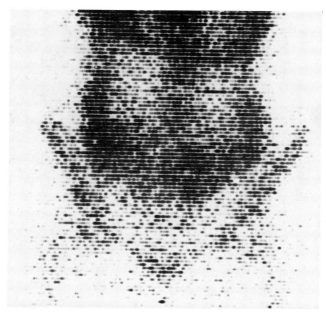

FIG. 5.—An anterior ⁶⁷Ga scan of the pelvis and abdomen of a 16-year-old girl with metastatic osteogenic sarcoma showing retention of radioactivity throughout the colon despite 2 days of laxatives and an enema prior to the scan.

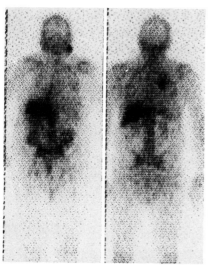

FIG. 6.—*Left*, a posterior whole body ⁶⁷Ga scan in a 58-year-old man with metastatic squamous cell carcinoma of the lung showing tumor in the left cervical lymph node and the right lower chest wall overlying the liver. The primary tumor had been excised prior to this scan. *Right*, a posterior whole body scan of a 66-year-old man with squamous cell carcinoma of the lung that had been treated with an inadequate dose of radiation. The scan shows a focus of radioactivity in the left hemithorax. After the lung was removed, assays showed the concentration of ⁶⁷Ga in tumor was 7 times that in the normal lung.

Table 2
Results of ^{67}Ga Scans in Cancer of
the Lung by Histopathologic Type*

Histopathologic Type	Scan Results†			%Positive
	Positive	Negative	Equivocal	
Squamous, moderately or well-differentiated	51	9	0	85
Squamous, large cell, undifferentiated	65	14	1	81
Adenocarcinoma, bronchoalveolar	25	2	7	74
Small cell, oat cell	17	6	1	71
Not otherwise specified	13	3	0	81
Total	171	34	9	80%

*DeLand *et al.*, in press.
†Sites of tumor proven at surgery or autopsy.

Simply reporting a higher incidence of positive scans in lung cancer is apt to be misleading and does not convey a true picture of the clinical usefulness of ^{67}Ga. From a clinician's point of view, the value of ^{67}Ga scanning for detecting lung cancers must be weighed against the fact that many, if not most, lung cancers can be detected more easily with a chest X-ray examination. Reports citing 85 per cent or more positive scans include many patients with large tumors located in distal parts of the lungs, well away from the mediastinum and hilar regions. In many, the ^{67}Ga scan provides no additional information about the primary tumor over that obtained from a chest X-ray examination—a quicker, easier, and less expensive test and one that exposes patients to less radiation. A more appropriate estimate of the clinical usefulness of ^{67}Ga scanning would be the frequency with which lesions are detected by scanning when they are either not detected or merely suspected on the X-ray studies.

For cancer of the lung, as for other tumors, the greatest value of ^{67}Ga scanning may be in the staging of the disease, *e.g.*, detecting metastases prior to the initial therapy. The CGSLR reported detecting lymph node metastases by scanning in more than 70 per cent of patients with histologically proven regional lymph node metastases (DeLand *et al.*, in press). This view is enhanced by the recent reports on the use of ^{67}Ga scanning for brain tumors (Jones Koslow, Johnston, and Ommaya, 1972; Henkin, Quinn, and Weinberg, 1973). In patients with negative or equivocal pertechnetate brain scans, with brain metastases, ^{67}Ga scanning may significantly increase the diagnostic accuracy of brain scanning.

LYMPHOMAS

Over-all, approximately 3 or 4 scans were positive in patients with lymphoma (Table 1). However, the percentage for individual lesions detected on scans depends greatly on their size, location, and histopathology. For reasons that are not entirely clear, lymphomas in the neck and chest are detected with greater reliability than those in other parts of the body (Table 3) (Greenlaw *et al.*, in press; Johnston *et al.*, in press). The mediastinum, abdomen, and pelvis are of particular importance as regions where ^{67}Ga scanning has considerable potential for aiding the clinician. Intra-abdominal lesions are apt to be overlooked if only standard diagnostic procedures are used. The region of the celiac group of nodes in the epigastrium, a frequent site for lymphomas, is particularly difficult to evaluate by physical examination or even with lymphangiography, although tumors in this area can be detected on scans (Fig. 7). Probably no other nonsurgical procedure is as effective in detecting lymphomas deep in the epigastrium.

Although there is as yet no unanimity on this matter, we believe that lymphomas with greater histiocytic cellularity generally give a higher percentage of positive scans. Lesions in which the lymphocyte is the predominant cell are positive much less often (Table 4) (Greenlaw *et al.*, in press). Likewise, a slightly higher rate of positive scans has been reported for Hodgkin's lesions of nodular sclerosis type than for the mixed cellularity type (Table 4) (Johnston *et al.*, in press).

When ^{67}Ga was first observed to concentrate in lymphomas, it was hoped that ^{67}Ga scanning would replace the arduous procedures called for in the staging of Hodgkin's disease. Because accurate stag-

Table 3
Results of ^{67}Ga Scans for Malignant Lymphomas
by Anatomic Area*

Tumor Sites	Results of Scans[†]			
	Positive	Negative	Equivocal	%Positive
Neck	109	41	4	70
Thorax	22	3	0	88
Axilla	11	15	2	39
Abdomen and Pelvis	117	98	26	48
Inguinal-femoral	21	17	1	53

*Greenlaw *et al.*, in press; Johnston *et al.*, in press.
[†]Sites of tumor proven at surgery or autopsy.

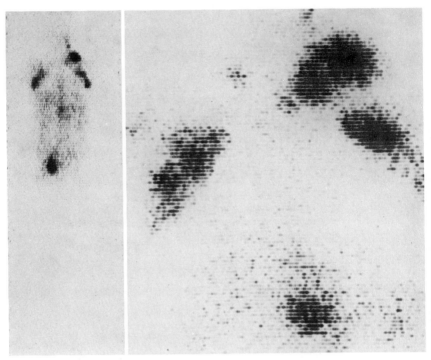

FIG. 7.—A posterior whole body ⁶⁷Ga scan *(left)* and an anterior ⁶⁷Ga chest scan *(right)* of a 40-year-old woman with widespread malignant lymphoma showing uptake of the radionuclide in tumors of both axillae, both sides of the neck, in the right groin, and in the midepigastrium.

ing is thought to be essential to optimum therapy, patients with Hodgkin's disease and certain other lymphomas are subjected to multiple biopsies of the marrow, extensive X-ray studies, lower extremity lymphangiography, exploratory abdominal surgery, and multiple visceral biopsies. If one test as safe and noninvasive as ⁶⁷Ga scanning could replace all of these, its clinical value would be indisputable. Unfortunately, it soon became apparent that there were inexplicable differences from patient to patient and even from lesion to lesion within the same patient, making it impossible to rule out the presence of tumor at any given site merely by a negative ⁶⁷Ga scan (Edwards and Hayes, 1972). The CGSLR reported failure to detect tumor in about one fourth of the surgically proven sites of Hodgkin's disease (Johnston *et al.*, in press). The detection of visceral involvement is of special interest and while there have been notable exceptions (Larson, Schall, and Johnston, 1971; Suzuki *et al.*,

Table 4
Results of ^{67}Ga Scans — Hodgkin's Disease* and Other Lymphomas† by
Histopathologic Type

Histopathologic Type	Results of Scans‡			%Positive
	Positive	Negative	Equivocal	
Hodgkin's, nodular sclerotic	94	31	7	71
Hodgkin's, mixed cell	35	24	6	53
Hodgkin's, lymphocyte depletion	4	6	0	—
Hodgkin's lymphocyte predominant	18	6	3	—
Hodgkin's, not otherwise specified	10	3	2	—
Hodgkin's Subtotal°	161	70	18	64%
Well-differentiated, lymphocytic lymphoma	6	7	0	—
Poorly differentiated, lymphocytic lymphoma	31	61	9	30
Mixed cell	28	23	2	52
Histiocytic	54	17	5	71
Burkitt's	5	0	0	—
Not otherwise specified	13	6	0	—
Malignant Lymphoma Subtotal†	137	114	16	51%
Total Lymphomas	298	184	34	57%

° Johnston *et al.*, in press.
† Greenlaw *et al.*, in press.
‡ Sites of tumor proven at surgery or autopsy.

1971; Lomas, Dibos, and Wagner, 1972), success in detecting Hodgkin's disease or other lymphomas in the liver or spleen has been poor. We are reluctant to interpret a scan as showing tumor involving either of these organs unless we see distinct hot spots of activity within the organ, as opposed to a diffuse increase of activity. Such a crucial decision as determining the stage of Hodgkin's disease prior to therapy cannot be entrusted to any single test with so high a false-negative rate. However, ^{67}Ga scans frequently disclose sites of unsuspected tumor that have eluded detection with other diagnostic procedures. Gallium-67 scans serve well as a complement to lymphangiography and other X-ray studies for staging (Turner *et al.*, 1972; Turner *et al.*, in press).

Therapy is known to affect a tumor's affinity for ^{67}Ga. When a tumor is completely ablated, whether by drugs or radiation, we cannot expect to see localization of ^{67}Ga. Even after radiation that is less than ablative, scans often show little or no ^{67}Ga localization where tumor uptake had been readily demonstrated before therapy. One is inclined to attribute such a decrease in ^{67}Ga uptake to the effectiveness of the therapy, and in some instances this association may be justified. However, neither the relationship between tissue lethality, radiation dose, and ^{67}Ga uptake nor the time course of the effect of radiation on the gallium uptake of tumors has been worked out. The amount of ^{67}Ga retained in irradiated normal tissues is also diminished (Swartzendruber and Hübner, 1973). Clearly, there is a need for such studies dealing with radiation and with chemotherapy. In the meantime, one should be very circumspect in evaluating a tumor's response to therapy from changes in its affinity for ^{67}Ga. It is well known that lymphomas and some other tumors undergo morphologic changes that require reclassification. Similarly, a tumor which at one time has concentrated ^{67}Ga may lose this affinity while retaining its malignancy and proliferative characteristics.

FIG. 8.—An anterior ^{67}Ga scan of the pelvis of a 45-year-old woman who had had total lymph node irradiation (4,000 R) for Stage III Hodgkin's disease. She had completed her radiation treatment only 6 weeks before this scan and was having some pain in the region of the left iliac crest where the scan shows a lesion (arrow). The broken lines indicate the location of the radiation ports and show that the lesion was just at the edge of the treatment field. Note also the decreased radioactivity in the normal structures within the radiation fields.

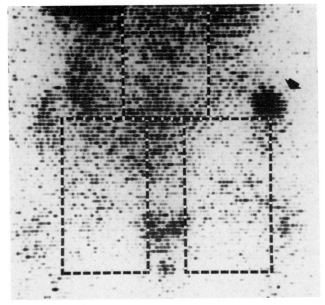

The nondestructive feature of ⁶⁷Ga scanning makes it especially applicable for periodic post-therapy evaluations. Because it is safe, relatively painless, and only moderately expensive (compared to lymphangiography or exploratory surgery) it can be repeated at fairly frequent intervals. Asymptomatic recurrences of lymphomas may thus be detected at a time when they can be treated effectively (Fig. 8). It may be that this application will prove to be the single most valuable contribution of ⁶⁷Ga scanning to clinical medicine.

BREAST CANCER

Our experience in detecting cancer of the breast with ⁶⁷Ga is neither extensive nor encouraging. The experience of other investigators has been contradictory (Table 1). Ito reported 4 positive scans in 4 patients (Ito *et al.*, 1971); Langhammer reported 3 positive scans in 9 patients (Langhammer *et al.*, 1972), but apparently all 3 positive scans were in treated patients. Fogh reported 15 positive scans for 19 patients (Fogh, 1971). Conversely, Lavender *et al.* (1971) reported only 5 patients with positive scans had advanced disease with either skin or chest wall involvement or metastases, while none of the 4 early primary carcinomas gave positive scans. Higasi reported 8 positive scans in 16 patients with breast cancer, although some of the tumors with negative scans were smaller than 2 cm. in diameter (Higasi *et al.*, 1972). Apparently, further experience with larger numbers of patients for whom the size of the tumors and the conditions of the scanning are defined will be necessary to find the true percentage of breast cancers detectable by scanning with ⁶⁷Ga.

Even with breast cancer, though, there are some points of agreement. First, the incidence of false-positive scans has been low for breast lesions. Higasi reported 1 positive scan in a patient with an inflammatory benign lesion, while 17 other patients with benign cystic and fibrocystic lesions failed to show ⁶⁷Ga uptake (Higasi *et al.*, 1972). Fogh and Edeling (1972) reported no positive scans for 12 benign breast lesions. None of these authors detected a difference in the scan results attributable to the histopathology of the malignant tumors.

Because of frequency of skeletal metastases of breast carcinoma, ⁶⁷Ga scanning may prove to be of special value in detecting early spread of this tumor. Gallium is known to be a bone-seeking element, and ⁶⁷Ga will localize at sites of skeletal metastases of a variety of tumors (Fig. 9) (Okuyama, Ito, Awano, and Sato, 1973). In our own

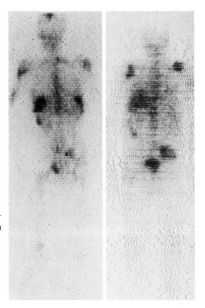

FIG. 9.—*Right*, a posterior whole body
^{67}Ga scan of a 17-year-old girl with
disseminated Ewing's sarcoma with
numerous skeletal metastases. *Left*, a
posterior whole body ^{67}Ga scan of a 62-year-
old man showing 4 skeletal metastases of an
adenocarcinoma from an undetermined
primary site. (Courtesy of Edwards and
Hayes, 1970.)

experience with 14 patients with metastatic breast cancer, in at least
8, only skeletal metastases were detected with ^{67}Ga scanning. Scans
alone do not indicate whether the radioactivity at sites of metastases
is in the neoplastic tissue, in the surrounding reactive bone, or in
both.

MISCELLANEOUS TUMORS

In addition to the tumors discussed above, ^{67}Ga scanning is reported to be of value occasionally in a variety of other tumors, including
colonic, rectal, renal, gynecological, and myeloid tumors, as well as
sarcomas. Nash and associates have shown that a number of colonic
and rectal cancers do concentrate ^{67}Ga equally as well as some other
tumors that are readily detectable on scans (Nash, Dance, McCready,
and Griffiths, 1972). Of 19 colonic and rectal carcinomas surgically
removed and assayed, 11 had tumor-to-normal uptake ratios of greater than 3:1 with a range of 1:1 to 83:1. They suggest that the difficulty others have in demonstrating colonic tumors may be because of
inadequate bowel preparation. We have used a mild laxative-enema
program (30 ml. of milk of magnesia with 5 ml. of cascara sagrada
given daily, plus saline enemas prior to the scan) to encourage bowel
evacuation, allowing some modification for patients whose bowels
are unusually resistant or sensitive to laxatives. In some patients, the

scans appear to show the entire colon full of ⁶⁷Ga-labeled feces (Fig. 5), while in others the bowel appears to be free of activity. Unfortunately, even a little retention can be very troublesome when there is a question of intra-abdominal tumors. Perhaps Dr. Nash's suggestion of a bowel cleansing program similar to that used for colonic surgery would be justified where the abdominal findings are of special interest.

Summary

The poorly understood affinity of tumors for ⁶⁷Ga has been widely but empirically applied to the clinical problem of detecting cancers. Gallium-67 scans are often difficult to interpret; the results are often ambiguous and have led to contradictory reports of clinical experience. Depending somewhat on histological type, most untreated primary lung cancers, untreated Hodgkin's tumors, and malignant lymphomas will be detected on scanning with ⁶⁷Ga. The incidence of false-positive results depends to a large extent on the skill of the interpreter at recognizing radioactivity in normal or non-neoplastic tissue. The clinical applications for which ⁶⁷Ga is best suited are: (1) the staging of Hodgkin's disease and certain other lymphomas that might be treated with radiation therapy; (2) the detection of early occult recurrences after therapy in Hodgkin's disease and other lymphomas; (3) the detection of occult metastases of lung and breast cancer (possibly others) prior to extensive surgical procedures aimed at curing the patient; and (4) the detection of metastases of known cancers in patients with symptoms not attributable to known sites of tumor.

Negative ⁶⁷Ga scans do not rule out cancer, not even the presence of additional metastases in a patient in whom the primary cancer showed ⁶⁷Ga uptake. Likewise, ⁶⁷Ga uptake in a lesion neither proves nor rules out malignancy of the lesion, nor can one reliably predict the histopathologic classification of a tumor on the basis of the scan findings.

With a better understanding of the mechanisms responsible for the uptake of gallium in normal and neoplastic tissues, additional clinical applications for ⁶⁷Ga scanning, such as the early assessment of therapy, may take on even greater importance.

Acknowledgments

Support for this work was received from Joint AEC-NIH Interagency Agreement No. 40-266-71 and American Cancer Society Grant No. CI-54.

The Medical Division of Oak Ridge Associated Universities is under contract with the U.S. Atomic Energy Commission.

REFERENCES

Berelowitz, M., and Blake, K. C. H.: 67Gallium in the detection and localization of tumours. South African Medical Journal, 45:1351–1359, December 11, 1971.

Brown, D. H., Swartzendruber, D. C., Carlton, J. E., Byrd, B. L., and Hayes, R. L.: The isolation and characterization of gallium-binding granules from soft tissue tumors. Cancer Research, 33:2063–2067, September 1973.

DeLand, F. H., Sauerbrunn, B. J. L., Boyd, C., Wilkinson, R. H., Jr., Friedman, B. I., Moinuddin, M., Preston, D. F., and Kniseley, R. M.: 67Ga-citrate imaging in untreated primary lung cancer: Preliminary report of Cooperative Group. Journal of Nuclear Medicine. (In press.)

Dige-Petersen, H., Heckscher, T., and Hertz, M.: 67Ga-scintigraphy in nonmalignant lung diseases. Scandinavian Journal of Respiratory Diseases, 53:314–319, June 19, 1972.

Edwards, C. L., and Hayes, R. L.: Tumor scanning with 67Ga citrate. Journal of Nuclear Medicine, 10:103–105, February 1969.

————: Scanning malignant neoplasms with gallium-67. The Journal of the American Medical Association, 212:1182–1190, May 18, 1970.

————: Localization of tumors with radioisotopes. In Goswitz, F. A., Andrews, G. A., and Viamonte, M., Jr., Eds.: Clinical Uses of Radionuclides: Critical Comparison with Other Techniques. (Proceedings of a Symposium Held at Oak Ridge Associated Universities, November 1971.) Oak Ridge, Tennessee, USAEC Symposium Series No. 27, CONF-711101, 1972, pp. 618–639.

Edwards, C. L., Hayes, R. L., and Nelson, B.: The "normal" 67Ga scan. (Abstract) Journal of Nuclear Medicine, 13:428–429, June 1972.

Fogh, J.: 67Ga-accumulation in malignant tumors and in the prelactating or lactating breast. Proceedings of the Society for Experimental Biology and Medicine, 138:1086–1090, December, 1971.

Fogh, J., and Edeling, C.: 67Ga scintigraphy of malignant tumours. Nuclear-Medizin, 11:371–395, December 30, 1972.

Greenlaw, R. H., Weinstein, M. B., Brill, A. B., McBain, J. K., Murphy, L., and Kniseley, R. M.: 67Ga citrate imaging in untreated lymphomas: Preliminary report of Cooperative Group. Journal of Nuclear Medicine. (In press.)

Haubold, V., and Aulbert, E.: 67Ga as a tumor scanning agent. Clinical and physiological aspects. In: Medical Radioisotope Scintigraphy, Vol. II, 1972. Proceedings of a Symposium, Monte Carlo, International Atomic Energy Agency, 1973, pp. 553–564.

Hayes, R. L., and Carlton, J. E.: A study of the macromolecular binding of 67Ga in normal and malignant animal tissues. Cancer Research, 33:3265–3272, December 1973.

Hayes, R. L., and Edwards, C. L.: New applications of tumour-localizing radiopharmaceuticals. In: Medical Radioisotope Scintigraphy, Vol. II, 1972. Proceedings of a Symposium, Monte Carlo, International Atomic Energy Agency, 1973, pp. 531–552.

Henkin, R. E., Quinn, J. L., and Weinberg, P. E.: Adjunctive brain scanning with ⁶⁷Ga in metastases. *Radiology*, 106:595–599, March 1973.

Higasi, T., Nakayama, Y., Murata, A., Nakamura, K., Sugiyama, M., Kawaguchi, T., and Suzuki, S.: Clinical evaluation of ⁶⁷Ga-citrate scanning. *Journal of Nuclear Medicine*, 13:196–201, March 1972.

Ito, Y., Okuyama, S., Awano, T., Takahaski, K., Sato, T., and Kanno, I.: Diagnostic evaluation of ⁶⁷Ga scanning of lung cancer and other diseases. *Radiology*, 101:355–362, November 1971.

Johnston, G., Benua, R. S., Teates, C. D., Edwards, C. L., and Kniseley, R. M.: ⁶⁷Ga-citrate imaging in untreated Hodgkin's disease: Preliminary report of Cooperative Group. *Journal of Nuclear Medicine*. (In press.)

Jones, A. E., Koslow, M., Johnston, G. S., and Ommaya, A. K.: ⁶⁷Ga-citrate scintigraphy of brain tumors. *Radiology*, 105:693–697, December 1972.

Kay, D. N., and McCready, V. R.: Clinical isotope scanning using ⁶⁷Ga citrate in the management of Hodgkin's disease. *The British Journal of Radiology*, 45:437–443, June 1972.

Langhammer, H., Glaubitt, G., Grebe, S. F., Hampe, J. F., Haubold, U., Hör, G., Kaul, A., Koeppe, P., Koppenhagen, J., Roedler, H. D., and van der Schoot, J. B.: ⁶⁷Ga for tumor scanning. *Journal of Nuclear Medicine*, 13:25–30, January 1972.

Larson, S. M., Milder, M. S., and Johnston, G. S.: Interpretation of the ⁶⁷Ga photoscan. *Journal of Nuclear Medicine*, 14:208–214, April 1973.

Larson, S. M., and Schall, G. L.: Gallium 67 concentration in human breast milk. (Letter to the editor) *The Journal of the American Medical Association*, 218:257, October 11, 1971.

Larson, S. M., Schall, G. L., and Johnston, S.: The value of ⁶⁷Ga scanning in the evaluation of liver involvement in Hodgkin's disease: Comparison with ⁹⁹ᵐTc-sulfur colloid. *Nuclear-Medizin*, 10:241–244, September 30, 1971.

Lavender, J. P., Lowe, J., Barker, J. R., Burn, J. I., and Chaudhri, M. A.: Gallium 67 citrate scanning in neoplastic and inflammatory lesions. *The British Journal of Radiology*, 44:361–366, May 1971.

Lomas, F., Dibos, P., and Wagner, H. N., Jr.: Increased specificity of liver scanning with the use of ⁶⁷gallium citrate. *The New England Journal of Medicine*, 286:1323–1329, June 22, 1972.

Nash, A. G., Dance, D. R., McCready, V. R., and Griffiths, J. D.: Uptake of gallium-67 in colonic and rectal tumours. *British Medical Journal*, 3:508–510, August 26, 1972.

Nelson, B., Hayes, R. L., Edwards, C. L., Kniseley, R. M., and Andrews, G. A.: Distribution of gallium in human tissues after intravenous administration. *Journal of Nuclear Medicine*, 13:92–100, January, 1972.

Okuyama, S., Ito, Y., Awano, T., and Sato, T.: Prospects of ⁶⁷Ga scanning in bone neoplasms. *Radiology*, 106:123–128, April 1973.

Suzuki, T., Honjo, I., Hamamoto, K., Kousaka, T., and Torizuka, K.: Positive scintiphotography of cancer of the liver with Ga⁶⁷ citrate. *The American Journal of Roentgenology, Radium Therapy and Nuclear Medicine*, 113:92–103, September 1971.

Swartzendruber, D. C., and Hübner, K. F.: Effect of external whole-body x-irradiation on gallium-67 retention in mouse tissues. *Radiation Research* 55:457–468, September 1973.

Swartzendruber, D. C., Nelson, B., and Hayes, R. L.: Gallium-67 localization in lysosomal-like granules of leukemic and nonleukemic murine tissues. *Journal of the National Cancer Institute*, 46:941–952, May 1971.

Turner, D. A., Gottschalk, A., Hoffer, P. B., Harper, P. V., Moran, E., and Ultmann, J. E.: Gallium-67 scanning in the staging of Hodgkin's disease. In: *Medical Radioisotope Scintigraphy*, Vol. II, 1972, Proceedings of a Symposium, Monte Carlo, International Atomic Energy Agency, 1973, pp. 615–630.

Turner, D. A., Pinsky, S. M., Gottschalk, A., Hoffer, P. B., Ultmann, J. E., and Harper, P. V.: The use of ^{67}Ga scanning in the staging of Hodgkin's disease. *Radiology*, 104:97–101, June 1972.

Viadya, S. G., Chaudhri, M. A., Morrison, R., and Whait, D.: Localisation of gallium-67 in malignant neoplasms. *The Lancet*, 2:911–914, October 31, 1970.

Van der Schoot, J. B., Groen, A. S., and de Jong, J.: Gallium-67 scintigraphy in lung diseases. *Thorax*, 27:543–546, September, 1972.

Winchell, H. S., Sanchez, P. D., Watanabe, C. K., Hollander, L., Anger, H. O., McRae, J., Hayes, R. L., and Edwards, C. L.: Visualization of tumors in humans using ^{67}Ga-citrate and the Anger whole-body scanner, scintillation camera and tomographic scanner. *Journal of Nuclear Medicine*, 11:459–466, July 1970.

Indium-111 Radiopharmaceuticals in Cancer Localization

DAVID A. GOODWIN, M.D.,* MICHAEL W.
SUNDBERG, Ph.D.,†‡ CAROL I. DIAMANTI, B.A.,*
and CLAUDE F. MEARES, Ph.D.‡§
*Department of Radiology, Division of Nuclear
Medicine, Stanford University School of Medicine,
Stanford, California, and Veterans Administration
Hospital, Palo Alto, California; †Department of
Chemistry, Stanford University, Stanford, California;
‡Present Address: Eastman Kodak Company, Rochester,
New York; and §Department of Chemistry, University
of California at Davis, Davis, California

TUMOR SCANNING often requires several days of delay following administration of the radiopharmaceutical to allow maximum tumor accumulation and elimination of unwanted background activity. In organs other than the brain, background activity is usually high. When radiolabeled proteins like ^{131}I albumin (Chou, Aust, Moore, and Peyton, 1951; Planiol, 1959; Hisada, Hiraki, and Ohba, 1966) and ^{131}I fibrinogen (Monasterio, Becchini, and Riccioni, 1964), and protein-bound metals like ^{67}Ga citrate (Hartman and Hayes, 1969; Edwards and Hayes, 1970) are employed, the blood background is high and drops slowly over a period of several days. A similar delay is also necessary for labeled antibodies to reach optimum target and background concentrations (McCardle et al., 1966; Hoffer et al., in preparation). A radiolabel with ideally matched physical characteristics for tumor scanning should therefore have a physical half-life of approximately 1 to 3 days in addition to suitable gamma emissions

57

(Wagner and Emmons, 1966). [111]Indium, with a half-life of 2.8 days, comes close to having optimum physical characteristics for providing scans up to 1 week following administration with a minimum of radiation exposure to the patient (Goodwin et al., 1969; Hunter and de Kock, 1969; Finston, Goodwin, Beaver, and Hupf, 1969; Hunter and Riccobono, 1970). These observations suggested an investigation of [111]Indium-labeled compounds and a study of their tumor-localizing properties.

Dosimetry

Since one of the most important factors in the use of [111]Indium is the large amount of information (photons) provided at low cost to the patient (rads) (Goodwin, Song, Finston, and Matin, 1973), it seems appropriate to present some of the pertinent dosimetry data first. [111]Indium decays by electron capture emitting gamma rays of 173 kev (87 per cent) and 247 kev (93 per cent). Internal conversion electrons and low energy X-rays result in a betalike energy deposition of 36 kev per disintegration. For delayed imaging (1 to 3 days), it is superior to ^{99m}Tc, ^{131}I, [198]Au, or ^{67}Ga in terms of photons per rad. Preliminary estimates of radiation dose for ^{111}In radiopharmaceuticals are shown in Table 1.

General Methods

The [111]InCl$_3$ used in these experiments was obtained from Medi-Physics, Inc., Emeryville, California, and New England Nuclear, North Billerica, Massachusetts, in 0.05 N HCl (pH 1.5), containing from 1 to 7 mc. per ml. (Brown and Beets, 1972). Radiochemical analysis of ^{111}In-labeled compounds was carried out by paper chromatography, column chromatography, and electrophoresis. In some experiments, protein binding was measured by means of perturbation of angular correlation (PAC) measurements utilizing the special decay characteristics of [111]Indium (Meares, 1972).

Table 1
Preliminary Estimates of [111]In Radiation Dose: Rads per Mc.

Organ	[111]InCl$_3$ (Transferrin)	[111]In Bleo
Total body	0.5	0.063
Marrow	3.6	0.45
Liver	4.5	0.56
Bladder	—	0.01 to 0.5
		(Depending on voiding)

Biological half-life studies were done in normal Balb/c white mice using whole body counting. Organ distribution studies and tumor uptake were done in specially prepared Balb/c white mice. A tumor line, KHJJ, derived from a primary mammary carcinoma arising in a mouse which had been maintained for more than 100 transplant generations was used for the assay (Rockwell, Kallman, and Fajardo, 1972). Transplantation was by subcutaneous implantation of tumor fragments about 1 mm. in diameter in the flank. The study was carried out after approximately 14 days growth, when the tumor had reached a size of about 1.0 cm.[3] (Fig. 1). On histological examination,

FIG. 1 *(top).*—KHJJ tumor after 16 days of growth, showing the size and location in the flank of a Balb/c mouse.

FIG. 2 *(bottom).*—Histological section of KHJJ tumor (×700). The generally undifferentiated carcinomalike pattern with round or polygonal cells with little stroma has not changed in over 3 years (>100 transplant generations). (Courtesy of Dr. Luis Fajardo, Department of Pathology, Veterans Administration Hospital, Palo Alto, California.)

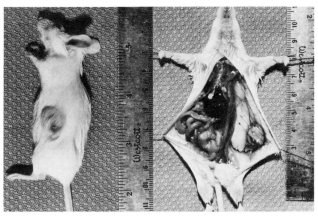

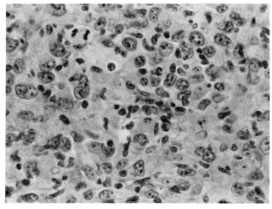

the tumor had a "carcinomalike" pattern with a predominance of islands of round or polygonal malignant cells with little stroma, and a generally undifferentiated appearance (Fig. 2). After transplantation, the tumor "took" in almost all animals and grew without metastasizing or killing the mice within 16 days. For the bioassay, a volume of 0.2 ml. containing 0.1 μc. of the compound was injected into the tail vein, and a minimum of 3 mice were injected with each compound. At 3 hours and 24 hours later, the mice were anesthetized with ether, the jugular vein cut, and the blood collected in 2 preweighed capillary tubes. Each mouse was then instantly killed by cervical dislocation and the major organs including a muscle sample, skin, bone (left femur plus marrow), tail, and a sample of tumor were excised. All organs including the tumor sample were washed with saline, lightly damped dry, and weighed immediately. Samples counted included the standard, blood, tail, and gauze with vena puncture blood, lungs, liver, spleen, kidneys, muscle, bone, and tumor. The results were expressed as per cent dose injected per gram of tissue, and as tumor-to-organ concentration ratios (Locksley, Sweet, Powsner, and Dow, 1954; Long, McAfee, and Winkelman, 1963).

The patient studies were performed at various times up to 1 week following intravenous injection of 1 to 5 mc. (average 2 mc.) of the ^{111}In-labeled compound. Images were obtained on the Anger Camera equipped with a dual spectrometer (Goodwin, Menzimer, and Del Castilho, 1970) and on the Ohio Nuclear dual 5-inch model 54D rectilinear scanner equipped with 5 to 1 minification capability.

Results and Discussion

When $InCl_3$ is injected intravenously at pH 1.5 to 3.0, the In^{3+} metal ion binds instantly and quantitatively to transferrin (Stern et al., 1967; Hosain et al., 1969). The distribution of this form of [111]Indium in the tumor-bearing mice at 24 hours showed tumor concentrations of about 5.0 per cent per gm. with tumor-to-organ ratios greater than 1 for muscle and blood (Table 2). The biological half-life of ^{111}In transferrin in normal mice was approximately 25 days, suggesting sequestration in the bone marrow. The bone-plus-marrow (distal femur) concentration was ~ 6.0 per cent per gm. With all of the compounds studied, there was some fraction of the injected activity which had a long biological half-life, similar to ^{111}In transferrin, suggesting a common final pathway of ^{111}In metabolism, probably in the bone marrow. The amount of label following this pathway varied with the compound injected.

Table 2
Distribution of ^{111}In in Mice after 24 Hours

Organ	% Dose / gm. Organ	%/gm. Tumor / %/gm. Organ
[111]InCl$_3$		
Tumor	5.03 ± 0.20	−
Muscle	1.41 ± 0.12	3.57 ± 0.17
Bone	5.7 ± 0.99	0.99 ± 0.22
Blood	1.78 ± 0.11	2.82 ± 0.07
Citrate (^{111}In)		
Tumor	4.73 ± 0.025	−
Muscle	1.18 ± 0.020	4.12 ± 0.42
Bone	6.0 ± 0.96	0.80 ± 0.14
Blood	1.82 ± 0.21	2.61 ± 0.11

Human studies with ^{111}In transferrin have shown a blood disappearance half time of about 10 hours, with increasing localization in the bone marrow at 24 and 48 hours seen on whole body scanning (Goodwin, Goode, Brown, and Imbornone, 1971) (Fig. 3). This observation, made on patients injected for the purpose of tumor localization, has suggested the use of ^{111}In transferrin for bone marrow visualization (Lilien, Berger, Anderson, and Bennett, 1973). Imaging of some tumors was possible with ^{111}In transferrin (Fig. 4), but the high background, especially in areas near or overlying bone marrow, has proven to be an insurmountable problem (Fig. 5). Indium was not excreted via the gastrointestinal tract, and no activity was seen in the bowel on the whole body scans. About 1 to 2 per cent of ^{111}In activity was excreted in the urine in the first 24 hours. The kidneys were only occasionally visualized on the whole body scan, despite consistently high concentrations demonstrated in the mouse kidney.

In an attempt to decrease the transferrin binding of [111]Indium and thus lower the background in muscle and bone, and because of reports of tumor uptake of [67]Gallium citrate (Edwards and Hayes, 1970), ^{111}In citrate was studied. It was found that the citrate forms a relatively weak chelate with Indium which quickly gives up the metal to the protein transferrin both in vitro and in vivo. The citrate, EDTA, and transferrin compounds could be clearly separated by column chromatography (Fig. 6). Chromatography was done following in vitro incubation of ^{111}In citrate in human serum for 3 hours (Fig. 7) and 24 hours after injection of tumor mice on soluble extract of the tumor

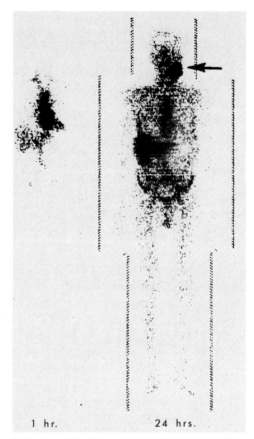

FIG. 3.—Whole body scan. ^{111}In-labeled transferrin is initially retained within the vascular space immediately following injection. Over the subsequent 24 hours, the activity leaves the blood pool and is deposited in the bone marrow. The vertebral column and pelvis are visualized well at this time. Metastatic carcinoma of the prostate is seen in the left side of the neck in this patient at 24 hours. (Courtesy of Goodwin, Goode, Brown, and Imbornone, 1971.)

(Fig. 8). As with $^{111}InCl_3$, most of the activity appeared in the transferrin peak following ^{111}In citrate incubation or injection (Table 3). A comparison of $^{111}InCl_3$ and ^{111}In citrate with $^{67}GaCl_3$ and ^{67}Ga citrate in the KHJJ tumor mice, showed about the same tumor concentrations with all 4 compounds (Fig. 9). However, the tumor-to-organ ratios were higher with ^{67}Ga citrate (Goodwin, Imbornone, and Song, 1971) (Fig. 10). As predicted by the animal model, there was little difference in the human scans using ^{111}In citrate as compared to $^{111}InCl_3$.

Indium forms stable chelates with EDTA and DTPA as well as

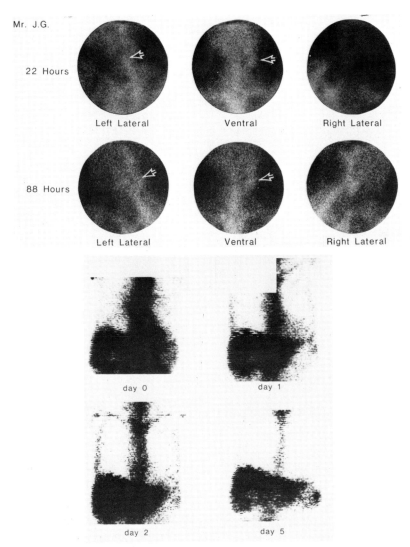

FIG. 4. *(top).*—Hodgkin's disease and palpable lymph nodes in left cervical chain in a 22-year-old male. These nodes concentrated ¹¹¹In transferrin sufficiently to visualize (arrows); sternal and cervical bone marrow also is evident.

FIG. 5 *(bottom).*—Failure to visualize a liver metastasis, and marrow distribution of ¹¹¹In transferrin.

several other chelating agents. These substances are all rapidly excreted in the urine and tumor concentrations are low (Fig. 9). Recently, it has been shown that ¹¹¹Indium also forms a stable chelate with the antitumor antibiotic bleomycin (Merrick *et al.*, 1973; Good-

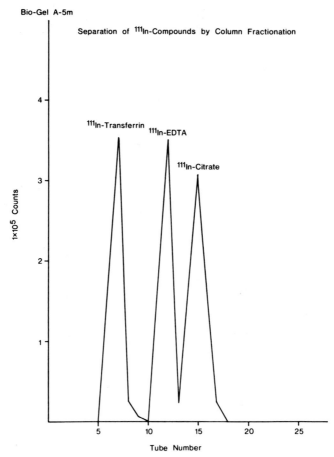

FIG. 6. — Clear separation of ^{111}In-labeled compounds by column chromatography.

win *et al.*, 1973). This offered a unique opportunity to study the distribution in vivo of an antitumor agent of proven effectiveness. The possibility that the antitumor agent might have greater specificity for tumor than other compounds was an exciting one and provided a rational approach to tumor imaging (Emerson, O'Mara, and Lilien, 1973; Grove, Eckelman, and Reba, 1973; Verma *et al.*, 1973). As obtained commercially (Bristol Laboratories, Syracuse, New York), the naturally occurring copper has been removed, and Renault and his colleagues have shown that this copper-free material readily chelates a variety of other cations (Renault, Rapin, and Wicart, 1971). As a result of this work, bleomycin labeled with ^{57}Co was given a prelimi-

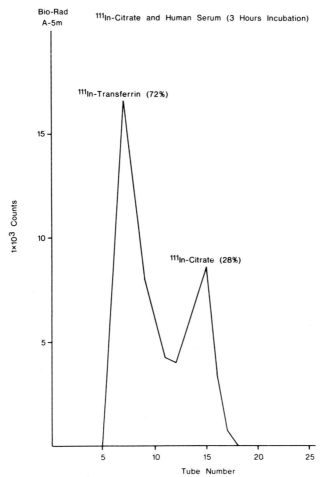

FIG. 7.—Seventy-two percent translocation of ^{111}In activity from citrate to transferrin following incubation of the labeled citrate with human serum for 3 hours. (Courtesy of Goodwin, Meares, and Song, Radiology, 105:699, Dec. 1972.)

nary clinical trial as a tumor-scanning agent by J. P. Nouel and his co-workers (Nouel *et al.*, 1972). Because of the more desirable physical characteristics of [111]Indium, Merrick and co-workers at Hammersmith Hospital have labeled bleomycin with this radionuclide. Their initial clinical reports have been encouraging (Merrick *et al.*, 1973).

Our method of labeling bleomycin with [111]Indium was done by simple chelation of added [111]InCl$_3$ (Goodwin, Lin, Diamanti, and Goode, in preparation). From 1 to 3 ml. of InCl$_3$ containing approximately 5 mc. was added directly to 15 mg. of lyophilized powdered

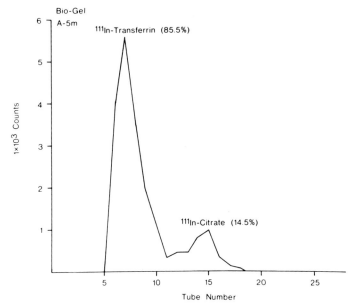

FIG. 8.—Chromatography of soluble extract of KHJJ tumor 24 hours after injection of ^{111}In citrate.

bleomycin obtained from Bristol Laboratories. After about 15 minutes of incubation, the pH was adjusted to approximately 6 to 7 with 1 ml. of phosphate buffer. This solution was transferred to a sterile multidose vial and was sufficient for 2 or 3 patients. Contrary to published reports (Thakur, 1973), we found that prolonged incubation or heating was not necessary, as chelation of ^{111}In^{+++} occurred very rapidly at room temperature. The preparation was carried out under aseptic conditions and no further sterilization was necessary. It was

Table 3
Column Fraction with Bio-Rad A-5m

Compound	Highest Peak	Tube No. of Activity	Recovery
I. In Vitro.			
^{111}In-Transferrin	7	5–9	98.7%
^{111}In-Citrate	15	13–17	99.6%
^{111}In-EDTA	12	10–14	89%
^{111}In-Citrate + Transferrin	7, 15	5–10, 12–17	72%, 28%
II. In Vivo. Tumor Assay (Injected to tumor mice)			
^{111}InCl$_3$ (Transferrin)	7	5–9	86%
^{111}In-Citrate	7, 15	5–10, 12–17	85%, 15%

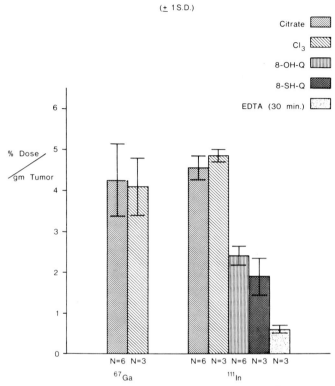

FIG. 9.—Comparison of ⁶⁷Gallium and ¹¹¹Indium compounds in tumor-bearing mice.

not necessary to refrigerate this preparation. Chromatography was carried out on 20 cm. strips of Whatman #1 paper, by the descending method, using 10 per cent ammonium chloride with the solvent adjusted to pH 5.5. In this system, more than 93 per cent of the activity appeared in 3 fractions. The largest amount (56 per cent) appeared in a peak corresponding to bleomycin B (Rf 0.75). Approximately equal amounts appeared as bleomycin A (18 per cent, Rf 0.95), and a third biologically active fraction (19 per cent, Rf 0.55) (Fig. 11) (Umezawa, Maeda, Takeuchi, and Yoshiro, 1966). In this chromotographic system, at pH 5.5, $InOH_3$ colloid and ¹¹¹In transferrin stayed close to the origin. ¹¹¹In bleomycin was stable for up to a week at room temperature and, unlike In citrate, did not show translocation of the Indium label to transferrin after 1 hour incubation with serum in vitro (Fig. 12). Other cations competed with In^{+++} for bleomycin labeling (Fig.

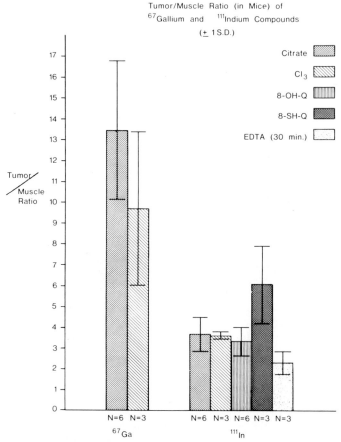

FIG. 10.—Comparison of [67]Gallium and [111]Indium compounds in tumor-bearing mice.

13), zinc (Zn^{++}) being the major contaminant at levels of about 200 μg. per ml. After removal of the zinc on Bio Rad (AGIX8) anion exchange resin, much higher specific activities are possible. With very high specific activity ^{111}In bleomycin (Medi-Physics, Inc., Emeryville, California), a shift in activity from bleomycin B to bleomycin A occurred on storage for 1 month at room temperature (Fig. 14).

The biological excretion following intravenous injection into normal Balb/c white mice had 2 major phases. Rapid excretion accounted for 80 to 85 per cent of the injected activity within the first 24 hours. The remaining 15 per cent was excreted very slowly, with a

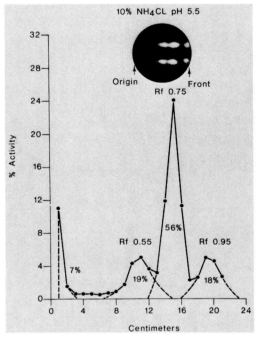

FIG. 11.—Paper chromatography of ¹¹¹In-labeled bleomycin. (Courtesy of Goodwin *et al.*, in preparation.)

T½B = 15.5 days, and represented a fraction which was firmly bound probably as ¹¹¹In transferrin in the bone marrow (Fig. 15).

The tissue distribution of ¹¹¹In bleomycin in Balb/c mice bearing KHJJ tumor in the flank is shown in Table 4. At 3 hours, tumor uptake was 1.32 per cent per gm., but blood levels were still 1.48 per cent per gm. There was little concentration in the liver or spleen, and muscle and bone background were low. The tumor-to-muscle ratio was 3.63 and the tumor-to-bone ratio was 1.59 at the early time. There was improvement in all of these parameters at 24 hours because of a slight increase in tumor concentration and a further decrease in background. Tumor concentration at 24 hours was 1.98 per cent per gm., and blood levels were 0.48 per cent per gm. Liver and spleen concentrations were still low, and bone (including marrow) showed a small increase. The tumor-to-muscle ratio had increased to 6.42 and the tumor-to-blood ratio also had gone up to 4.60. By comparison, InCl₃ showed a different distribution at 24 hours. The absolute tumor concentration was higher, 5.03 per cent per gm., but so

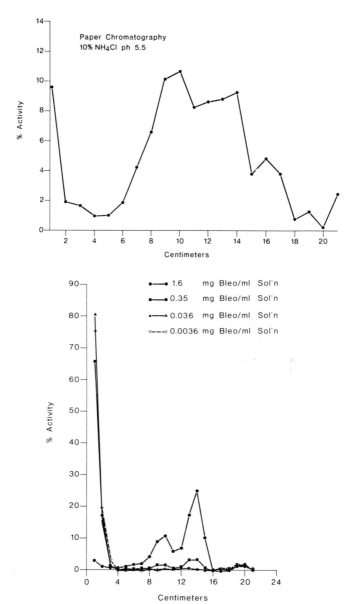

FIG. 12 *(top).* — Paper chromatography of ¹¹¹In bleomycin after incubation in human serum 1 hour at room temperature. (Courtesy of Goodwin, Lin, Diamanti, and Goode, in preparation.)

FIG. 13 *(bottom).* — Effect of competing cations in the ¹¹¹InCl solution (principally Zinc, Zn⁺⁺) on bleomycin labeling. (Courtesy of Goodwin, Lin, Diamanti, and Goode, in preparation.)

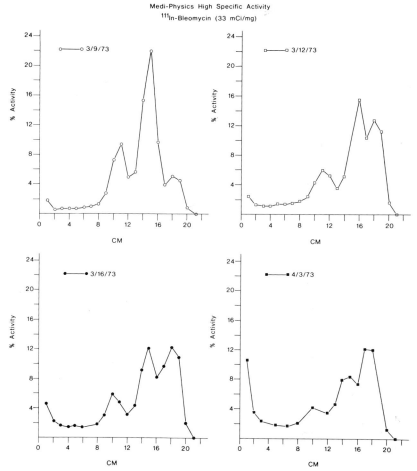

Medi-Physics High Specific Activity
^{111}In-Bleomycin (33 mCi/mg)

FIG. 14.—Effect of very high specific activity on stability of ^{111}In bleomycin stored at room temperature. A shift of activity from the B peak to the A peak occurred over a period of days and weeks. (Courtesy of Goodwin, Lin, Diamanti, and Goode, in preparation.)

were all the other tissue concentrations, producing inferior tumor-to-organ rations. Most significantly, the tumor-to-muscle ratio was only 3.57 and the tumor-to-bone (plus marrow) ratio was 0.99 (Table 2).

Patient studies were performed at 18 to 72 hours following intravenous injection of 1 to 5 mc. of ^{111}In bleomycin (average 2 mc.). Following injection into patients, the labeled material was rapidly excreted as ^{111}In bleomycin in the urine (Fig. 16). A suggestion of a shift in serum activity from the bleomycin B peak to the bleomycin A

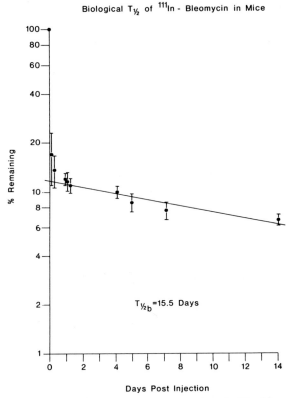

FIG. 15.—Whole body counting of 3 mice injected with ^{111}In bleomycin shows a rapid excretion phase comprising about 85 per cent in the first 24 hours and a subsequent slow phase, $T^{1/2}B = 15.5$ days, suggesting relatively firm fixation of this activity in the bone marrow.

peak occurred over 24 hours with an accompanying increase in origin activity, probably transferrin (Fig. 17). In those tumors which could be visualized, ^{111}In bleomycin was rapidly concentrated in the tumor within the first hour following intravenous injection, and the tumor retained this activity up to 48 hours (Fig. 18). Some tumors did not concentrate ^{111}In bleomycin at all. The bone marrow became increasingly labeled from 24 to 48 hours and caused most of the background interference. The liver and kidneys were also visualized at 24 hours.

In general, the scans showed a low target (tumor)-to-background ratio. In one case of cancer of the base of the tongue, this was measured by in vitro well scintillation counting on biopsy samples to be

Table 4
Balb/c Mice with KHJJ Tumor: ^{111}In-Bleomycin*

	% Dose/gm. Organ Mean ± Standard Deviation	
	3 Hours 3 Mice	24 Hours 6 Mice
Blood	1.48 ± 0.15	0.48 ± 0.20
Lungs	1.50 ± 0.060	1.22 ± 0.58
Liver	1.34 ± 0.17	2.77 ± 1.03
Spleen	1.00 ± 0.035	1.93 ± 0.40
Kidneys	7.47 ± 0.48	8.98 ± 2.24
Tumor	1.32 ± 0.076	1.98 ± 0.38
Muscle	0.37 ± 0.076	0.31 ± 0.026
Bone	0.86 ± 0.21	1.26 ± 0.087
Brain	0.066 ± 0.0050	0.054 ± 0.017
Skin	0.80 ± 0.12	1.18 ± 1.02

	Tumor/Organ Mean ± Standard Deviation	
	3 Hours 3 Mice	24 Hours 6 Mice
Blood	0.91 ± 0.12	4.60 ± 1.74
Lungs	0.88 ± 0.078	1.80 ± 0.60
Liver	0.99 ± 0.095	0.80 ± 0.34
Spleen	1.32 ± 0.036	1.05 ± 0.22
Kidneys	0.18 ± 0.012	0.23 ± 0.079
Tumor	—	—
Muscle	3.63 ± 0.62	6.42 ± 1.40
Bone	1.59 ± 0.41	1.58 ± 0.33
Brain	20.29 ± 2.68	41.35 ± 19.62
Skin	1.67 ± 0.18	2.31 ± 0.97

*Goodwin *et al.*, in preparation.

about 3 to 1. This necessitated a careful study of the scan images for small differences in uptake. In one patient, a metastatic tumor of the liver was visualized where the colloid scan demonstrated a focal defect (Figs. 19 and 20). Another patient with metastatic seminoma had received 600 rads to his chest for radiotherapy just prior to study with ^{111}In bleomycin. His tumor was visualized (Fig. 21), and the scan also demonstrated a significant decrease in marrow uptake of ^{111}In within the irradiated area.

The optimum dose-to-scan interval varied depending on the region of interest. Early studies performed from 1 to 6 hours after injection demonstrated high blood and tissue background. Bone marrow uptake was evident at 24 hours and increased at 48 and 72 hours, while the blood levels continued to fall. Regions overlying active bone marrow were best studied at 24 hours, while other areas had the

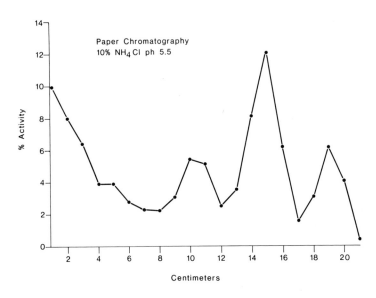

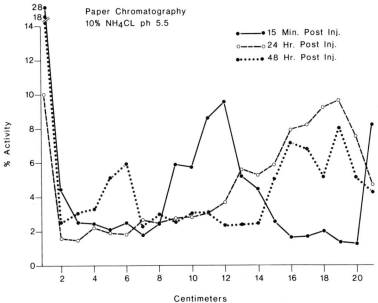

FIG. 16 *(top).*—A 24-hour urine sample of a patient following 1.62 mc. [111]In bleomycin containing 6.74 mg. bleomycin shows the majority of the activity is excreted as ^{111}In bleomycin, with a small unidentified fraction at the origin. (Courtesy of Goodwin, Lin, Diamanti, and Goode, in preparation.)

FIG. 17 *(bottom).*—Serum activity shows a shift of activity from the B peak to the A peak with a small increase in origin activity over 48 hours. (Courtesy of Goodwin, Lin, Diamanti, and Goode, in preparation.)

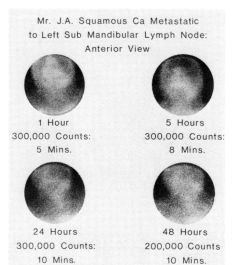

Mr. J.A. Squamous Ca Metastatic
to Left Sub Mandibular Lymph Node:
Anterior View

1 Hour
300,000 Counts:
5 Mins.

5 Hours
300,000 Counts:
8 Mins.

24 Hours
300,000 Counts:
10 Mins.

48 Hours
200,000 Counts
10 Mins.

Fig. 18. — Rapid accumulation of activity in the tumor following 1.9 mc. [111]In bleomycin; the activity remained relatively fixed in the tumor over 48 hours. (Dual peak.) (Courtesy of Goodwin, Lin, Diamanti, and Goode, in preparation.)

lowest background activity at 48 to 72 hours. If uncertainty existed about the region of interest, whole body scans were done at 24, 48, and 72 hours. A summary of the cases studied is shown in Table 5.

Nine of 29 (31 per cent) proven malignancies were not visualized on the scan with ^{111}In bleomycin. Of these, 2 were small primary carcinomas of the larynx, and 1 was a small tonsillar carcinoma. A bladder carcinoma metastatic to a rib also failed to be visualized. All 4 of these lesions were small, less than 3 cm. in diameter. Two other false-negatives had prior radiotherapy; one of these cases was an end-stage carcinoma of the larynx (also postlaryngectomy) and the other case was a carcinoma of the lung. The other 3 false-negatives were much larger and might have been expected to be visualized (carcinoma of the prostate with bone metastasis, squamous carcinoma of the larynx with a palpable lymph node metastasis, and a lymphoma with large neck nodes).

Of 29 patients, 20 (69 per cent) had positive visualization of their lesions by scan. Mr. P. D. (Fig. 22) had carcinoma of the stomach with a metastatic lesion in the upper humerus which visualized well, since it was situated away from erythropoietic marrow; he also had a second metastasis to the right pubic bone which was missed on first reading of the scan but seen well in retrospect. Mr. L. D. (Fig. 23) had a squamous carcinoma of the lip with a recurrent right submandibular mass well outlined on the right lateral view.

It is of interest that the animal model correctly predicted the bio-

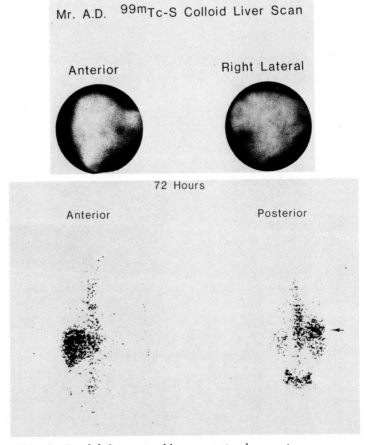

FIG. 19 *(top).* — Focal defects caused by metastatic adenocarcinoma.
FIG. 20 *(bottom).* — Concentration of ^{111}In bleomycin in metastatic adenocarcinoma of the liver (same patients as Fig. 19).
(Courtesy of Goodwin, Lin, Diamanti, and Goode, in preparation.)

logical distribution subsequently demonstrated on the human scans. The kidneys excreted 70 to 80 per cent of the material in the first 24 hours. The remaining activity had a long biological half-life. Increasing marrow activity with time, demonstrated on the scans, suggested that the labeled bleomycin which was initially fixed in the tissues was slowly metabolized, releasing the [111]Indium which was carried on transferrin to the bone marrow. The marrow uptake was much less notable with ^{111}In bleomycin than with [111]InCl$_3$ (transferrin).

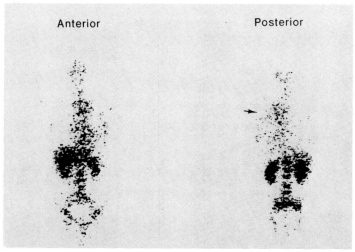

FIG. 21.—Metastatic seminoma to the lung visualized 18 hours following 1.77 mc. [111]In bleomycin. Note marked suppression of bone marrow uptake on posterior view where patient had just received 600 rads for radiotherapy. (Courtesy of Goodwin *et al.*, in preparation).

Tumor uptake was initially rapid, occurring within the first 3 hours, and this activity became relatively fixed in the tumor. The background activity fell over the next 24 hours or longer, improving the tumor-to-background ratio at the later times. As predicted by the animal studies, the absolute uptake of activity by the tumor on the positive patient scans was not high. We found marrow activity a definite disadvantage, especially when searching for tumor in the thorax or over the axial skeleton.

Both false-positive and false-negative results demonstrated a lack of specificity of ^{111}In bleomycin, and in this respect, it is similar to all other previously studied agents. Our series is too small to establish an accurate estimate of the incidence of false-positive and false-negative results, but it does suggest that this will be a serious problem in the general use of this agent for tumor diagnosis by scanning. However, ^{111}In bleomycin may find a useful clinical role in certain specific cases such as elucidating a focal defect on a colloid liver scan or determining the site and extent of certain tumor types. The suitability of ^{111}In as a label for studies which concentrate only a very small fraction of the activity in the target and require waiting periods of up to 72 hours prior to imaging has been clearly demonstrated.

Table 5
^{111}In-Bleomycin Clinical Results in 32 Patients*

Diagnosis	Positive	Negative	Comments
Malignant Lesions (Biopsy Proven)			
Squamous cancer, Head + Neck Cancer	10	5	1 postradiotherapy missed 3 small lesions < 3 cm. missed
Lung cancer	2	1	18 months after 6,000 rads to chest No evidence of recurrence
Stomach cancer	2	0	Metastatic lesions
Seminoma	1	0	Lung metastasis
Prostatic cancer	1	1	Bony metastasis ^{99m}Tc Poly-PO$_4$ Bone Scan Positive (+++) in both cases
Malignant melanoma	1	0	
Bladder cancer	0	1	Small bone metastasis < 3 cm. Poly-PO$_4$ bone scan positive
Adenocarcinoma (Primary unknown)	2	0	
Fibrous histiocytic sarcoma of leg	1	0	Recurrence postsurgery
Lymphoma: neck nodes	0	1	Mixed lymphocytic histiocytic type
Totals	20	9	
Benign Lesions			
Granuloma lung	1	0	Not proven
Paget's disease	0	1	Biopsy prostate: benign hypertrophy Bone scan (Poly-PO$_4$) positive
Cirrhosis of the liver	0	1	No biopsy: clinical diagnosis
†Osteomyelitis of the jaw	0	1	Biopsy proven
Totals	1	3	

°Goodwin *et al.*, in preparation.
†Same case as lung cancer, 18 months after 6,000 rads to mediastinum.
‡Same case as lung cancer, 18 months after 6,000 rads to mediastinum.

New Labeling Techniques

In our search for other ^{111}In-labeled compounds which might show promise as tumor-imaging agents, the major limitation has been in labeling technique. It has been impossible to use ^{111}Indium as a label for biologically interesting molecules because of its limited ability to form stable organometallic compounds under physiological conditions. In an effort to broaden the labeling capabilities of ^{111}Indium to include organic compounds other than chelates, Sundberg (1973) has developed a new method using a covalent label based on a metal chelate. This bifunctional chelate utilizes the covalent metal binding molecule, 1(*p*-benzenedrazonium)-ethylene-diamene-N, N, N′N′-tetra-acetic acid (azoϕEDTA) (Fig. 24). With this compound, a link is formed between the EDTA-^{111}In chelate and the

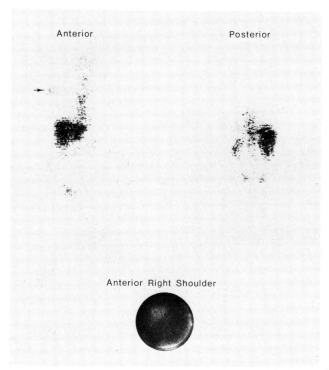

Anterior   Posterior

Anterior Right Shoulder

FIG. 22—A patient with adenocarcinoma of the stomach with a metastasis to the upper right humerus and right pelvis which was visualized 24 hours following 3.5 mc. ¹¹¹In bleomycin containing 7.5 mg. bleomycin. (Courtesy of Goodwin *et al.*, in preparation.)

protein, by means of the diazo bond. Following metabolism of the complex, rapid excretion of the azoφEDTA-¹¹¹In fragment by the kidneys should lower the blood background. We have used human serum albumin (HSA) and bovine fibrinogen labeled with ¹¹¹In in this way for studies of their distribution and metabolism in normal and tumor-bearing mice and in dogs (Goodwin, Meares, Diamanti, and Sundberg, in press).

The labeling was carried out as follows: To a solution of 100 mg. of fibrinogen (bovine fibrinogen 65 per cent clottable Sigma) (~200 nMole) in 10 ml. of a 0.01 M borate buffer pH 8.3 at 4° C was added to a solution containing approximately 200 μc. of ¹¹¹InCl₃ and 5 μl. of a 5.7 mM. solution of azoφEDTA (28.5 nMole). The pH was readjusted to 8.5 and the solution stirred slowly overnight. The coupling reaction was then dialyzed against a frequently changed buffer containing 0.1 N sodium chloride until radioactivity was no longer present

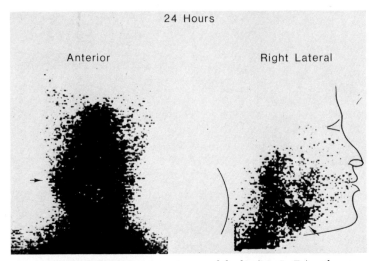

FIG. 23.—Resection of squamous carcinoma of the lip (Mr. L. D.) with a recurrence in a right submandibular node. This metastasis is well seen, especially on the right lateral view, following 2.04 mc. [111]In bleomycin containing 9 mg. of bleomycin. (Courtesy of Goodwin *et al.*, in preparation.)

in the dialysate. Human serum albumin (HSA) (25 per cent salt-poor human serum albumin, U.S.P. Cutter Laboratories) and one batch of fibrinogen were prepared similarly with the exception of the dialysis. For the albumin labeling, a solution of 250 mg. (3.8 μMole) HSA in 1 ml. of 0.1 N NaCl was combined with 4 ml. of a 0.01 M borate buffer, pH 9 at 4° C. A solution containing 200 μc. of ^{111}In and 0.14 μMole of azoϕEDTA was added, the pH readjusted to 9.0, and the solution allowed to stir in the cold overnight. The pH of both of these solu-

FIG. 24.—Covalent metal binding molecule which forms a link between the EDTA ^{111}In chelate and the protein by means of a diazo bond. (Courtesy of Sundberg, 1973.)

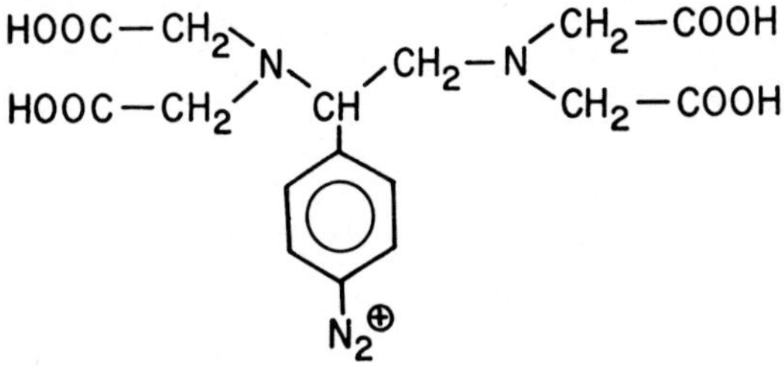

$$HOOC-CH_2 \diagdown N-CH_2-N \diagup CH_2-COOH$$
$$HOOC-CH_2 \diagup \quad CH \quad \diagdown CH_2-COOH$$

1-(p-Benzenediazonium)-ethylenediamine-N,N,N',N'-tetraacetic

acid (azoϕEDTA).

tions was readjusted to 7.0 prior to injection. Formation of diazonium coupling to proteins was confirmed by ultraviolet spectrometry and angular correlation measurements (Sundberg, 1973).

The clotting ability of the ^{111}In-labeled fibrinogen was tested by adding 1 unit of thrombin to 1 ml. of the dialyzed ^{111}In fibrinogen solution. After 3 hours, a visible clot had formed which was wound out of the solution on a wooden stick and the radioactivity in the clot was compared with that remaining in the solution. The clot contained 53 per cent of the radioactivity or about 80 per cent of theoretical value, assuming the material was initially 65 per cent clottable.

For intravenous injection into mice, the labeled protein solution was adjusted to a specific activity of $1\mu c./ml.$ with 0.1 N NaCl. Each mouse received 0.2 ml. of the solution containing 0.2 $\mu c.$ of ^{111}In. For organ distribution, Balb/c mice with a 16-day-old KHJJ tumor transplant were again used. The biological half-life of the labeled proteins in normal Balb/c mice was determined by whole body counting, correcting for physical decay. The biological half-lives of ^{111}In-labeled fibrinogen and ^{111}In-labeled HSA (both dialyzed and undialyzed) are shown in Table 5, along with the results of control experiments performed with ^{131}I-labeled HSA, ^{111}In azoϕEDTA, and ^{111}InCl$_3$ (transferrin). Three mice were used for each compound and they were followed up to 16 days. The ^{111}In azoϕEDTA was very rapidly excreted; T$^{1}/_{2}$B $\cong$ 4 hours. Plotted in a semilogarithmic way, the protein curves could be analyzed into 3 exponential components. The first phase was an initial rapid drop caused by mixing and rapid excretion of unreacted azoϕEDTA. The second phase had a medium and the third phase a long biological half-life. This was in contrast to the ^{131}I HSA curve which had a single exponential drop over a 4-day period of observation with a T$^{1}/_{2}$B of 1.2 days. The terminal long half-life portion of the ^{111}In-labeled HSA and fibrinogen curves represented a fraction equal to approximately 40 to 50 per cent of the total injected activity when extrapolated back to zero time. We interpret this to be the result of formation of slowly exerted metabolites, probably ^{111}In transferrin which is sequestered in bone marrow. The second portion of these curves probably represents a composite disappearing fraction. This requires correction to determine the true protein half-life. This was done by extrapolating the third phase of the curves back to zero time and using these values as a continuously changing baseline for the protein disappearance estimation. The distance above the extrapolated line for each point in the second phase was calculated and the line replotted on semilog paper using the least-squares method. The derived T$^{1}/_{2}$'s are shown in Table 6. Both

Table 6. — Biological Half-Life Whole Body Counting

Semi-Log Plot (Least-Squares)	^{111}In-Fibrinogen (Undialyzed)	^{111}In-Fibrinogen (Dialyzed)	^{111}In-Albumin (Undialyzed)	^{131}I-Albumin	^{111}InCl$_3$ (Transferrin)	^{111}In azoφEDTA (Control)
Phase I	~4 H	—	~4 H	—	—	4.22 H
Phase II	14.9 H	20.9 H	28.08 H	28.8 H	46.3 H	—
^{111}In-derived Phase III	22.7 D	19.7 D	20.7 D	—	27.0 D	—

Abbreviations: H = Hours; D = Days. Dotted line indicates absence of Phase.

dialyzed and undialyzed ^{111}In fibrinogen values agree fairly well, indicating rapid early excretion of unbound label. ^{111}In-albumin had a somewhat longer T½, and this value agreed with the ^{131}I-albumin control experiment. These values are different from either ^{111}In azoφEDTA or ^{111}InCl$_3$ injected alone. The T½ of the third phase was similar in all ^{111}In-labeled protein experiments, suggesting a final common pathway for the ^{111}In label.

The absolute tumor uptake of both ^{111}In-labeled albumin and fibrinogen was high (Table 7)—7.28 ± .78 per cent per gm. and 7.75 ± .17 per cent per gm. The background activity in other organs at 24 hours also was high; however, the tumor-to-organ ratios compared favorably with the other agents studied and exceeded 1 in all organs except liver, spleen, and kidneys. In contrast, the control group, injected with azoφEDTA labeled with ^{111}In, had very little concentration of activity in any of the organs except the kidney, by which route it is rapidly excreted. The absolute tumor uptake (per cent per gm.) of ^{111}In-labeled HSA and fibrinogen was significantly higher than the concentrations attained in a large number of the experiments in our laboratory with ^{67}Gallium citrate (4.2 ± .8), ^{67}Gallium chloride (4.1 ± .7), ^{111}Indium citrate (4.7 ± .4), ^{111}Indium chloride (5.0 ± 0.2), ^{111}Indium bleomycin (2.0 ± 0.4), and ^{131}I-labeled HSA (3.31 ±.1) using the same tumor model.

Preliminary experiments using serial dog scintiphotography following intravenous ^{111}In-labeled HSA and ^{111}In transferrin showed identical intravascular distribution of label initially. Images taken 2 days later showed significantly less bone marrow uptake with ^{111}In-labeled HSA (Fig. 25). The serial images also showed renal excretion of activity with this label which was not evident with ^{111}In transferrin.

A modification in the ^{111}In HSA labeling technique was also used for a similar dog study (Meares, unpublished data). The HSA was diazotized with the azoφEDTA using a citrate buffer, and this mixture was extensively dialyzed for 48 hours. The ^{111}InCl$_3$ solution was then prepared by passing it over a Bio-Rad (AGI-X8) anion exchange resin. The desired amount of activity (4 mc.) was evaporated to dryness in a Nalgene container and labeling was accomplished by simply adding the diazotized HSA citrate buffer solution and stirring for 5 minutes. This method allows very high specific activities as well as the possibility of using short half-lived radionuclides. The ease of this technique for labeling HSA with 4 mc. of ^{111}In demonstrates the feasibility of the method for use in human scintigraphy.

It is possible to label the plasma proteins albumin and fibrinogen using a covalent label based on a metal chelate. An advantage for radiopharmaceutical preparation is that the choice of radioactive label may be made after diazotization with azoφEDTA and other time-consuming steps like dialysis or column chromatography. This technique also allows the use of short-lived radionuclides such as ^{113m}In

Table 7
Absolute Uptake of ^{111}In-Labeled Albumin and Fibrinogen

	Control azoφEDTA-^{111}In 3 Tumor Mice 24 Hours % Dose/gm		Bovine Fibrinogen azoφEDTA-^{111}In 3 Tumor Mice 24 Hours % Dose/gm		Human Serum Albumin azoφEDTA-^{111}In 3 Tumor Mice 24 Hours % Dose/gm	
	Mean	S.D.	Mean	S.D.	Mean	S.D.
Blood	0.14	0.072	3.64	0.66	3.03	0.51
Lungs	0.17	0.21	4.89	1.33	5.94	0.73
Liver	0.19	0.053	14.74	3.10	9.70	0.73
Spleen	0.11	0.033	9.87	1.66	9.16	0.43
Kidneys	1.00	0.17	27.26	7.47	30.48	4.07
Tumor	0.28	0.040	7.28	0.78	7.75	0.17
Muscle	0.044	0.034	0.81	0.13	1.57	0.33
Bone	0.11	0.055	5.97	1.52	6.70	0.62
Brain	0.0073	0.0081	0.21	0.041	0.30	0.025
Skin	0.12	0.026	2.00	0.14	3.81	0.19

	Tumor/Organ		Tumor/Organ		Tumor/Organ	
	Mean	S.D.	Mean	S.D.	Mean	S.D.
Blood	2.48	1.26	2.03	0.29	2.60	0.40
Lungs	1.63	0.27	1.55	0.35	1.32	0.18
Liver	1.53	0.32	0.50	0.062	0.80	0.061
Spleen	2.78	0.70	0.74	0.045	0.84	0.0404
Kidneys	0.29	0.050	0.28	0.040	0.25	0.032
Muscle	15.80	19.72	9.19	1.72	5.09	1.09
Bone	2.95	0.99	1.26	0.26	1.16	0.12
Brain	21.67	2.35	35.06	9.24	25.68	2.44
Skin	2.46	0.40	3.64	0.38	2.04	0.075

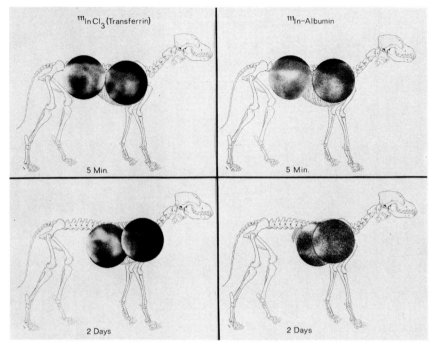

FIG. 25—Comparison by scintiphotography of the distribution of ^{111}In transferrin and ^{111}In-labeled albumin in a dog. Initially, more activity is seen in the kidney and later, less in the bone marrow with ^{111}In albumin. At 5 minutes, the heart pool is well visualized with both agents.

($T\frac{1}{2}$ 100 minutes). The behavior in vitro and in vivo of the labeled proteins showed only some minor alterations in function when compared to similar studies using other labels. The technique represents an extension of general radioactive tagging which allows nearly any protein or polypeptide to be labeled with any metal strongly chelated by EDTA.

Summary

^{111}In has optimum decay characteristics for tumor imaging by scintillation scanning. We have explored several ^{111}In-labeled compounds in vitro and in vivo to assess their tumor-imaging potential; ^{111}In bleomycin is the most useful at the present time. A new labeling technique has opened the way for synthesis of a variety of organic compounds labeled with ^{111}Indium, as well as for other radionuclides strongly chelated by EDTA. Studies carried out in mice and dogs show this is an effective method for labeling serum albumin and fibrinogen and that these compounds show promise for tumor imaging.

Acknowledgments

The authors gratefully acknowledge the secretarial assistance of Mrs. Alice Koenig, the expert technical help of Miss Carol White-leather, Mrs. Gertrude Ward, and Mr. Chung Song, the generous gift of bleomycin from Dr. Karl Agre of Bristol Myers, Inc., and the dosimetry calculations performed by Dr. Roland Finston of Stanford University, Department of Health Physics. The authors also acknowledge the helpful advice from and discussions with Dr. Max S. Lin.

This work was supported by Veterans Administration Program, Grant No. 3204, National Institutes of Health Grant No. GM-14752, and National Science Foundation Grant No. GP-4924.

REFERENCES

Brown, L. C., and Beets, A. L.: Cyclotron production of carrier-free Indium-111. *International Journal of Applied Radiation and Isotopes,* 23:57–63, February 1972.

Chou, S. N., Aust, J. B., Moore, G. E., and Peyton, W. T.: Radioactive iodinated human serum albumin as tracer agent for diagnosing and localizing intracranial lesions. *Proceedings of the Society for Experimental Biology and Medicine,* 77:193–195, June 1951.

Edwards, C. L., and Hayes, R. L.: Scanning malignant neoplasms with Gallium 67. *The Journal of The American Medical Association,* 212:1182–1191, May 18, 1970.

Emerson, D. A., O'Mara, R. E., and Lilien, D. L.: [111]Indium-bleomycin as a tumor imaging agent. (Abstract) *Journal of Nuclear Medicine,* 14:625, August 1973.

Finston, R. A., Goodwin, D. A., Beaver, J. E., and Hupf, H. B.: [111]In: Production, radionuclidic purity, and dosimetry of a new radiopharmaceutical for lymphatic scanning. (Abstract) In *Second International Conference on Medical Physics.* 1969, p 118.

Goodwin, D. A., Finston, R. A., Colombetti, L. G., Beaver, J. E., and Hupf, H.: 2.8-Day ^{111}In-colloid for lymphatic scintiphotography. (Abstract) *Journal of Nuclear Medicine,* 10:337, June 1969.

Goodwin, D. A., Goode, R., Brown, L., and Imbornone, C. J.: ^{111}In-labeled transferrin for the detection of tumors. *Radiology,* 100:175–179, July, 1971.

Goodwin, D. A., Imbornone, C. J., and Song, C. H.: Comparative study of tumor and organ distribution of ^{111}In and ^{67}Ga-labeled compounds in mice (Abstract) *Journal of Nuclear Medicine,* 12:434, June 1971.

Goodwin, D. A., Lin, M. S., Diamanti, C. I., and Goode, R. L.: [111]Indium labeled bleomycin for tumor localization by scanning. (In preparation.)

Goodwin, D. A., Lin, M. S., Diamanti, C. I., Goode, R. L., and Meares, C. F.: ¹¹¹In labeled bleomycin for tumor localization by scintiscanning. (Abstract) *Journal of Nuclear Medicine*, 14:401, June 1973.

Goodwin, D. A., Matin, P., and Finston, R. A.: ¹¹¹In—A new radiopharmaceutical for extended studies. (Abstract) *Journal of Nuclear Medicine*, 11: 388, June 1970.

Goodwin, D. A., Menzimer, D., and Del Castilho, R.: A dual-spectrometer for high-efficiency imaging of multi-gamma-emitting nuclides with the Anger camera. *Journal of Nuclear Medicine*, 11:221–223, May 1970.

Goodwin, D. A., Song, C. H., Finston, R., and Matin, P.: Preparation, physiology, and dosimetry of ¹¹¹In labeled radiopharmaceuticals for cisternography. *Radiology*, 108:91–98, July 1973.

Goodwin, D. A., Meares, C. F., Diamanti, C. I., and Sundberg, M.: Chelates for radiopharmaceutical labeling. Proceedings of the First World Congress of Nuclear Medicine, Tokyo, Japan, 1974. *International Journal of Nuclear Medicine*. (In press.)

Grove, R. B., Eckelman, W. C., and Reba, R. C.: Preparation, distribution, and tumor imaging properties of ¹¹¹In, ⁵⁷Co, ⁶⁷Ga, and ⁵⁹Fe labeled bleomycin. (Abstract) *Journal of Nuclear Medicine*, 14:627, August 1973.

Hartman, R. E., and Hayes, R. L.: The binding of Gallium by blood serum. *The Journal of Pharmacology and Experimental Therapeutics*, 168:193–198, July 1969.

Hisada, K. I., Hiraki, T., and Ohba, S.: Positive delineation of human tumors with ¹³¹I human serum albumin. *Journal of Nuclear Medicine*, 7:41–49, January 1966.

Hoffer, P. B., Lathrop, K., Bekerman, C., Fang, V. S., and Refetoff, S.: Use of ¹³¹I-CEA antibody as a tumor scanning agent. *Journal of Nuclear Medicine*, 15:323–327, May 1974.

Hosain, F., McIntyre, P. A., Poulose, K., Stern, H. S., and Wagner, H. N.: Binding of trace amounts of ionic indium-113m to plasma transferrin. *Clinica Chimica Acta*, 24:69–75, April 1969.

Hunter, W. W., Jr., and de Kock, H. W.: ¹¹¹In for tumor localization. (Abstract) *Journal of Nuclear Medicine*, 10:343, June 1969.

Hunter, W. W., Jr., and Riccobono, X. J.: Clinical evaluation of ¹¹¹Indium for localization of recognized neoplastic disease. (Abstract) *Journal of Nuclear Medicine*, 11:328, June 1970.

Lilien, D. L. Berger, H. G., Anderson, D. P., and Bennett, L. R.: ¹¹¹In-Chloride: A new agent for bone marrow imaging. *Journal of Nuclear Medicine*, 14:184–186, March 1973.

Locksley, H. B., Sweet, W. H., Powsner, H. J., and Dow, E.: Suitability of tumor-bearing mice for predicting relative usefulness of isotopes in brain tumors. *American Medical Association Archives of Neurology and Psychiatry*, 71:684–698, June 1954.

Long, R. G., McAfee, J. G., and Winkelman, J.: Evaluation of radioactive compounds for the external detection of cerebral tumors. *Cancer Research*, 23:98–108, January 1963.

McCardle, R. J., Harper, P. V., Spar, I. L., Bale, W. F., Andros, G., and Jiminez, F.: Studies with Iodine-131 labeled antibody to human fibrinogen for diagnosis and therapy of tumors. *Journal of Nuclear Medicine*, 7:837–847, November 1966.

Meares, C. F.: The Application of Perturbed Angular Correlation Studies to Biological Problems, Ph.D. Dissertation, Stanford University, Stanford, California, 1972, 234 pp.
_____: Unpublished data.
Merrick, M. V., Gunasekera, S. W., Lavender, J. P., Nunn, A. D., Thakur, M. L., and Williams, E. D.: The use of ^{111}Indium for tumor localization. In Medical Radioisotope Scintigraphy. Vienna, Austria, 1973, International Atomic Energy Agency, Vol. II, pp. 721–729.
Monasterio, G., Becchini, M. F., and Riccioni, N.: Radioiodinated I^{131} and I^{125} fibrinogen for the detection of malignant tumors in man. In Medical Radioisotope Scanning. Vienna, Austria, 1964, International Atomic Energy Agency, Vol. II, pp. 159–171.
Nouel, J. P., Renault, H., Robert, J., Jeanne, C., and Wicart, L.: La bléomycine Marquée au Co^{57}. Nouveau Presse Médicale, 1:95–98, January 8, 1972.
Planiol, T.: Diagnosis of intracranial lesions by gammaencephalography, using human serum albumin labelled with Iodine-131. In Medical Radioisotope Scanning, International Atomic Energy Agency, and World Health Organization Seminar, Vienna, Austria, 1959, pp. 189–211.
Renault, H., Rapin, J., and Wicart, L.: Toxicologie Analytique. La chélation de divers cations radioactifs par certains polypeptides, utilisée comme méthode de marquage. Application á la bléomycine. Comptes Rendu Academie Des Sciences, Serie D, 2013–2015, November, 1971.
Rockwell, S. C., Kallman, R. F., and Fajardo, L. F.: Characteristics of a serially transplanted mouse mammary tumor and its tissue-culture-adapted derivative. Journal of the National Cancer Institute, 49:735–749, September 1972.
Serafini, A. N., Dunning, W., Charyulu, K., and Weinstein, M. D.: Concentration of ^{111}In-chloride and ^{67}Ga-chloride in the irradiated rat lymphosarcoma. (Abstract) Journal of Nuclear Medicine, 12:464, June 1971.
Stern, H. S. Goodwin, D. A., Scheffel, U., Wagner, H. N., and Kramer, H. H.: $In^{113m}$for blood-pool and brain scanning. Nucleonics, 25:62–68, February 1967.
Sundberg, M. W.: Bifunctional EDTA Analogues with Applications for the Labeling of Biological Molecules, Ph.D. Dissertation. Stanford University, Stanford, California, 1973, 212 pp.
Thakur, M. L.: The preparation of Indium-111 labelled bleomycin for tumour localisation. International Journal of Applied Radiation and Isotopes, 24: 357–358, 1973.
Umezawa, H., Maeda, K., Takeuchi, T., and Yoshiro, O.: New antibiotics, bleomycin A and B. Journal of Antibiotics, Ser. A.: 200–209, September 1966.
Verma, R. C., Bennett, L. R., Touya, J. J., Morton, D. L., and Witt, E.: ^{111}Indium-Bleomycin: A new radiopharmaceutical for tumor scintigraphy. (Abstract) Journal of Nuclear Medicine, 14:8, August 1973.
Wagner, H. N., Jr., and Emmons, H.: Characteristics of an ideal radiopharmaceutical. In Radioactive Pharmaceuticals. Oak Ridge, Tennessee, United States Atomic Energy Commission, Division of Technical Information, 1966, pp. 1–32.

Quality Control of Nuclear Imaging Devices

M. F. JAHNS, Ph.D., and T. P. HAYNIE, M.D.
Departments of Physics and Medicine, The University
of Texas System Cancer Center M. D. Anderson
Hospital and Tumor Institute, Houston, Texas

NUCLEAR IMAGING DEVICES are of 2 main types: rectilinear scanners and gamma cameras. Figure 1 shows the essential components of a rectilinear scanner. A sodium iodide detector crystal moves in a raster pattern, as shown by the arrows, to scan over the organs of interest in the patient. This crystal detects the penetrating radiation emitted from a radionuclide distributed within the patient. A phototube and associated electronics amplify the signal from the crystal and cause the emission of visible light from a light source whose intensity is proportional to the intensity of radiation detected. The light source is fixed to the detector crystal and moves in a raster pattern with respect to the film, thus forming a developable image on the film. Lead shielding and a collimator between the detector crystal and the patient assure that the radiation detected at any time is from activity within a relatively small volume within the patient. Figure 2 shows the essential components of a gamma camera. This instrument is stationary with respect to the patient. Radiation from the patient passes through a collimator and is detected by a sodium iodide crystal, generally $1/2$ inch thick and about 11 inches in diameter. The signal from the crystal is detected and amplified by some of the 19 phototubes arranged in hexagonal array. From the intensities of the signals from the various phototubes, a coordinate computer generates x- and y-position pulses corresponding to the position with-

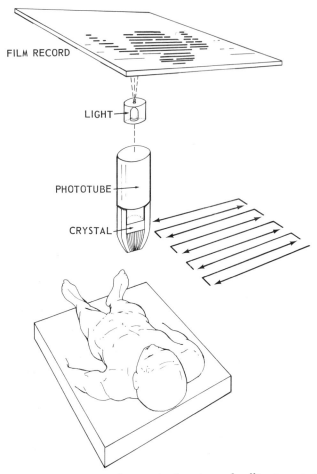

FILM RECORD

LIGHT

PHOTOTUBE

CRYSTAL

FIG. 1.—Rectilinear scanning device. As detector and collimator move in a raster pattern over the distribution of radioactivity in the patient, the light exposes photographic film to produce an image of the distribution.

in the patient from which the radiation originated. When the energy analyzer determines that the detected photon energy was within a preselected energy range, a z-signal permits a flash of light to be generated on the screen of the read-out oscilloscope, the position on the screen being determined by the x-axis and the y-axis signals. Thus, radiation from a particular region in the patient causes a flash of light at a corresponding point on the oscilloscope. A photographic camera integrates these signals on the scope to form an image of patient radio-

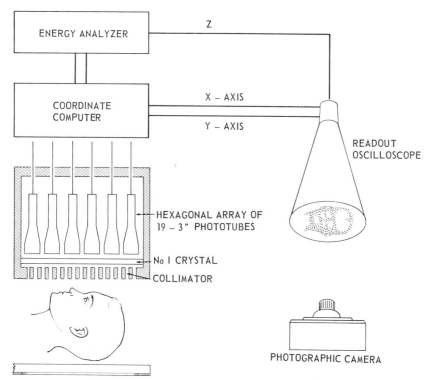

Fig. 2.—Gamma camera. Collimated gamma rays from the patient form an image of scintillations in the NaI crystal. Phototubes detect these scintillations and produce electronic pulses which are processed by the coordinate computer to produce x- and y-axis position pulses. When the total detected energy is analyzed and found to lie within a range of interest, a z-pulse from the analyzer permits the x- and y-pulses to position a flash of light on the oscilloscope screen. A great number of such flashes form an image of the radioactivity distribution on film in the photographic camera.

activity. In an instrument as complex as a scanner or camera, many components are subject to the possibility of malfunction or failure. Additionally, some of the components' characteristics change slightly with changes in their environment, resulting in a change in the over- all performance of the instrument. To obtain optimum performance from an instrument and to detect incipient or actual failure as early as possible, a quality control program should be instituted and followed.

Imaging devices, both moving and stationary, thrive in an environ- ment that also would be pleasant to humans. Maintaining a cool, constant temperature, low radioactivity, a dust-free environment, and a stable power supply are the first steps in achieving quality performance from an instrument. These factors should be given scheduled periodic reconsideration, and particularly at a time when a new imaging procedure is introduced. In particular, one must be sure that a new procedure does not place radioactivity in the field of view of another instrument.

A minimum of interruption of power to scintillation counting instrumentation will yield the best results in terms of consistency. We believe that all imaging instruments, both vacuum-tube type and solid state, should be left turned on at all times except when being repaired. In particular, the high voltage to a photomultiplier tube should be altered only when absolutely necessary.

Rectilinear Scanners

Rectilinear scanners should be calibrated at least once each day with a long-lived source. The energy calibration generally matches the energy scale of the instrument to the known gamma ray energy of the calibration source. Some newer instruments are equipped with preset windows for commonly used nuclides. While these are convenient, the count rate from such a window should be periodically checked against a manually set window. Again, unless the instrument does not have an amplifier gain control, do not calibrate by varying the high-voltage supply. After the energy scale of the instrument has been calibrated, a timed count of the source in a fixed, easily repeated geometry, using a wide analyzer window, should also be made. In the calibration, failure to observe a sharp peak, or observing a count rate differing from measurements on previous days by more than what may be attributed to statistical variations, indicates a change in instrument performance that may not be noticed on the image produced by the instrument. A permanent record should be made of the results of the calibration, including the measured count rate from the standard source. Each entry to this permanent record should be analyzed each day for indications of incipient failure. When trouble is suspected, gray-scale readings should be made. These may be obtained from a source in a fixed relationship to the detector and varying the count rate by changing the window setting, or from a pulse generator, or by scanning a standard object such as a wedge phantom. Scanning a wedge phantom has the advantage that the entire system is being checked simultaneously.

After the rectilinear scanner has been calibrated using a standard source, the instrument energy analyzer window should be peaked on the radionuclide to be used in the patient scan. The source used in this procedure should be placed within the field of view of the detector crystal and should not be strong enough to cause misleading sum peaks in the radiation spectrum. The control setting determined to peak the instrument best on the radionuclide to be scanned also should be recorded and analyzed daily.

Gamma Cameras

While a properly calibrated rectilinear scanner will most likely have a uniform sensitivity throughout the scan area, the gamma camera, which views its entire field at all times, requires that special attention be given to assure maximum uniformity of sensitivity. The camera performance should be studied using a point source placed on the crystal axis at a distance of at least 4 feet from the face of the crystal. The source activity should cause a count rate not in excess of 10,000 counts per second. The resulting flood picture should be carefully inspected and compared with similar pictures made on previous days. This picture should be displayed in a convenient location for reference by the physician when he is interpreting patient images. Besides using a point source, flood field images can be obtained using an extended source. At M. D. Anderson Hospital, we alternately use a source containing a ¼-inch thick, 14-inch square volume of radioactive solution placed directly in contact with a camera collimator. Other studies using this source will be discussed later.

A permanent record should be kept of the optimum energy analyzer window setting, the number of counts used in making the flood image, and the intensity setting of the oscilloscope being photographed. This is also a convenient time to note and record the minimum intensity setting at which light flashes can be seen on the oscilloscope screen.

When a patient with a radionuclide different from the previous study is imaged, the camera analyzer is of course reset for the appropriate energy. In setting the analyzer window, care must be exercised to assure that the primary photopeak is being observed. If an extended source is used in setting the analyzer, many photons will be stopped in the collimator material and may thereby produce a larger count rate from lead X rays than the count rate obtained from unscattered photons reaching the crystal. Such a prominent X-ray peak may be obtained when a patient containing radioactivity or a strong point source outside the collimator field of view is used for calibrating the instrument. A uniform flood image can be obtained with the analyzer window set on an X-ray peak, but a patient image

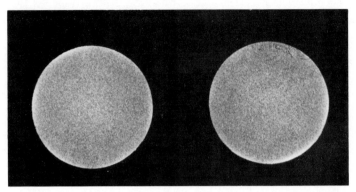

Fig. 3.—Camera images of a flood field source. Right: nonuniform image in upper right quadrant. Left: image from same source and camera settings obtained after cleaning face of oscilloscope.

obtained with this setting would show very little detail. Analyzer windows always should be set by using a weak source located within the collimator's field of view. In Figure 3, the flood field image on the right shows reduced activity near the upper right quadrant. When an image such as this is obtained, it is good practice to repeat the exposure after resetting the oscilloscope orientation controls to rotate the image 90° on the display. If the nonuniformity in the next image then appears in a new location, its cause probably is associated with the photubes or the position computer network in the camera. If the uniformity does not change position, it is probably caused by the display oscilloscope or its camera. The improved flood field on the left in Figure 3 was obtained by removing a smudge from the face of the oscilloscope. The scope face, the photographic camera lenses, *etc.*, should be carefully checked and cleaned each time they are exposed to the operator's hands.

Occasionally, flood field image nonuniformity will be caused by nonuniform photographic film. Film nonuniformity usually extends into nonexposed regions of the film which may be detected by careful examination under a bright light.

Harris (1973) reported that flood field image nonuniformity may result from a poorly focused light spot on the oscilloscope screen. Although this effect could not be reproduced on instruments in our laboratory, we have seen that a properly focused light spot improves contrast. Oscilloscope focus should be checked at the beginning of each day, and particularly at times when the intensity level is changed.

Sanders and Sanders (1971) have advocated the use of an asymmetric energy analyzer window to improve image contrast by increased scatter rejection, particularly when a high count rate is easily attained. Figure 4 shows flood images and spectra of detected radiation. In each spectrum, the vertical axis represents the count rate of

FIG. 4 *(top).* — Flood field images of ^{99m}Tc for various energy windows. The brighter points in the spectrum indicate pulses accepted by the pulse-height analyzer. Note increased image nonuniformity for the more asymmetric windows.

FIG. 5 *(bottom).* — Flood field images of ^{99m}Tc for various energy windows. The flag-shaped display beside each image shows the distribution of pulses, with higher energy events causing a trace at a higher position on the oscilloscope. The energy range of pulses contributing to the image is indicated by the blanked rectangle. To obtain image *A*, a 5 per cent centered window was opened to 20 per cent. Image *B* was obtained with a symmetric 15 per cent window.

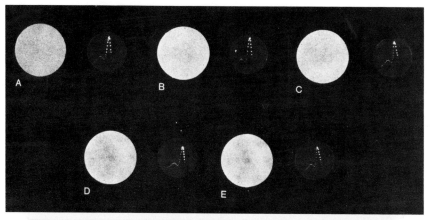

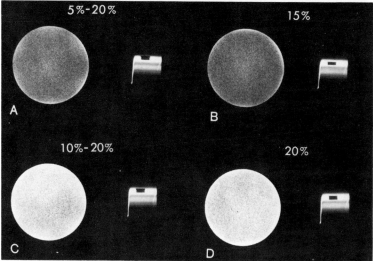

pulses per energy interval and the horizontal axis represents the energy or pulse-height of the counts. The analyzer window position for each of the flood images is indicated by the brighter dots seen in the corresponding spectrum. Figures 4B, C, D, and E show how image nonuniformity increased as a more asymmetric window is used. Note that the brighter points in the spectrum are shifted to the high-energy side, corresponding to fewer counts from scattered radiation.

Figure 5 shows flood field images obtained from another camera. The small picture to the right of each image shows the energies of the pulses detected, with the horizontal lines which appear higher on the picture corresponding to higher energy pulses. The darkened rectangle indicates the position of the analyzer window. To obtain Figure 5A, a 5 per cent window centered on the ^{99m}Tc peak was opened to 20 per cent. A 15 per cent symmetrically placed window gave essentially the same count rate and produced the improved flood field image shown in Figure 5B. A symmetrically placed 20 per cent window shown in Figure 5D yields the same count rate and a more uniform flood field image than the 10 per cent centered window widened to 20 per cent seen in Figure 4C. It seems quite likely that artifacts introduced by using an asymmetric window would more than offset any improvement in image contrast obtained by scatter rejection.

In addition to the daily instrument calibrations and uniformity checks, a more extensive check of camera performance should be made on a weekly basis. This should include a study of the resolving ability and spatial distortion as well as the uniformity of sensitivity that is checked on other days. In our laboratory, a lead strip bar phantom is used for resolution checks. Figures 6A and 6B show an image obtained from a point source irradiating the detector crystal without a collimator and the image obtained from a point source when the bar phantom is placed directly over the camera detector crystal. This phantom consists of sets of lead bars 3/16 in., 1/4 in., 3/8 in., and 1/2 in. wide, separated by their own width. In Figures 6C through 6F, the bar phantom has been imaged using a collimator with phantom-to-collimator distances of 0, 1, 2, and 4 inches. For these images, the extended flood source described earlier is placed in direct contact with the bar phantom. By carefully examining these images and comparing them with earlier results, spatial distortion or a gradual loss of resolution can be detected at an early stage. The image obtained when the bar phantom is in contact with the collimator should be repeated with the phantom rotated to different azimuthal positions with respect to the face of the camera. For some

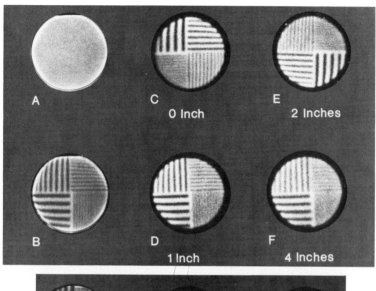

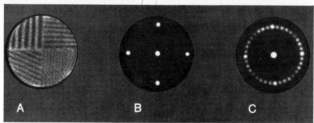

FIG. 6 *(top).*—*A,* image obtained from point source with uncollimated crystal. *B,* same source, lead strip bar phantom placed directly over detector (see text). *C-F,* images from extended flood source in contact with bar phantom separated from high resolution collimator by 0, 1, 2, and 4 inches.

FIG. 7 *(bottom).*—*A,* distorted image of bar phantom caused by a particular orientation of bars relative to rows of collimator holes. *B,* image of 4 point sources equally spaced on 20 cm. circle. *C,* same as *B,* except display orientation rotated in 15 per cent increments.

orientations, a highly regular distortion similar to that seen in Figure 7A will appear. Such an image appears for certain orientations between the lead bars and rows of collimator holes and is not caused by camera distortion. It occurs most frequently when a high energy collimator is used. Spatial distortion is further checked by imaging 4 point sources equally spaced on a 20 cm. diameter circle placed in contact with the collimator. Such a source is easily contructed by drilling holes in a piece of lucite and placing a small piece of cotton in each hole to absorb a small amount of radioactive solution. An image from such a source is seen in Figure *7B*. The extent of spatial distortion can be determined by measuring the length of the sides and diagonals of the square on the image. This image also is used to measure image minification by the gamma camera. From this, a scale is contructed for measuring the size of objects appearing in patient images. The image shown in Figure *7C* was obtained from the 4-point source by rotating the display orientation in 15° increments and counting for a fixed time interval in each position.

The contamination of collimators by long-lived nuclides and light leaks onto photographic film should be checked periodically by leaving the camera in the record mode overnight. This may also reveal an irregularly functioning display oscilloscope.

Conclusions

Again, the importance of keeping good records on each imaging instrument in the laboratory cannot be overemphasized. Daily and weekly calibration records and records of any intermittent malfunction should be reviewed and fully discussed with the instrument serviceman. Such action may well avert a prolonged breakdown at a later time. The personnel who operate nuclear imaging devices and the physician who interprets such images can, if they are willing to make the effort, determine how near optimum a device is functioning and also become capable of detecting incipient or actual failures. While efforts to maintain quality of images do not yield exciting break-throughs, they may in the long run yield more improvement in the physician's receiver operating characteristics than any other effort.

REFERENCES

Harris, C. C.: The care and feeding of nuclear medicine instrumentation. *Seminar in Nuclear Medicine*, 3(3):225–238, July 1973.

Sanders, T. P., Sanders, T. D., and Kuhl, D. E.: Optimizing the window of an Anger camera for ^{99m}Tc. *Journal of Nuclear Medicine*, 12:703–706, November 1971.

Physical Principles of Diagnostic Ultrasound

J. M. HEVEZI, Ph.D.
Program in Diagnostic Radiology, The University of
Texas Medical School at Houston, Houston, Texas

SINCE THE DISCOVERY of X rays, radiologic diagnosis has been the modality of choice in assessing abnormal internal structural and functional anatomy. Radionuclide imaging has provided additional information concerning these parameters, often unobtainable by other means. In recent years, the techniques of ultrasonic and thermographic imaging have received widespread attention because their application does not involve the use of ionizing radiation and the information provided by these methods is in a different form than that presented by radiographic techniques. As experience is gained in the use of diagnostic ultrasound and as the equipment becomes more technically sound, the physician will have at his disposal a unique combination of diagnostic tools. A basic understanding of the strengths and weaknesses of the newer modalities is crucial to their further exploitation in the diagnostic arena.

Ultrasound is acoustic energy propagated in the form of longitudinal waves. Unlike electromagnetic waves which are transverse in nature and can travel in a vacuum, acoustic waves require matter for propagation and may be viewed as alternating compression and rarefaction of the propagating medium in the direction of the ultrasonic beam. Acoustic frequencies utilized in medical diagnosis have been limited to the range from 1–15 MHz. — values far above the audible range. These waves travel through matter with a velocity characteristic of the medium; the average value for tissue is 1,540 meters per second. Hence, the acoustic wave length in tissue is limited to the range from 1.5–0.1 mm. These values correspond to the theoretical limit of resolution in acoustic imaging. Proportionately better resolution is achieved by using higher frequencies, but the depth of penetration of the beam decreases as the frequency is increased, and a compromise between resolution and depth of visualization must be accepted. Table 1 shows the relationship between frequencies and wave length in tissue.

Pulse-echo ultrasound is the most common modality employed in diagnosis. As its name implies, a short burst of acoustic energy at a fixed frequency is emitted from an acoustic transducer into the structure to be examined. The same transducer is used as a receiver to "listen" to the return echoes from structures within the body. These echoes occur at tissue interfaces within the body and are displayed as voltage pulses on an oscilloscope. Since the arrival time of an echo to the transducer in contact with the surface is proportional to the depth of the interface beneath the surface, the correct spatial relationship of echo-producing interfaces will be preserved on the display. This method of presentation is the so-called A-mode (Amplitude modulation), a term adopted from radar terminology. The echo amplitudes increase with the proximity of the echo-producing interfaces to the transducer and the disparity of tissue density on either side of the interface. In pulse-echo work, the amplitide of the return echo is greatest when the interface is perpendicular to the direction of travel of the ultrasonic beam. Indeed, if the angle that the tissue interface makes with the direction of the beam is too great, no echo will be recorded for that interface.

As alluded to previously, echoes will be returned to the transducer if there is a disparity of tissue characteristics on either side of the interface. These characteristics are the acoustic impedance values for

Table 1
Relationship* between Acoustic Frequencies Used in Medical Diagnosis and Their Corresponding Wave Lengths

f(MHz)	λ(mm)
1.0	1.5
2.5	0.6
5.0	0.3
7.5	0.2
10.0	0.15

*Assuming an average velocity of sound in tissue of 1,540 meters per second.

tissues on either side of the interface. The acoustic impedance is the product of the density and the velocity of sound in the medium. Table 2 gives the percentage of acoustic energy returned to the transducer when various substances interfaced to muscle are insonified. Note that the air-muscle boundary reflects most of the incident acoustic energy, leaving little transmitted energy for echo-producing information beyond this interface. Hence, air-filled body cavities present difficult structures to study ultrasonically.

In order to produce 2-dimensional images of structures, some electronic manipulation of the A-mode presentation is necessary. This begins with displaying the echoes as bright dots in a line (corresponding to the acoustic beam direction) on the display. The brightness of the dots is proportional to the amplitide of the return echoes, and the display forms the so-called B-mode (Brightness modulation) presentation. B-mode is not used alone in ultrasonic imaging, but the particular manipulation of the echo-produced dots

Fig. 1.—Schematic demonstration of the steps involved in producing an M-mode image, beginning with A-mode.

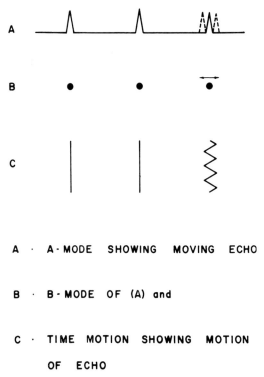

A · A-MODE SHOWING MOVING ECHO

B · B-MODE OF (A) and

C · TIME MOTION SHOWING MOTION OF ECHO

determines the type of scan. Table 3 lists the hierarchy of scan modes available with pulse-echo ultrasound systems.

In the M-mode (Motion mode) presentation, the bright dots are swept across the display face such that moving echoes trace a curved path during the sweep. The display may be "frozen" on a storage oscilloscope and photographed for interpretive analysis. Figure 1 demonstrates schematically the steps involved in producing an M-mode image, beginning with A-mode. The chief application of M-mode operation is in cardiac studies where valve and other cardiac motions may be displayed and analyzed for departures from normalcy. The diagnosis of pericardial effusion is generally made at many institutions using M-mode.

With the advent of good commercial scanning equipment, compound B-mode scans are destined to be the most frequently utilized ultrasound examination because they produce a direct 2-dimensional map of interfaces in the body which may be correlated with normal cross sectional anatomy. This scanning technique also begins with the basic B-mode presentation or a line of bright dots on the display corresponding to echo-producing interfaces encountered within the body by the ultrasonic beam. In this method of imaging, however, the location (position and angle) of the acoustic transducer is electronically computed and displayed on the oscilloscope along with the B-mode presentation. As the transducer is moved across the

FIG. 2.—Schematic diagram of compound B-mode ultrasonic scanning system. Along with B-mode presentation, transducer position information is input to the storage oscilloscope from which permanent film recordings may be made.

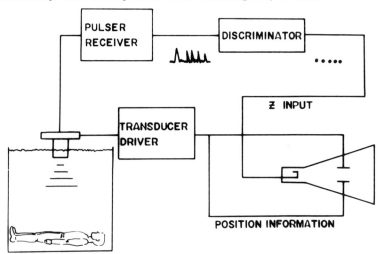

Table 2
Values of Acoustic Impedance for Various Tissue Systems

	$Z \times 10^{+5}$	R %
Saline	1.51	0.28
Air	0.00004	99.95
Muscle	1.68	0.00
Fat	1.37	1.04
Liver	1.65	0.028
Kidney	1.62	0.032
Blood	1.61	0.045
Bone	6.8	36.1

Abbreviations: Z = acoustic impedance; R = corresponding percentage of reflected acoustic intensity with the various systems interfaced to muscle.

body, a new set of B-mode dots will be displayed on the oscilloscope in a different position. In this way, a 2-dimensional map of acoustic interfaces in the body may be built up by constantly changing the position and angle of the transducer. In order that information be preserved at previous transducer positions, the image is displayed on a storage oscilloscope and subsequently photographed for permanent recording. Figure 2 is a schematic diagram illustrating the operation of compound B-mode scanning. Echoes returned from the patient are presented as B-mode dots which modulate the electron beam on the oscilloscope, while the position of the transducer electronically modulates the deflector plates on the oscilloscope. Patients do not require complete submersion in a water bath for a successful compound B-mode scan, but the figure emphasizes an important point: Some coupling medium between the transducer face and the patient's skin is necessary for good transmission and reception of the ultrasound beam. Indeed, without this coupling medium, the first interface encountered by the ultrasound beam is the air-skin interface which, as was pointed out in Table 2, returns most of the ultrasonic energy back to the transducer. Coupling gel and common mineral oil are good coupling media applied directly to the skin.

Table 3
Types of Ultrasonic Scans Presently Employed

I. A(mplitude) Mode
II. B(rightness) Mode
  A. M(otion) Mode
  B. Compound Scan
    1. Linear
    2. Sector
    3. Complex

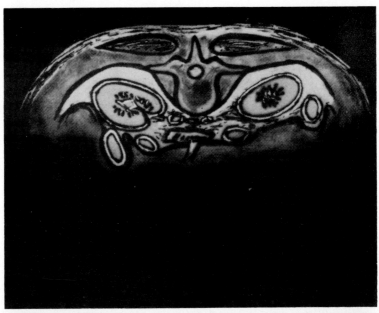

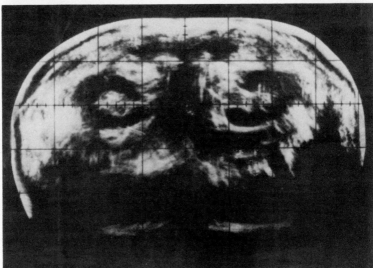

FIG. 3 *(top).* — Schematic representation of partial transverse section through renal bodies.

FIG. 4 *(bottom).* — Compound B-mode scan of section shown in Figure 3. Note outline of renal bodies and collecting ducts.

B-mode scans are commonly made by moving the transducer in contact with the surface of the body along transverse or sagittal planes. By obtaining scans at 1 to 2 cm. intervals in these planes, 3-dimensional information may be extracted. In contact scanning, one has freedom in positioning the transducer so that the maximum number of interfaces are intercepted in a perpendicular direction to the beam. Noncontact scans are less common but have the advantage that the scanned object is held rigidly throughout the scan, thus improving reproducibility and accuracy. Water is used as a coupling medium in noncontact scans and, as described in Table 3, motion of the transducer may either be of linear, sector (sweeping the transducer through a given angle), or a combination of these motions.

Figure 3 is a diagram of a partial transverse section through the kidneys. In Figure 4, the corresponding compound B-mode scan is presented. Note the good outline of renal bodies and echoes produced by the collecting systems. Further clinical applications of compound B-mode scanning are presented by others elsewhere in this volume.

In summary, some of the methods of extracting and presenting ultrasonic information from the body have been presented. The field of ultrasound has progressed to the point that pulse-echo ultrasound systems are in routine use in major institutions both as an adjunct to other diagnostic modalities, and frequently as the sole method of extracting useful information. As the technology of such systems becomes more refined and our knowledge of the interaction of acoustic energy with matter increases, the future holds great promise for this diagnostic modality.

Physical Principles of Thermography

A. ZERMENO, Ph.D.

*Department of Diagnostic Radiology, The University of
Texas System Cancer Center M. D. Anderson Hospital
and Tumor Institute, Houston, Texas*

THERMOGRAPHY MAY BE DEFINED as the technique of imaging or mapping the infrared radiations emitted by an object. In the early 1800's, Sir William Herschel, while studying the properties of prisms and their ability to disperse light according to wave length, noted the manifestation of heat associated with the electromagnetic radiations lying just below the red end of the visible spectrum. With the development of more sophisticated heat measuring devices, such as the thermopile and the bolometer, the spectral distribution of wave lengths emitted from a heated body was determined experimentally.

Figure 1 illustrates the distribution of wave lengths emitted from a body at 310° K, or human body temperature. It is important to note that the peak emission occurs at 9 μm. wave length and that essentially no emission takes place below 1 micron. This is the region commonly employed in infrared photography.

It was later shown experimentally as well as theoretically that the total radiated energy of all wave lengths emitted per second and per centimeter of area from such a body varies as the fourth power of the absolute temperature. This relationship is called the Stefan-Boltzman law.

$$W = \epsilon \sigma T^4$$
$$W\lambda = 8\pi c^2 \, h\lambda^{-5}(e^{hc/\lambda kT}-1)^{-1}$$

The constant ϵ is called the emissivity of the object and is found dependent upon the physical nature of its surface. The latter equa-

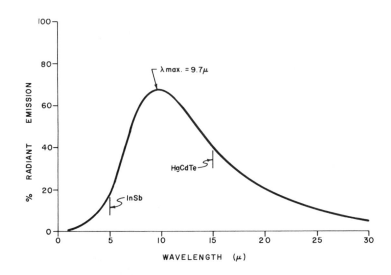

EMISSION OF A BLACKBODY AT 310°K

FIG. 1.—The distribution of wave lengths emitted by the human body. Note the maximum emission to occur at 9.7 μm. Also illustrated is the long wave length limit of response of InSb as compared to HgCdTe detectors.

tion was derived by Max Plank, to describe the shape of the wave length distribution, and hence referred to as the Plank distribution. It was at this time that he introduced the concept of photons of infrared energy as implied by use of the term "h," called "Plank's constant," which was to play a very important role in the subsequent development of atomic theory. Experimentally, the total emission from a body was found to be enhanced when the surface of this body was blackened with soot from a burning candle. Thus the name "black body" was probably coined to describe a body which most efficiently emits infrared radiation or mathematically possesses an emissivity (ϵ) of unity.

Later work by the French proved the emissivity of human skin to be very near unity and thus closely representing an ideal black body radiator. This property also was shown to be independent of skin pigmentation within the infrared region. Once the emissivity of an object is known, measurement of the total energy emitted per unit area and solid angle allows us to calculate the temperature of the object. This technique of temperature determination is called infrared radiometry.

A thermograph machine may therefore be thought of as a scanning radiometer which, by means of mirrors, scans the heat-sensing detector in a systematic fashion across the patient and in this serial manner, records temperatures. Figure 2 is a simplified drawing of a mirror system illustrating the method of horizontal and vertical scanning most commonly used in present-day thermographic scanners. Important here is the concept of the resolution element size (r) shown on the right of the figure. The resolution element is simply the image of the detector projected into space by the optical system. This image comes to focus in the focal plane. The size of the resolution element determines the spatial resolution of the system and thus the image detail. The smaller the element, the higher the resolution of the image. Many factors affect the size of this element, and these will be discussed later.

A closer examination of thermographic scanners reveals 3 basic components. First the detector, its size and characteristics; second the optomechanical scanner; and third the display device or means of recording the thermal image.

Detectors are categorized basically as being 1 of 2 types: thermal

FIG. 2.—A simplified mirror scanning system. The resolution element size (r) is the image of the detector projected into the plane of the patient. This element size ultimately determines the spatial resolving capability of the scanner.

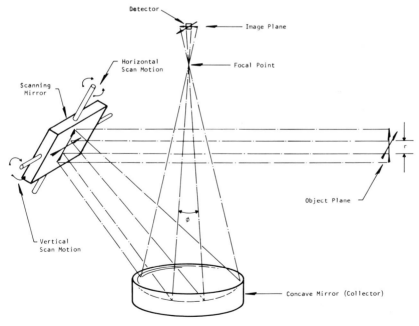

detectors or photon detectors. The bolometer is an example of a thermal detector. Here, the infrared radiation is first absorbed by a blackened surface which results in a rise in temperature of the absorber. This heat is then conducted to a heat-sensitive material such as a strip of platinum foil which changes electrical conductivity with temperature. The spectral response of such detectors is extremely wide; however, as would be expected, the response time is long, requiring a much longer scan time to synthesize a thermal image. The photon detector, however, is usually a semiconductor type device in which the initial absorption of an infrared photon results in an ionization or creation of extrinsic charge carriers. Photon detectors

FIG. 3.—A comparison of the detectabilities of InSb and HgCdTe as a function of wave length. The ideal curves represent the theoretical limits of detectability for both the photoconductive and photovoltaic mode of operation.

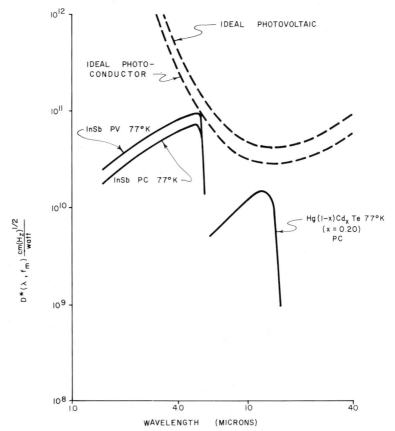

are designed to operate in 1 of 2 modes: photoconductive or photo-voltaic. The 2 modes are similar in that the charge carriers are extrinsic, *i.e.* caused by doping. However, the photovoltaic detector employs a junction similar to that of a diode. Response times are much shorter for photon detectors compared to thermal detectors; however, their spectral response is much more limited, being sensitive principally to the higher energy photons.

The sensitivity of all infrared detectors is specified in terms of their $D°$ (deé-star) which simply relates the inverse number of watts of infrared energy required to produce a signal equal to the noise content of a detector of unit area per cycle of bandwidth. Expressed in this manner, we may calculate the theoretical limit of detectivity called $D°$ (blip).

Figure 3 illustrates the $D°$ of 2 types of detectors as a function of

FIG. 4.—A graphic solution to the system equation, relating frame rate to resolution element size for various numbers of detectors. Note that in excess of 7 HgCdTe detectors in an array are required to obtain real-time viewing at the desired resolution if other parameters considered ideal for medical applications are maintained.

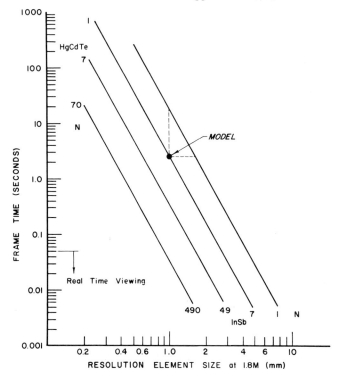

wave length and their proximity to the blip limit. The response of InSb (indium antimonide) is noted for both the PV (photovoltaic) and PC (photoconductive) mode. It is important to note the spectral response of the Hg:Cd:Te (mercury-cadmium-teluride) detector in comparison to that of InSb and the similarity to those wave lengths emitted by the human body at normal body temperature.

Concerning optomechanical scanners, we find a number of the design parameters to be dependent upon clinical requirements. The user must specify such parameters as desired frame-rate, number of scan lines per frame, field of view, depth of field, and thermal sensitivity. Very often the chosen design parameters are incongruent with physical limitations as imposed by detector characteristics, technological know-how, or perhaps, as is most often the case, available funds. System equations can be derived which express explicitly the interrelation of these parameters. An example of such an equation in

FIG. 5.—Graphic relationship of angular resolution to structures resolvable at specified patient distances.

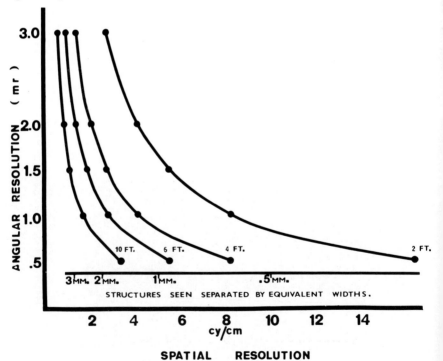

simplified form, relating frame time to resolution element size, diameter of mirror, f/, detector size, *etc.*, is:

$$FF' \simeq \frac{f^2 \lambda c^2 D^4 10^8}{2r^4 \, N\eta \, \int_0^{\lambda_c} Q_B{}^{d\lambda}}$$

where: F = frame time (recording time) (secs.); F' = duty cycle = recording time/scanning time; f = focal length of collector (cm.); λc = detector cut-off wave length; D = object distance (cm.) r/ϕ, and assorted constants; r = resolution element size; N = number of detectors; η = system efficiency; and Q_B = radiation flux from the background. A plot of this equation appears in Figure 4 for the parameters specified above. The point labeled "model" characterizes the properties of currently available equipments using the Hg:Cd:Te detectors. Note also the number of detectors required in an array to attain real-time viewing with resolution comparable to that currently available. Here resolution is specified in terms of the resolution element size. Another expression for this parameter is in terms of the instantaneous field of view or angular resolution. Figure 5 relates this parameter to other measures such as object size and spatial frequency resolvable. One method of measuring the resolution of a scanner is illustrated in Figure 6. This is a thermal test target consisting of a heated copper plate masked by a Mylar sheet containing slits of various widths and spacings, thus producing a thermal silhouette. Measurements made of these thermal images with a microdensitom-

FIG. 6.—Photograph of a termal test target designed for use in determining the spatial resolving capability of a thermographic scanner.

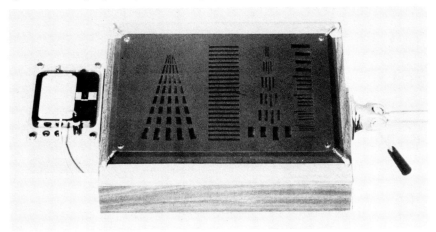

eter allow us to calculate the modulation transfer functions for various machines and thus compare their image-forming capability. Figure 7 is a plot of such functions for systems now commercially available. The unit labeled proposed TI is that of the Texas Instruments Thermiscope. Figure 8 is a sample breast thermogram using the high-resolution Thermiscope.

Various methods of displaying the thermal image have been used in the past. The most popular is the CRT (cathode ray tube). Permanent photographs may be made of the CRT using a variety of films. The 2 most widely used are Polaroid and 70-millimeter roll film. Polaroid film, although expensive, affords the user a developed film within seconds after exposure. The 70-mm. film technique is much less expensive and thus suitable for high-volume work, but it does require routine development procedures. The hazards of this tech-

FIG. 7.—The modulation transfer functions of existing thermographic scanner presently available. The 10 per cent amplitude response level is empirically derived as the resolving capability of the eye to changes in density.

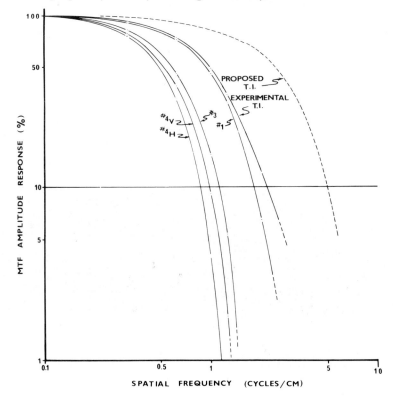

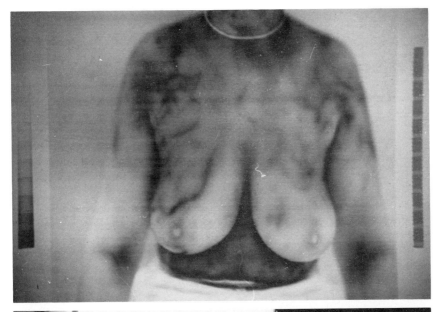

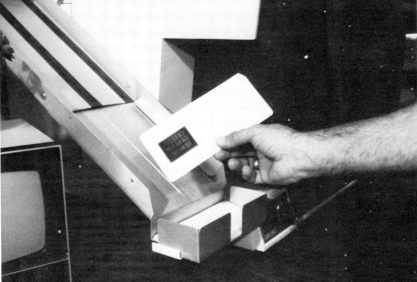

FIG. 8 (*top*).—A typical breast thermogram as produced on a high-resolution thermographic scanner. Note dark areas representing areas of increased heat.

FIG. 9 (*bottom*).—An aperture card containing multiple exposures thus capable of storing complete patient studies. The application of this camera/processor to thermography and other medical areas is presently under development.

nique lie in not knowing whether one has a satisfactory exposure until long after the patient has been discharged.

The latest in recording techniques presently under development employs the 3M aperture card which is a microfilm technique. By using the 3M Model 2000 camera/processor, microfilms may be obtained, within seconds after exposure, which contain all views permanently mounted on a data card which is computer compatible. Figure 9 is a photograph of such an image card. The advantages of this technique are: (1) low cost (cheaper than 70 mm.), (2) immediate access, (3) efficient storage, and (4) computer retrievable. All of these are desirable in the operation of a mass-screening installation.

Physical Aspects of Xeroradiography of the Breast

DAVID D. PAULUS, M.D.
*Department of Diagnostic Radiology, The University of
Texas System Cancer Center M. D. Anderson Hospital
and Tumor Institute, Houston, Texas*

XERORADIOGRAPHY is a relatively new process of recording the radiographic image and when applied to radiography of the breast is called xeromammography. Xeromammography differs from film mammography primarily in the utilization of an electrostatically charged selenium-coated plate to record the radiographic image instead of the familiar radiographic film. A brief explanation may help to provide a basic understanding of the xeroradiographic recording process.

The xerographic plate which replaces the X-ray film in recording the image has an aluminum base upon which is deposited a thin layer of vitreous selenium. Selenium is a photoconductor which will retain a positive charge placed upon it in the dark. A positive charge is placed upon the surface of the selenium within the conditioner as the first step in the process. This is accomplished during passage of the plate underneath a high voltage (7,000 – 10,000 volts D.C.) wire grid which emits ions directed towards the moving plate (Fig. 1). The charged selenium plate is automatically sealed within a light-tight cassette which protects the charged surface from discharging in ambient light as well as from pressure or contact with extraneous objects.

The charged plate is placed under the breast and exposed to an X-ray beam in the conventional manner just as X-ray film would be

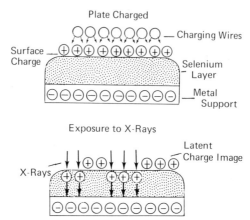

FIG. 1 *(top)*.—Charging of the selenium plate by a high-voltage wire grid.
FIG. 2 *(bottom)*.—Exposure of the charged plate to X rays. Plate partially discharged.

used in producing a mammogram (Fig. 2). X rays discharge the photoconductor in amounts proportional to the variation in intensities of X rays striking the plate. The plate is partially discharged leaving a latent electrostatic pattern of the part examined.

In order to make this latent pattern of charges visible, the cassette is inserted into the developing unit where the plate is automatically removed and placed into a closed chamber. A finely divided and charged blue plastic powder or toner is sprayed on the surface (Fig. 3). The negatively charged blue toner is attracted to the image of positive charges, producing a blue image of the part examined. This powder image is transferred to a special plastic-coated paper where it is permanently fixed by the application of heat; it is then ready for interpretation. The residual toner is removed from the plate by a revolving brush, and any remaining charges on the plate are neutralized by a brief 15 sec.—140° F heating process. The plate then is ready to be charged and used for another exposure.

The selenium plate will retain its full charge for only a relatively short period of time before the charges will begin to leak away. Therefore, in order to obtain the best possible image, the plate must be exposed and developed shortly after charging. Delays in developing of 30 to 60 minutes or longer will result in a rapidly diminishing density of the final image.

In summary, xeroradiography involves the production of an image utilizing a photoconductor (selenium), electrostatic charges, X rays, and pigmented developing powder (toner).

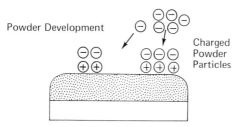

Powder Development

Charged
Powder
Particles

FIG. 3.—Development. Negatively charged blue toner powder attracted to latent image of positive charges. Image reproduced in blue.

There is a notable difference between the characteristics of the xeroradiographic image and those of the conventional X-ray film image. Xeroradiographs are like photogaphic positives, *i.e.*, the thicker sections of the breast appear darker, whereas film mammograms are negative and the thicker areas appear lighter, Since the toner of choice in xeroradiography is blue, the denser areas of tissue appear as a deeper blue against the white background of the paper base. The less dense areas will appear lighter since they allow passage of more X rays with greater exposure of the photoconductor surface which discharges and attracts less blue toner. A positive image of a normal breast is illustrated in Figure 4.

There are 2 types of contrast in xeroradiography: one between relatively large areas of uniform density, and another at local margins of discontinuity such as lines, edges of masses, veins, trabeculae, or points such as microcalcifications. Small-area contrast is caused by fringing electrostatic fields being strongest at the margins of such boundaries and having a greater attraction for the blue developing powder (Fig. 5). This results in an increase in thickness of the blue toner at the edges of a charged area, compared with that on either side, and gives rise to the adjacency or edge enhancement effect (Fig. 6). The edge enhancement effect occurs whenever there is an abrupt difference in density, and the magnitude of the effect on the image is proportional to the density difference and its abruptness of change. This is responsible for the local contrast at discontinuities being greater in xeroradiographic images when compared with X-ray film images.

The following illustration shows the effect that edge enhancement has on the visibility of local margins of discontinuity, in particular, edges of masses and small densities such as tiny masses or calcifications (Fig. 7). A phantom was constructed composed of lucite cylinders of varying diameters and thicknesses. There is a 5- to 10- per

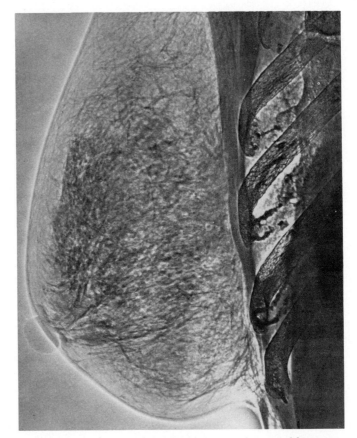

FIG. 4.—Positive xeroradiographic image of a normal breast.

cent ransmittal difference in thickness between each of the vertical rows numbered 1 through 5. Within each vertical row, the cylinders are the same thickness, but they vary in diameter down to the smallest of approximately 1.5 millimeters.

The appearance of the phantom on a xeroradiographic image taken directly overhead shows this variation in thickness and diameter between the rows of cylinders. Notice how each cylinder, which might simulate a breast mass, is clearly visible against the background density. This visibility is not the result, to any great extent, of its difference in thickness from the background but primarily of the edge enhancement effect—the attraction of excessive powder or toner to the margin of the cylinder, regardless of its thickness or diame-

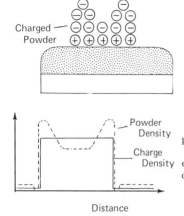

Powder Density

Charge Density

Distance

FIG. 5 *(top)*. — Negatively charged blue toner powder builds up at margins of charged area.
FIG. 6 *(bottom)*. — Diagrammatic illustration of edge enhancement effect — powder (toner) density distribution over charged area.

ter (Fig. 8). How little the thickness or transmittal difference from the background contributes to visibility is demonstrated if we take a cutout of background density and obliterate the margin of the largest central cylinders, or in essence eliminate the effect of edge enhancement on their margins. Although, unfortunately, the margins of the background cutout are themselves enhanced, note now how much more difficult it is to distinguish between the transmittal density of this cylinder and the surrounding background. This might be compared to a mass lying within a dense breast, its margins obscured by the background glandular stroma with resultant poor broad-area contrast.

Conversely, note that the smallest diameter cylinders just above the numbers appear much denser than their larger companions, although they have the same thickness. This is because their margins are so close together; their visibility is caused entirely by edge enhancement. This illustrates the increase in small-area contrast and the apparent greater visibility of small structures such as tiny masses and calcifications on xeroradiographic images.

In comparison, resolution obtained with a xerographic image, although considerably less than can be obtained with fine-grain mammography film, is still acceptable. Resolution, although difficult to specify precisely, lies in the range between screen film and fine-grain industrial film. Together with the characteristic edge enhancement of xeroradiography, the image allows clear visualization of much of the internal architecture of the breast such as individual ducts, veins, trabeculae, small masses, and microcalcifications. It is vital that changes in these small structures be visualized and careful-

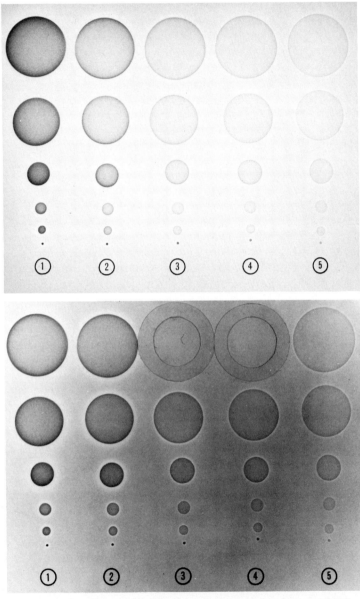

FIG. 7 *(top)*. — Phantom of lucite cylinders; 5 to 10 per cent transmittal difference in thickness between each vertical row. All cylinders within each vertical row are same thickness. Edge enhancement of margins is primary factor in cylinder (mass) visibility.

FIG. 8 *(bottom)*. — Background cutouts obliterate margins of large cylinders in rows 3 and 4 making transmitted density of these cylinders difficult to distinguish from background density. Margins visible are those of the cutout, not the cylinders.

ly studied if we are to have any significant success in the diagnosis of minimal breast cancer before it becomes clinically apparent.

The xerographic exposure within wide limits of technical factors will produce a grossly acceptable image but may fail to record all of the significant structures of the breast. However, the image content is accurate only within a narrow technical range, or, in other words, all significant structures of the breast architecture may not be recorded over the wide technical range that will produce a grossly acceptable image. The failure to recognize the relationship of broad radiographic latitude to the narrow technical corridor required to produce a good xerographic image has resulted in undue criticism of this technique.

Our measurements also have shown that the sensitivity of a xerographic plate lies between medium-speed screen film and nonscreen film. In essence, the production of a high-quality xerographic image requires a smaller dose rate of radiation than fine-grain industrial film or its medical equivalent used in routine mammography.

The molybdenum target tube is generally accepted as being superior to the tungsten target tube in film mammography. Although the physical aspects differ considerably, we have found the tungsten spectrum to be better suited to the production of the xerographic image than that of molybdenum.

In summary, the primary image characteristics of xeroradiography as compared with X-ray film imaging are: (1) wide radiographic latitude, (2) inherent edge enhancement, (3) low broad-area contrast, (4) less sensitivity than screen film, and (5) more sensitivity than nonscreen film.

These image characteristics must be considered, however, in the context of what has been discussed previously. The change from films to xerographic imaging does not eliminate the necessity of continued care in positioning the patient and following the recommended technical factors. Such care will produce consistently good xeroradiographic images. The change from interpretation of film images to xeroradiographic images with their edge enhancement and low-area contrast also requires visual adaptation which is usually more difficult than anticipated.

Xeroradiography is still a relatively new process of image production. The selenium plates used in xerography are delicate and technically difficult to produce, and they frequently contain undesirable artifacts. The processing equipment is complicated and, on occasion, prone to malfunction. Some initial design and mechanical defects should not be unexpected. However, there are continuing technological advances in equipment design and reliability which should improve the efficiency of the examination. The relative insensitivity of the selenium plate compared with standard screen film has so far prevented routine use of xeroradiography in the examination of many thicker and denser portions of the body without delivering excessive amounts of radiation. However, this too should gradually improve and in the future, we may expect greater and more comprehensive use of xeroradiography, together with its advantages, in diagnostic radiology.

REFERENCES

Dodd, G. D.: Personal communication.

Hevezi, J. M.: Personal communication.

Wolfe, J. N.: *Xeroradiography of the Breast.* Springfield, Illinois, Charles C Thomas, 1972, 175 pp.

————: Xeroradiography: Image content and comparison with film roentgenograms. *The American Journal of Roentgenology, Radium Therapy and Nuclear Medicine,* 117:690–695, March 1973.

A Systematic Approach to the Diagnosis of Primary Tumors of Bone

JACK EDEIKEN, M.D.
Department of Radiology, Thomas Jefferson University Hospital, Philadelphia, Pennsylvania

ROENTGENOGRAPHICALLY, bone tumors are a most interesting and complicated subject, confused by disagreements over their nomenclature and by arguments as to their benign or malignant nature, and even their actual existence. Not only do experienced radiologists differ, but pathologists differ as well.

Often, the final diagnosis rests with neither the pathologist nor the radiologist, but with the final outcome of the case; whether the patient lives or dies determines the true nature of the lesion. A good example is some giant cell tumors, which only in retrospect may be classified as benign or malignant.

Evaluation of the suspected bone tumor should be a cooperative effort of the radiologist, the pathologist, and the orthopedic surgeon.

The role of the radiologist has changed somewhat in the last 25 years. At one time, there were very few sophisticated bone pathologists, and roentgenographic interpretation was often more accurate than the histologic findings; the pathologist realized that accurate histological diagnosis could not be achieved reliably without the consulting radiologist.

Today, the radiologist's role is to discover and demonstrate the tumor, to estimate the extent of the lesion, to pinpoint the most appropriate biopsy site, and, most important, to indicate the compatibility of the histologic and radiologic diagnoses.

The roentgen demonstration of most tumors usually is easy because of the presence of pain and a mass indicating the site, and the roentgen features are often dramatically portrayed on the initial examination. Occasionally, however, the lesions are not obvious even when extensive involvement is present, as when, in a long bone, cortical destruction must occur before the radiolucency is apparent. Without cortical destruction, extensive medullary cavity invasion will not be demonstrated roentgenographically. This often occurs with round cell tumors (Ewing's sarcoma, reticulum cell sarcoma, and multiple myeloma), lymphomas, and metastatic disease. In the spine and other trabecular bones, almost half of the spongy bone must be destroyed before osteolytic roentgen features occur, so that there may be extensive disease throughout the osseous structures with little or no roentgenographic evidence.

The presence of calcification assures roentgen demonstration even without bone destruction. Calcification occurs most frequently in mesenchymal tumors, such as osteosarcoma and chondrosarcoma, and in some of their benign counterparts. Tomography is useful in evaluating the character of the calcification and defining it when it is not obvious in the survey roentgenograms. Tomography should be used in most examinations, since the characteristics and extent of the lesion often are not clarified in the survey study, and it helps to define extraosseous soft tissue masses and determine the biopsy site.

Arteriography has limitations in distinguishing benign from malignant tumors and in defining the histologic type, but it is useful in outlining the extent of the lesion and often helps the surgeon determine the type and extent of surgery needed.

The most important function of the radiologist is to help the pathologist toward a diagnosis. Although some histologic patterns are plainly characteristic, some occur with both benign and malignant disease. This is particularly true of cartilaginous lesions. The pathologist may receive only a small biopsy specimen, either not representative of the entire lesion or from the wrong site, so that the true pattern of the tumor will not be reflected in the histologic slides. It is then the role of the radiologist to either confirm a correlation or, if there is doubt, indicate a rebiopsy or re-evaluation of the histologic section.

In his consultant role, the radiologist must be able to evaluate the clinical and radiologic features and either arrive at a diagnosis or present a differential diagnosis compatible with the histologic impression. Various features must be critically evaluated.

The transition zone is the zone between the tumor and the host bone. In the past, the features of this zone were used for distinguishing benign from malignant tumors; however, they are more useful as an indication of degree of aggressiveness than of benignancy or malignancy. The transition zone may be well defined or ill defined. The well-defined zone (narrow) with a sclerotic margin indicates the least aggressive of all lesions (Figs. 1 and 2). If it is well defined (short transition) but without a sclerotic rim, it is, while still nonaggressive, more so than that with the sclerotic margin (Figs. 3 and 4). If the transition zone is ill defined (wide), aggressiveness is indicated (Fig. 5).

The reasons for these distinctions are fairly clear. Slowly growing lesions give the host bone a chance to protect itself; the slower the growth the more likely a narrow transition and a sclerotic margin.

FIG. 1 *(left).*—Fibrous dysplasia. Well-defined thick sclerotic margin indicates a lack of aggressiveness in a long-standing inactive lesion.

FIG. 2 *(center).*—Chondromyxoid fibroma. Osteolytic lesion containing a well-developed sclerotic margin not as thick as in Figure 1. This indicates a lack of aggression, but slightly more aggression than the lesion in Figure 1. A small calcification is present within the lesion which indicates cartilaginous tissue. Calcification is infrequent with chondromyxoid fibroma.

FIG. 3 *(right).*—Unicameral bone cyst with pathologic fracture. Transition zone is well defined (short transition zone), but there is no sclerotic margin. This indicates a nonaggressive lesion, but one more aggressive than the lesions in Figures 1 and 2.

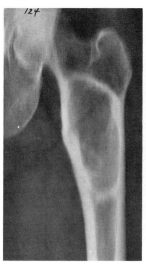 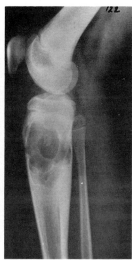 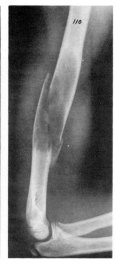

Most lesions with a sclerotic margin or a well-defined transition zone are benign, except for chondrosarcomas, fibrosarcomas, and giant cell tumors. Agressive lesions are usually malignant, except for infections, eosinophilic granuloma, aneurysmal bone cyst, and giant cell tumor. However, these exceptions are not invariable, and fibrosarcomas and chondrosarcomas may appear very aggressive, while eosinophilic granuloma and aneurysmal bone cysts may be nonaggressive.

Cortical break-through does not usually occur in benign lesions unless there is superimposed trauma. However, the cortex may be so thin (*i.e.* aneurysmal bone cyst) that it is not visible roentgenographically and this may be mistaken for a malignant characteristic. When infection penetrates the cortex, multiple gaps of normal cortex continue to exist between the areas of erosion. Neoplasms, however, when breaking through the cortex usually create large single defects with no normal intervening cortex (Fig. 6). Extraosseous extensions of the tumor bone are usually apparent.

Periosteal reactions may be described as either solid or interrupt-

FIG. 4 *(left).* — Giant cell tumor. Cortex is unbroken and the transition zone between the tumor and the host bone is short, although not as short as in Figure 3. This indicates a greater degree of aggressiveness, although this is a benign giant cell tumor.

FIG. 5 *(center).* — Reticulum cell sarcoma. Ill-defined destructive lesion in the upper end of the tibia with penetration of the cortex and soft tissue mass anteriorly. The transition zone is ill defined (long transition zone) and indicates a very aggressive lesion.

FIG. 6 *(right).* — Metastatic carcinoma. Ill-defined but circumscribed destructive lesion in the midportion of the fibula, as well as a large single destruction of cortex on the lateral aspect with no normal intervening cortex. The long transition zone indicates aggressiveness.

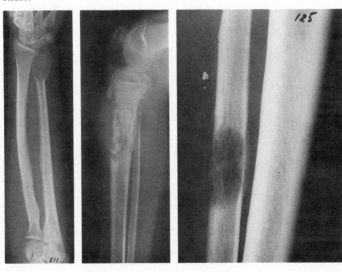

ed. Solid periosteal reactions may be defined as a single layer of new bone greater than 1 mm. in thickness (Fig. 7). It is uniform in density, and the entire sheath of periosteal new bone looks the same, with a uniform, solid appearance, although remarkable differences may be seen from patient to patient. This is a hallmark of a benign process.

Essential in the recognition of a solid periosteal reaction is its persistence, relatively unchanged, for weeks. It may increase in size, but the uniformity of its roentgen density changes little. Here, the importance of roentgen technique cannot be overemphasized: Roentgenograms of a uniform quality must be consistently produced so that reliable comparisons may be made in successive follow-up studies.

Solid periosteal reactions vary from patient to patient depending upon the nature and course of the illness. As an example, eosinophilic granuloma may produce a minor periosteal reaction with only a thin layer of periosteal new bone, or the reaction may be more aggressive with a thicker periosteal response. Yet in both, the periosteal new bone is solid and uniform. New bone may vary remarkably in density as well as thickness. It is the uniformity and solidarity that are significant, not the thickness or density which indicate only the progress and age of periosteal response.

Morphologically, solid uniform periosteal new bone may be thick or thin, of any degree of density, and have an even or undulating sur-

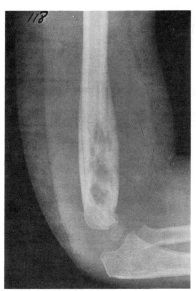

FIG. 7.—Eosinophilic granuloma. Destructive lesion in the lower end of the humerus that is ill defined and aggressive. However, there is solid periosteal reaction on both sides of the lesion that consists of a single layer of periosteal new bone greater than 1 mm. in thickness. In spite of the aggressive nature of the destructive lesion, the solid periosteal reaction indicates benignancy.

face. Thickness and density seem related to the aggressiveness of the irritant, but duration may also play a part. Thus, low levels of irritants acting for long periods, or more aggressive irritants acting for shorter periods, may produce similar roentgen changes. Regardless of time or intensity, the periosteal response to benign conditions usually will be even and uniform.

Among the conditions that frequently cause solid periosteal new bone are eosinophilic granuloma, fractures, osteomyelitis, hemorrhage, hypertrophic pulmonary osteoarthropathy, osteoid osteoma, vascular disease, and the storage diseases.

Although solid uniform periosteal reactions indicate benignancy, benign lesions may not always express themselves in this classic manner. They may instead cause periosteal responses highly suggestive of malignant disease.

Dense, undulating periosteal reactions often occur with long-standing varicosities or arterial disease. The periosteal reaction is often a centimeter or more thick and the outer surface is rough and undulating. The mechanism of production is unknown.

Thin undulating periosteal reactions are located on the concave aspects of long bones. Pulmonary osteoarthropathy is the best example. The reactions which are not densely ossified are associated with benign or malignant tumors of the thoracic cavity. The mechanism of growth is unknown, but after thoracotomy (with or without removal of the tumor) the reaction subsides within 6 months.

Dense elliptical periosteal reactions vary from 2 mm. to 1 cm. in thickness. They are thickest near the center and taper toward both ends. They occur in long-standing cortical osteoid osteomas. Occasionally, round cell tumors (Ewing's or reticulum cell), when treated by radiation, may cause elliptical reactions but these often are permeated by the osteolytic areas characteristic of malignant growth.

Periosteal cloaking is found in long-standing, benign conditions such as storage disease and chronic osteomyelitis. It is usually several millimeters thick and irregularly dense. The free margin is straight, which does not occur with malignancy.

Codman's triangle was first described by Ribbert in 1914; he believed it was the result of periosteal elevation caused by an expanding mass. The significance of the triangular Codman's cuff merits particular mention. Previously considered a manifestation of malignant bone disease, it is now appreciated that it may result from anything benign or malignant lifting the periosteum. Under microscopic consideration, tumor cells are not present within the cuff. Indeed, when invaded by tumor, Codman's triangle disappears. In contrast, collections of pus and blood notoriously elevate the periosteum, producing these periosteal triangles. Therefore, the presence of a Codman's triangle is not an indication of malignancy, but the result of an elevation of the periosteum which may occur with either benign or malignant conditions.

The interrupted periosteal reactions are not uniform but pleomorphic with varying roentgen patterns. Lamellated (onion skin) (Fig. 8) or perpendicular (sunburst) periosteal reactions (Fig. 9) are classic examples. Caused by periosteal elevation in active conditions (malignant tumor, infection, repeated hemorrhage), the interrupted pattern indicates an active, rapidly progressive process.

Characteristic of interrupted periosteal reactions is their lack of stability; radiographically they change constantly. The more aggressive the irritant the greater the degree of periosteal change from week to week, sometimes from day to day.

Lamellated periosteal reactions occur in active conditions such as acute osteomyelitis and malignant tumors. The lamellations are caused by intermittent growth. According to Sissons (1949), single lamellations may form within 1 week. Brunschwig and Harmon

FIG. 8 *(left)*.—Osteosarcoma. Extensive destructive lesion throughout the lower end of the femur with lamellated periosteal reaction present on the anterior surface. These small lamellations indicate an aggressive nature but not necessarily malignancy.

FIG. 9 *(right)*.—Metastatic carcinoma. Extensive destructive lesion throughout the upper end of the humerus. Periosteal reaction noted in the lateral margins is perpendicular and indicates an active aggressive lesion.

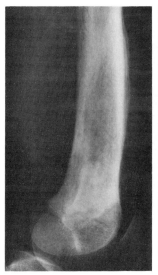
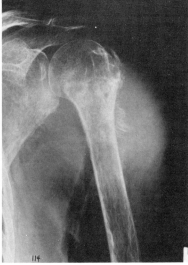

(1935) believe lamellations are the result of alternating periods of rapid and slow growth. During slow growth, the periosteum has time to form a layer of bone analogous to the involucum of infection while during rapid growth, no new bone is formed. Bleeding under the periosteum also influences these roentgen appearances.

Perpendicular (sunburst) reactions are the result of new bone growth at right angles to the shaft of the host bone, usually caused by malignant tumor which elevates the periosteum. In Brunschwig's opinion, the new bone formation lies along fibrous bands (Sharpey's fibers) which extend between periosteum and cortex. Very likely, perpendicular bone growth also takes place along these vascular channels. Microradiography and serial histopathologic sections support this concept.

Osteosarcomas and Ewing's tumors tend to stimulate sunburst reactions, while chondrosarcomas and fibrosarcomas cause much less periosteal reaction. At times, Ewing's tumor and osteosarcoma will elevate the periosteum without provoking reaction. Occasionally, a single lamellated reaction may appear with a solid reaction superimposed. This is an excellent sign of a benign process, usually resulting from an infection or eosinophilic granuloma. The small lamellation should not lead one to the diagnosis of malignancy; the heaping up or presence of a solid reaction above it indicates benignancy although aggressiveness.

AMORPHOUS REACTIONS. — Malignant tumors, in addition to causing lamellations and perpendicular striations, with or without interspersed deossified areas, often cause amorphous calcification. Lying mainly between periosteal new bone and its parent bone cortex, these amorphous deposits may represent extension of tumor bone rather than periosteal response to the tumor. Often oval or spherical in shape, they range in size from millimeters to centimeters in cross section. These amorphous deposits usually denote bone malignancy; rarely do they accompany benign bone tumors. Usually, they help differentiate primary from metastatic bone tumors, the latter being far less likely to cause periosteal reaction or extraosseous amorphous deposits, except in the presence of an associated pathologic fracture.

Some malignant tumors tend to provoke more periosteal reactions than others, a difference not related to the degree of periosteal elevation. Fibrosarcomas notoriously invade the periosteum at a considerable height from the parent bone yet produce little periosteal new bone formation. The microscopic evidence suggests that a periosteal response does occur, but it is destroyed almost as soon as it forms. This happens with some chondrosarcomas, while, in contrast, osteosarcomas and Ewing's tumors usually tend to stimulate new bone formation; however, at times, while they elevate the periosteum, they may not provoke demonstrable periosteal new bone response. This may be related to the rate of tumor growth.

Periosteal reactions more commonly accompany malignant bone tumors than benign ones; however, they do not provide a reliable distinction, since benign lesions may also produce them. Experience shows that almost any type of periosteal reaction may be present with any type of bone tumor. The one notable exception is the solid type of periosteal reaction which, occurring almost exclusively in benign conditions, is of great diagnostic aid. Only rarely will a malignant lesion, a slow-growing tumor, or an asymptomatic tumor, produce a solid periosteal reaction. Treated tumors may also manifest this solid appearance. However, the presence of a solid periosteal reaction on the initial roentgenograms of a bone lesion is usually an indication of benignancy.

In general, the following line of thought may be reasonably applied to bone lesions with particular reference to the periosteum: Osteoblastic lesions confined to the host bone, unaccompanied by changes beyond the bone, may be benign or malignant. If, in the absence of infection or trauma, interrupted periosteal new bone is manifest beyond the parent bone, the lesion is far more likely to be a primary bone malignancy than a metastatic one, unless the primary lesion is of bone origin.

The patient's age plays an important role in the evaluation of malignant bone tumors and may lead to the diagnosis even when the tumor is roentgenographically atypical. The age distribution of a large number of patients with tumors reveals some interesting facts. During the first year of life, malignant bone tumors are almost exclusively neuroblastomas. Occasionally, Ewing's sarcoma may be found, but rarely before 6 months of age. A malignant tumor in the first 6 months of life, statistically, must be considered a neuroblastoma.

During the second decade, osteosarcoma and Ewing's sarcoma have their peak incidences. The roentgen and clinical features of these 2 tumors permit their differentiation, as does the fact that Ewing's tumors tend to arise in the diaphysis whereas osteosarcomas usually originate in the metaphysis.

During the third decade of life, reticulum cell sarcoma shows its peak incidence. In its histologic characteristics and pathophysiology, it is so similar to Ewing's sarcoma that they often cannot be differentiated. The course and the patient's age may be the deciding factors. Patients with Ewing's sarcoma live but a short time, whereas it is not unusual for patients with reticulum cell sarcoma to live comfortably for many years. Also, patients with Ewing's sarcoma are usually ill, with elevated temperatures. They look pale and sick and have lost weight, whereas patients with reticulum cell sarcoma primary in the bone appear well, even though the tumor may be large. During the third decade, lymphoma also most commonly affects bone. Hodgkin's disease or any other type of lymphoma may primarily manifest within the bone and it must be a consideration in this decade.

During the fourth decade, fibrosarcoma, parosteal sarcoma, and malignant giant cell tumors have their peaks. Fibrosarcoma and malignant giant cell tumors have similar histologic and clinical features but usually are easily differentiated radiographically from parosteal sarcoma.

In the fifth to the eighth decades, the most frequent bone tumors are metastatic tumors or multiple myeloma. Therefore, in older patients, bone lesions, whether polyostotic or monostotic, are considered metastases until proven otherwise. Chondrosarcoma tends to occur in older individuals.

To recapitulate: neuroblastoma is most common during the first six months of life; osteosarcoma and Ewing's tumor, in the teens and early twenties; fibroscarcoma, parosteal sarcoma, and malignant giant cell tumor during the third and fourth decades; and metastatic malignant disease and myeloma, with an occasional chondrosarcoma, above 40 years of age. Experience has shown that approximately 80 per cent of malignant tumors may be correctly determined on the basis of age alone.

Other statistical approaches to bone lesions have validity, and merit recall to supplement careful roentgen analysis. For example, it is extremely rare for tumor of the sternum to be benign, no matter what its appearance or the age of the patient. In generalized bone disease of children, when one or more vertebral bodies is collapsed, leukemia, neuroblastoma, and eosinophilic granuloma are the important considerations. With widespread epiphyseal lesions, increased density, and destruction, one must consider collagen disease or congenital anomaly.

Primary malignant tumors generally may be divided into 3 major categories: round cell tumors, mesenchymal tumors, and metastatic tumors. These 3 groups have certain characteristics which are usually sufficiently well defined.

The round cell tumors include Ewing's sarcoma, reticulum cell sarcoma, and multiple myeloma. Other secondary round cell tumors are leukemia, lymphoma, and neuroblastoma. These are more likely to arise in the midshaft of tubular bones than in the ends. They tend to be osteolytic, and new bone formation is reactive (Fig. 10). Tumor new bone is not produced, *i.e.*, there is an absence of new bone in the perifocal soft tissues.

The malignant mesenchymal tumors are osteosarcoma, fibrosarcoma, and chondrosarcoma. These tumors are capable of forming tumor matrices which, as their names imply, may be osteoid, chondroid, or fibroid. Osteoid and chondroid matrices almost invariably calcify, and this is their most characteristic roentgen feature. Usually, the calcified matrix extends into the soft tissues (Figs. 11 and 12). The chondroid matrix has a distinct, densely calcified snowflake pattern (Figs. 13 and 14), and the osteoid matrix is homogeneously dense. The fibroid matrix does not calcify, making fibrosarcomas difficult to differentiate from metastatic disease. Fibrosarcomas, like most mesenchymal tumors, occur at the ends of a long bone.

FIG. 10 *(left).*—Reticulum cell sarcoma. Multiple small permeations with normal intervening cortex in the lower third of the femur. Round cell tumors tend to occur in the shaft and to be osteolytic; if there is new bone formation, it is reactive and not tumor new bone. No new bone formation occurs in the soft tissue mass.

FIG. 11 *(right).*—Ewing's sarcoma. Osteoblastic lesion in the horizontal ramus of the left symphysis pubis, as well as periosteal reaction. The increased density is the result of reactive bone rather than calcified tumor matrix which does not occur with round cell tumors. An uncalcified soft tissue mass is present.

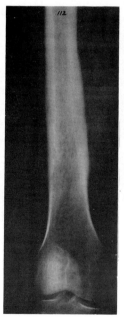

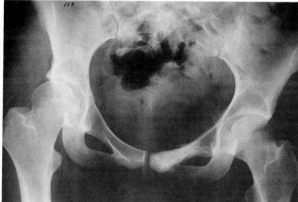

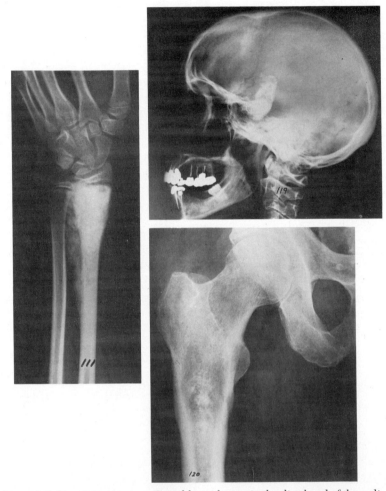

FIG. 12 *(left).* — Osteosarcoma. Osteoblastic lesion in the distal end of the radius extending to the epiphyseal line. The cartilage acts as a barrier to the tumor. In the soft tissues medially, there are tumor calcifications within the soft tissue mass. This indicates that this is a matrix-producing tumor. The increase in density in the radius itself could be the result of either reactive bone or tumor new bone, but the extension into the soft tissues indicates the true nature.

FIG. 13 *(top right).* — Chondrosarcoma of dorsum sella. Calcification is heterogenous and characteristic of cartilage calcification. This indicates the true nature of the condition.

FIG. 14 *(bottom right).* — Chondrosarcoma. Osteolytic lesion in the upper end of the femur with flocculent calcifications within it. This indicates that it is a matrix-producing tumor due to cartilage. The thickening of the endosteal surface of the cortex below the calcification is characteristic of chondrosarcoma.

Metastatic bone lesions are frequently osteoblastic. This is the result of reactive bone response to the tumors and not a manifestation of tumor new bone formation.

In summary, with careful roentgenographic and clinical evaluation, the pathologist and the radiologist can often come to a definite diagnosis. Both the isolated radiologic approach and the isolated histologic approach are full of pitfalls and cooperation is essential. However, in the last analysis, the patient's treatment is in the orthopedic surgeon's hands. Whatever the thoughts on the biopsy or the roentgen appearance, it is the orthopedic surgeon who is presented with the problem at the operating table, and he must be able to rely on sound input from both radiologist and pathologist to improve his chances of success.

REFERENCES

Brunschwig, A., and Harmon, P. H.: Studies in bone sarcoma; An experimental and pathological study of the role of the periosteum in formation of bone in various primary bone tumors. *Surgery, Gynecology, and Obstetrics*, 60:30–40, January 1935.

Sissons, H. A.: Intermittent periosteal activity. *Nature*, 163:1001–1002, June 25, 1949.

Tomography and Angiography in the Evaluation of Bone Lesions

J. BARNETT FINKELSTEIN, M.D.
Department of Diagnostic Radiology, The University of
Texas System Cancer Center M. D. Anderson Hospital
and Tumor Institute, Houston, Texas

TOMOGRAPHY AND ARTERIOGRAPHY are well established radiographic techniques currently available almost routinely to the referring physician (Beranbaum and Meyers, 1964; Daves and Loechel, 1962; Potter, 1971). The use of these procedures in skeletal radiography has not been as well emphasized as in the evaluation of other organ systems. At M. D. Anderson Hospital and Tumor Institute, we have accumulated considerable experience with these techniques in the evaluation and management of skeletal diseases. It is the purpose of this communication to illustrate with specific cases under what circumstances these procedures have proven worthwhile.

The initial radiographic evaluation of a patient suspected of having a bone tumor consists of chest radiography, a complete bone survey, and coned-down views of the specific area of interest. Tomography and/or arteriography are performed only if additional information regarding the diagnosis or treatment can be obtained. The tomograms are done with a polytome device utilizing hypocycloidal motion. Anatomic positioning as well as the number of laminograms and the distance between laminograms are tailored to the individual patient. Usually, multiple exposures are obtained at 0.5 cm. intervals in at least 2 projections which often include oblique views. In contrast to tomography, arteriography requires hospitalization and entails a minimal risk for the patient which must be carefully weighed against

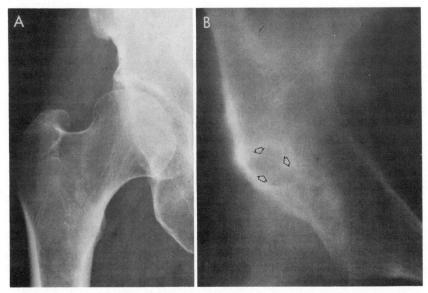

FIG. 1.—*A*, film of patient with known carcinoma of prostate and pain in right hip. Routine film is normal. *B*, tomogram clearly demonstrates a small osteolytic metastasis in the superolateral aspect of the acetabulum (arrows).

FIG. 2.—*A*, film of patient with known Ewing's sarcoma of the sacrum. Anteroposterior (AP) view of pelvis is difficult to interpret because of overlying gas and fecal shadows. *B*, tomogram clearly defines a large area of destruction in the right sacrum and ilium.

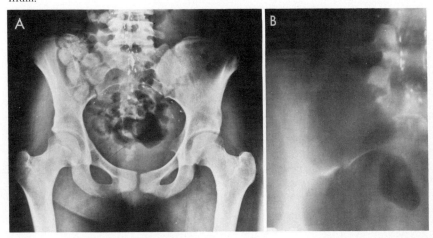

the potential value of the information to be derived. Arteriography is done with standard percutaneous catheterization of the appropriate peripheral vessel. The specific vessel catheterized, the position of the patient, the amount and rate of contrast material injected, and the

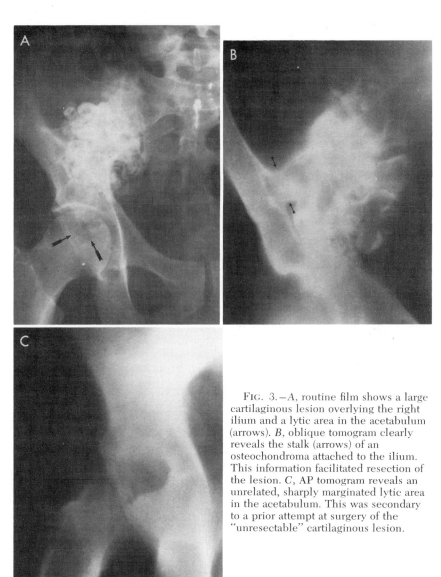

FIG. 3.—*A*, routine film shows a large cartilaginous lesion overlying the right ilium and a lytic area in the acetabulum (arrows). *B*, oblique tomogram clearly reveals the stalk (arrows) of an osteochondroma attached to the ilium. This information facilitated resection of the lesion. *C*, AP tomogram reveals an unrelated, sharply marginated lytic area in the acetabulum. This was secondary to a prior attempt at surgery of the "unresectable" cartilaginous lesion.

number of films exposed are all highly variable and again must be individualized (Bron, 1971; Chiappa, Galli, and Gennari, 1964; Jacobson and Shapiro, 1964; Koskinen, Roukkula, Ryoppy, and Vankka, 1970).

Tomography has proven to be of most value in the detection or confirmation of the presence of a bone lesion in the case of negative or equivocal routine films (Fig. 1). The yield to be expected from tomography is directly proportional to the anatomic complexity of the region examined. Excluding the skull and facial bones, tomographic exploration of the spin will be the most rewarding. If a patient has clinically significant signs or symptoms referrable to the spine, negative routine films should never be accepted as positive proof that a

FIG. 4.—A, radiograph of the humerus shows lytic lesions of the cortex in association with increased density within the bone. B, tomography more clearly defines the cartilaginous nature of the mineralization within the bone as well as the extensive nature of the lesion. Arrow indicates proximal extent of mineralized cartilage. A chondrosarcoma was resected and replaced with a bone graft.

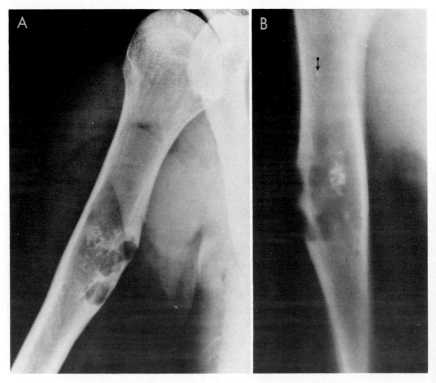

significant bone lesion does not exist. This is especially true in the sacrum (Fig. 2).

Decisions regarding the optimal biopsy site, the feasibility of resection, and the size of radiotherapy portals are all best made prior to surgical therapy or radiotherapy (Fig. 3). In this regard, we have found that the second most important use of tomography is in mapping the intraosseous extent of disease. Bone lesions frequently are considerably more extensive than they appear on routine films, so that every effort should be made to define the precise anatomic boundaries (Figs. 4 and 5).

In addition to detecting an abnormality and defining its boundaries, significant information regarding a specific diagnosis also can be obtained with tomography. Margins favoring a benign or malignant process are more clearly delineated than on plain films. Unsuspected

FIG. 5–*A*, adamantinoma of the tibia. AP view reveals one lytic area. *B*, tomogram shows extension of lesion inferomedially (arrows). This was not evident on multiple routine views.

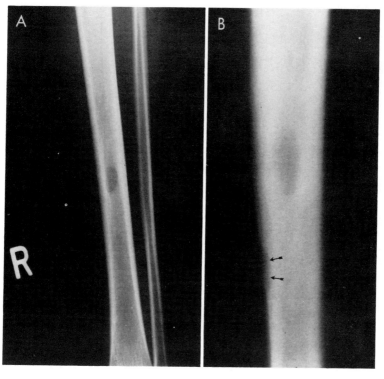

fractures and sequestra may be identified, and the presence of small amounts of mineralized osteoid or chondroid tumor matrix can be recognized (Fig. 4B). In short, tomography can better define a multitude of details about the internal architecture of a bone lesion which are of prime significance in making a radiographic diagnosis.

Arteriography has not proven to be as practical as tomography in the day-to-day evaluation of bone abnormalities. We use tomograms and arteriograms in a ratio of approximately 100 to 1. However, in properly selected cases, arteriography yields valuable information not obtainable by any other means. The procedure is most rewarding in the identification of soft tissue extensions of bone disease not evident on routine films or tomograms (Figs. 6, 7, and 8). While tomograms define the anatomic extent of disease within the bone, an arteriogram can show extension beyond the bone. If the bone lesion is hypervascular, the soft tissue extension may be visualized directly, while in cases where the primary lesion is hypovascular, vessel displacement serves to indicate the boundaries of a soft tissue mass.

In certain cases, especially osteochondromas, it is desirable simply

FIG. 6.—A, recurrent giant cell tumor of the distal femur. B, arteriogram with subtraction technique directly visualizes unsuspected soft tissue infiltration by the tumor (arrows).

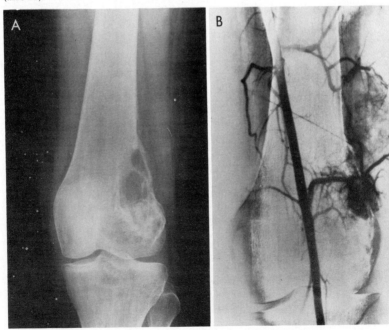

to visualize the anatomic relationship between major blood vessels and the obvious bone tumor in order to better plan the surgical approach and avoid vascular injury (Fig. 9).

While our experience is limited, an obvious use of arteriography is in the diagnosis of vascular disorders secondarily involving bone. The direct visualization of an aneurysm, arteriovenous fistula, or congenital arteriovenous malformation is essential for proper surgical planning (Fig. 10). Except in the diagnosis of these vascular diseases and in the identification of a nidus in osteoid osteomas, we have not found arteriography to be of value in making a specific histologic

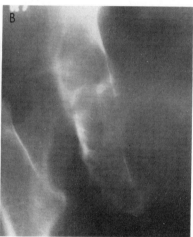

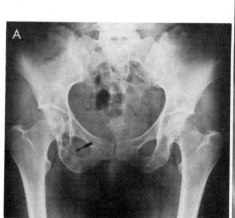

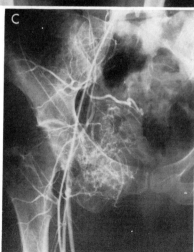

FIG. 7.—*A*, giant fibroxanthoma. AP view of pelvis shows lytic area in the right ischium (arrow). *B*, tomography indicates that the destruction extends superiorly into the acetabular region. *C*, arteriogram directly visualizes a huge, unsuspected intrapelvic component extending into the obturator foramen.

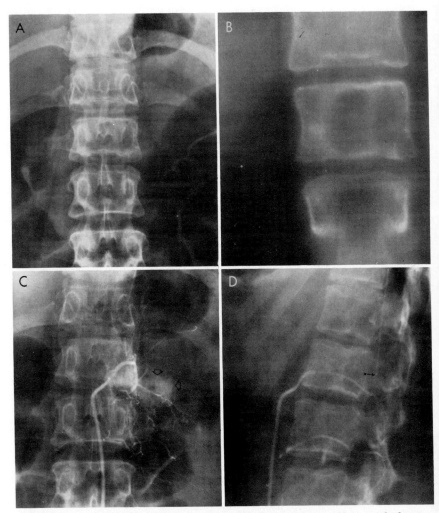

FIG. 8.—*A*, osteoblastoma of the first lumbar vertebra. Routine film reveals destruction of the body, pedicle, and transverse process. *B*, tomogram more clearly defines the extensive destructive process. *C*, AP arteriogram directly visualizes unsuspected hypervascular soft tissue extension of tumor (arrows). This area was selected for biopsy. *D*, lateral anteriogram demonstrates slight posterior displacement of the anterior spinal artery by soft tissue mass (arrow).

diagnosis or in differentiating benign from malignant conditions (Fig. 11). Occasionally, arteriography can be used to indicate the best site for biopsy (Fig. 12).

In summary, both tomography and arteriography are valuable diag-

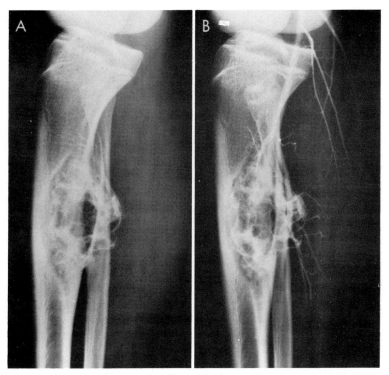

FIG. 9.—*A,* osteochondroma arising from the tibia. *B,* the relationship between major arteries and the bony lesion was visualized prior to operation as a precautionary measure.

nostic procedures in the evaluation of skeletal diseases. Tomography serves best to confirm the presence of a lesion not obvious on routine films and to define the anatomic extent of the abnormality prior to biopsy, resection, or radiation therapy. Less frequently, information regarding the specific histologic diagnosis is obtained. Arteriography is most useful for demonstrating soft tissue extension of a primary bone lesion. Visualization of major blood vessels prior to operation, and identification of vascular disorders affecting bone are additional uses. In our opinion, arteriography is rarely of value in making a specific histologic diagnosis or in differentiating benign from malignant disease.

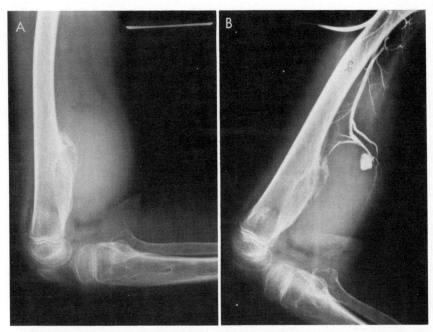

FIG. 10.—A, lateral view of the femur reveals a posterior soft tissue mass in a patient with osteochondromatosis. Malignant transformation was suspected. B, arteriogram clearly demonstrates a huge false aneurysm to be the cause of the mass.

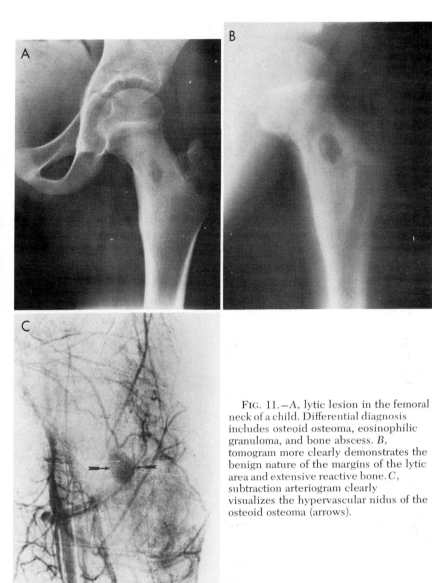

FIG. 11.—*A*, lytic lesion in the femoral neck of a child. Differential diagnosis includes osteoid osteoma, eosinophilic granuloma, and bone abscess. *B*, tomogram more clearly demonstrates the benign nature of the margins of the lytic area and extensive reactive bone. *C*, subtraction arteriogram clearly visualizes the hypervascular nidus of the osteoid osteoma (arrows).

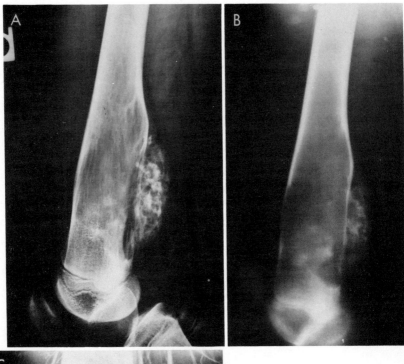

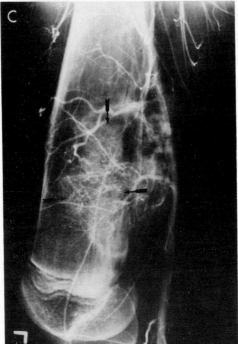

FIG. 12.—*A,* routine film shows a peculiar pattern of increased bone density at the posterior aspect of the femur. *B,* tomogram permits better appreciation of areas of increased density within the bone, a benign type of expansion posterosuperiorly, and a faint benign margin superiorly. *C,* arteriogram reveals a localized region of hypervascularity within the bone (arrows). This area was selected for biopsy and the final diagnosis was osteosarcoma arising within a bone cyst.

REFERENCES

Beranbaum, S. L., and Meyers, P. H.: *Special Procedures in Roentgen Diagnosis.* 1st Edition. Springfield, Illinois, Charles C Thomas, 1964, 597 pp.

Bron, K. M.: Femoral arteriography. In Abrams, H. L., Ed.: *Angiography.* Boston, Massachusetts, Little, Brown and Co., 1971, pp. 1221–1299.

Chiappa, M D., Galli, G., and Gennari, L.: Arteriography in bone and soft-tissue tumors. In Schebinger, R. A. and Ruzicka, F. F., Eds.: *Vascular Roentgenology.* New York, New York, Macmillan Co., 1964, pp. 469–478.

Daves, M. L., and Loechel, W. E.: *The Interpretation of Tomograms of the Head.* 1st Edition. Springfield, Illinois, Charles C Thomas, 1962, 248 pp.

Jacobson, H. G., and Shapiro, J. H.: Femoral arteriography. In Schebinger, R. A. and Ruzicka, F. F., Eds.: *Vascular Roentgenology.* New York, New York, Macmillan Co., 1964, pp. 426–446.

Koskinen, M. R., Roukkula, M., Ryoppy, S., and Vankka, E.: The value of angiography in the diagnosis of bone and soft tissue tumors of the extremities. In Jelliffe, A. M. and Strickland, B., Eds.: *Symposium Ossium.* London, England, E. & S. Livingstone, 1970, pp. 40–44.

Potter, G. D.: *Sectional Anatomy and Tomography of the Head.* New York, New York, Grune & Stratton, Inc., 1971, 334 pp.

Nuclear Techniques in Skeletal Neoplastic Disease

ROBERT E. O'MARA, M.D.
Division of Nuclear Medicine, University of Arizona
College of Medicine, Tucson, Arizona

DURING THE PAST DECADE, there has been a rapid advance in the use of radionuclide evaluation of the skeletal system in patients suffering from primary and secondary neoplasms. The radioisotopic bone study is a simple, safe technique that is useful for determining the presence and extent of disease, choosing sites for biopsy purposes, and obtaining an objective evaluation of the effect of various modes of therapy.

Radiopharmaceuticals

The radionuclides currently used for bone scanning are summarized in Table 1. ^{85}Sr was the first widely used agent. It has the main advantage of a long shelf-life. However, the relatively slow blood clearance of this nuclide and excretion via the colon necessitate a delay from injection to scanning of at least 2 days. The long physical and biological half-life results in a radiation dose that is somewhat high. This factor limits the amount injectable, resulting in poor counting statistics, suboptimal resolution, and long patient study times.

The introduction of shorter-lived radionuclides with higher doses injected has resulted in improved counting statistics. Shorter scanning times and relatively lower skeletal, marrow, and total body ra-

Table 1
Radionuclides for Bone Scanning

Radionuclide	Half-Life	Photon Energy (kev)	Recommended Dose (mCi)	Skeletal Dose (Rads)	Marrow Dose (Rads)
[85]Sr	64 days	513	.100	3.6	1.1
[87m]Sr	2.7 h	388	1 – 10	0.71	0.21
[18]F	1.85 h	511	1 – 10	1.5	0.40
[99m]Tc PP	6.0 h	140	10	0.45	0.10

Abbreviations: [85]Sr, 85-Strontium; [87m]Sr, 87m-Strontium; ^{18}F, 18-Fluorine; ^{99m}Tc PP, 99m-Technetium polyphosphate; h, hours; kev, Kiloelectron volts; mCi, millicuries; Rads, radiation absorbed dose.

diation doses also are a result. [87m]Sr, with a half-life of 2.8 hours and a gamma emission of 388 kev, was the first of this group of agents. Unfortunately, the short half-life of this radionuclide necessitates scanning within an hour or 2 after injection. This allows little time for excretion and results in high body background and a low target-to-background ratio. [18]F has a half-life of 1.8 hours with rapid blood clearance. This results in an improved target-to-background ratio. Its use is somewhat limited because of the short half-life. As a result, the user must be close to a nuclear reactor or cyclotron where this radiopharmaceutical is produced.

More recently, a variety of bone-seeking complexes of ^{99m}Tc have been introduced (Subramanian et al., 1971; Subramanian et al., 1972; Yano, McRae, VanDyke, and Anger, 1972). These include ^{99m}Tc polyphosphate, diphosphonate, and pyrophosphate. The tagging radionuclide, ^{99m}Tc, is readily available and relatively inexpensive. Its low gamma energy emission offers advantageous scanning characteristics in that it may be used with either rectilinear scanners or stationary camera devices. An early report indicates that ^{99m}Tc diphosphonate is more sensitive than ^{18}F in depicting metastatic disease to bone (Silberstein et al., 1973). As experience with these agents is gained, one of this class will become the agent of choice for bone scans.

All of the bone scanning agents in use at present are concerned with the mineral phase of bone. Bauer has defined the range of turnover rates in normal bone and has shown that an increase in turnover rate occurs in regions of insult where healing is taking place (Bauer and Wendeberg, 1959). The repair mechanisms include increased vascularity at the site, altered exchange processes, and new bone formation, all of which contribute to an area of increased radioisotopic activity signifying pathology on the bone scan. Identification of an area of positive involvement is independent of the net calcium bal-

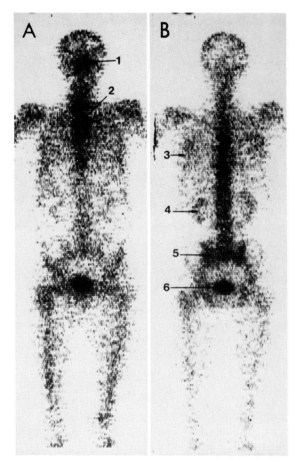

FIG. 1.—*A,* normal anterior bone scan accomplished 2 hours after intravenous injection of 5 mCi. ^{18}F. Note normal activity in base of skull (1) and sternum (2). *B,* posterior bone scan done simultaneously with Figure 1*A* on a dual-probed rectilinear scanner. Note normal activity in scapulae (3), kidneys (4), sacral alae (5), and bladder (6). These areas should not be confused with areas of abnormally increased activity.

ance and consequently, both osteolytic and osteoblastic lesions and regions which are normal radiographically may appear as positive areas on a scintiscan. An example of a normal bone scan is shown in Figure 1.

INSTRUMENTATION

With the relatively high gamma photon energy emissions of ^{85}Sr (513 kev) and ^{18}F (511 kev), one is limited to rectilinear scanning for the most part. Thin crystal, rapid-imaging devices such as the Anger Camera give poor resolution with such high energy emissions, even when special collimators are utilized. One of the main advantages of the newer radiopharmaceuticals utilized in bone imaging is that they may be used with any type of device.

Total body scanning is now possible with existing rectilinear scanners or camera device systems. One should not accept studies which include only the vertebral column and pelvis.

PATIENT STUDY

No patient preparation is necessary. Medication for pain relief may be administered for patient comfort during the scanning procedure which lasts approximately 1 hour.

The radiopharmaceutical is administered intravenously. Ten millicuries of ^{99m}Tc-diphosphonate is the dose currently employed in our laboratory. The study is begun 3 hours after injection. The patient voids immediately before the start of the study in an effort to clear as much activity as possible from the bladder and kidneys. Total body scanning is performed in both the anterior and posterior projections. Lateral and oblique views of selected areas may be obtained if necessary.

Metastatic Disease

Skeletal involvement by metastatic carcinoma is a fairly common autopsy finding, exceeded only by the incidence of metastases to lymph nodes, lungs, and liver (Abrams, Spiro, and Goldstein, 1950). The occurrence rate of such involvement has been reported to range from 27 to 70 per cent in autopsy series (Abrams, Spiro, and Goldstein, 1950, Jaffe, 1958). The rate appears to be dependent upon the thoroughness of the postmortem examination. In malignant tumors which commonly metastasize to the skeletal system (breast, prostate, thyroid, lung, and kidney), osseous involvement at the time of death is approximately 50 to 85 per cent (Abrams, Spiro, and Goldstein, 1950; Willis 1967). Detection of such metastatic disease to bone is crucial in the management of cancer patients. Both isotopic and radiographic skeletal surveys are being used currently as means to reach such detection.

There is general agreement that roentgenographic identification of secondary neoplastic deposits in bone frequently appears late in the clinical course. The reason for the relative insensitivity of the standard roentgenographic examination in demonstrating early lesions is that a minimum of 30 to 50 per cent of bone mineral has to be lost before such lesions become roentgenographically visible (Borak, 1942). Metastases to the spinal column are even more difficult to demonstrate, with estimates of 50 to 75 per cent of bone destruction being necessary before visualization is possible (Edelstyn, Gillespie, and Grebell, 1967). Frequently, a destructive lesion in a vertebral body must be greater than 1½ centimeters in size to be seen (Bachman and Sproul, 1955).

Many series now in the literature compare the results of bone scanning and roentgenographic studies. Some of these are summarized in Table 2. It is well documented that scintiscanning techniques frequently will demonstrate skeletal metastases before they are appreciated on radiographs. This also has been our experience at the University of Arizona. An example of such a case, involving a single metastatic deposit in the lumbar spine, is shown in Figure 2. Several studies have shown an estimated time between the appearance of a lesion on scintiscans and first demonstration on X-ray films to be from 3 to 6 months (DeNardo and Volpe, 1966; Greenberg *et al.*, 1968).

In patients with positive roentgenograms, the scan will frequently show that the amount of metastatic tumor present is far greater than considered radiographically (Fig. 3). This is of importance to the radiotherapist because it helps him plan treatment portals more efficiently. In addition, a discovery of multiple metastases may totally change the treatment plan from local therapy, such as radiation therapy, to systemic therapy with hormones or other drugs. Scanning techniques will also allow for optimization of sites for biopsy purposes. Scans are also quite useful in evaluating areas such as the sternum and scapulae that are difficult to study by radiographic techniques.

Visualization of the total skeleton is the only acceptable form of study at the present time. Often, metastatic deposits are found in peripheral bones (22 per cent in our experience) (O'Mara, unpublished data). This corresponds to the series reported by Shirazi, in which one fourth of solitary lesions were found in the extremities (Shirazi, Rayudu, and Fordham, in press). In that series of 100 solitary lesions, 55 were metastatic deposits on scanning.

Scanning techniques do contain a small percentage (3 to 8 per cent) of false-negatives. These usually occur in patients with highly anaplastic tumors or in patients with indolent, slow-growing lesions where reactive bone does not form or is not detectable. As a result, the scan should never be interpreted without corresponding radiographs.

Table 2
Comparison of Bone Scan and Radiograph in Detection of Metastatic Disease

Author	Number of Cases	+Scan +X-Ray #(%)	+Scan - or ± X-Ray #(%)	-Scan -X-Ray #(%)	- or ± Scan +X-Ray #(%)
Harmer et al., 1969	112	17(15%)	35(31%)	57(51%)	3(3%)
DeNardo and Volpe, 1966	84	29(34%)	32(38%)	18(21%)	3(4%)
Sklaroff and Charkes, 1964	40	18(45%)	3(8%)	16(40%)	3(8%)
Spencer et al., 1967	38	10(26%)	15(39%)	12(32%)	1(3%)
Legge et al., 1970	186	29(15%)	25(13%)	130(70%)	2(1%)
Total	460				
Average		22%	24%	51%	3%

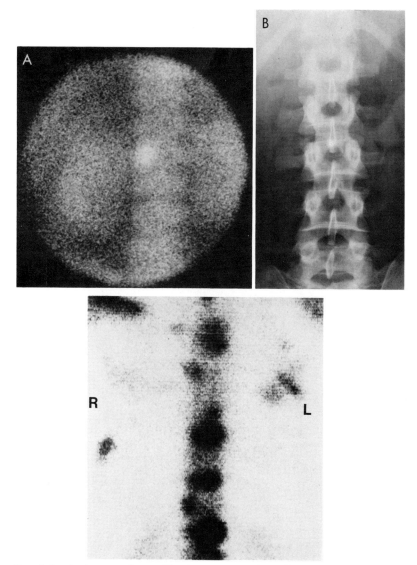

FIG. 2 *(top)*—*A*, scintiphoto of lumbar spine performed 3 hours after intravenous injection of 10 mCi. ^{99m}Tc polyphosphate. Note single area of increased activity at right pedicle of the second lumbar vertebral body in this 54-year-old man with lymphoma. *B*, radiograph of lumbar spine from same patient interpreted as normal. Biopsy of L_2 revealed osseous metastasis of the primary.

FIG. 3 *(bottom)*.—Posterior scan of the thorax performed in a 64-year-old male with primary prostatic carcinoma. This study was done 3 hours after the intravenous injection of 10 mCi. ^{99m}Tc polyphosphate. Note the multiple foci of abnormal activity present in the spine, ribs, and right shoulder. Corresponding radiographs of these areas demonstrated metastases at T_8 and T_{10} and the right shoulder only.

Frequently, scanning techniques will demonstrate metastatic disease in patients at the time of the initial discovery of a primary lesion. Sauerbrunn and co-workers have reported a prospective study of 82 patients suffering from carcinoma of the lung (Sauerbrunn, Hansen, and Napoli, 1972). Of the 82 patients studied, 29 had positive ^{85}Sr bone scans at the time of discovery of the malignant disease. Of these 29, only 4 had positive changes radiographically, and 14 presented histological evidence of metastases on biopsy of the posterior iliac crest alone. Sklaroff and Charkes (1968) demonstrated positive findings in 10 of 64 women who had just undergone radical mastectomy for cancer. Sharma and Quinn (1972) reported finding abnormal scans with ^{18}F in 46 of 88 patients with primary breast tumors. Of

Table 3
Normal and Benign Conditions Resulting in Positive Bone Scans*

A. Normal structure and variations:
Base of skull
Scapulae, sternum
Ala of sacrum
Kidneys and bladder
Epiphyses
GI tract with IV and oral administration
Asymmetric development of sternum, scapulae, clavicles, pelvis
Thyroid
B. Soft-tissue abnormalities:
Calcific tendinitis
Hydroureter and hydronephrosis
Healing postoperative scar
Soft-tissue osseous metaplasia
Dental abscess without bony involvement
Breast carcinoma
C. Osseous abnormalities:
Fracture
Arthritis
Osteomyelitis
Regional migratory osteoporosis
Postoperative osseous changes
Eosinophilic granuloma
Paget's disease
Renal osteodystrophy
Osteitis pubis
Fibrous dysplasia
Hyperostosis frontalis interna
Aseptic necrosis
Osteoid osteoma
Melorrheostosis
D. Abnormal regional decrease in activity:
Radiation suppression

*Adapted from O'Mara and Baker, 1973.

their total series of 160 patients, 81 had abnormal scans. A definite need still exists, however, for a prospective study outlining the limitations and advantages of scanning techniques in patients with a variety of primary malignant diseases.

It is important to emphasize that an area of increased activity on a scan does not necessarily depict tumor cells. A wide variety of normal variants and benign diseases will result in positive bone scans with this sensitive, but hardly specific, procedure. A summary of such conditions is presented in Table 3.

More will be said later concerning the use of secondary scanning agents to circumvent some of the confusing findings in patients who may have either benign or malignant disease.

PRIMARY MALIGNANT DISEASES

Bone scanning techniques will frequently show that the extent of bony involvement is far greater than originally suspected from routine radiographs. In addition, scanning techniques may be quite useful in demonstrating metastatic lesions elsewhere in the osseous system. An example of this is shown in Figure 4. Bone scanning is useful in depicting areas which offer greatest potential yield for biopsy purposes in the case of primary osseous neoplasm as well as in metastatic disease. These techniques also are useful for establishing radiotherapy portals.

In addition, in patients suffering from primary osteosarcoma of bone, scanning techniques with bone-seeking radionuclides such as ^{85}Sr and ^{18}F will occasionally demonstrate soft-tissue metastatic deposits (O'Mara, Brettner, Danigelis, and Gould, 1971; Samuels, 1968; Woodbury and Beierwaltes, 1967). At times, these lesions may not be evident by clinical or radiographic examination. Such information of spread of the original lesion is of great value in planning therapy for these patients.

NONSPECIFICITY

As noted before, the bone scan is a highly sensitive but totally nonspecific procedure. Frequently, patients in whom a search for metastatic disease is being carried out will harbor benign lesions. At present, many centers are placing emphasis on finding agents which will be tumor-specific in the detection of skeletal lesions. Currently used so-called "tumor scanning agents," such as ^{67}Ga-citrate and ^{111}In bleomycin, have proven fruitless in this type of effort since these ra-

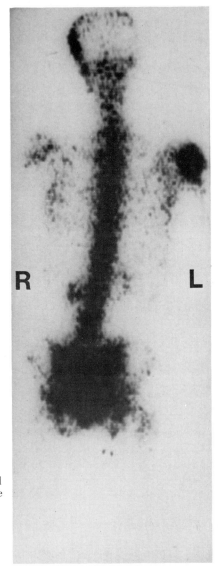

FIG. 4.—Posterior scan in a 14-year-old girl suffering from Ewing's sarcoma of the left hip demonstrates unsuspected metastatic deposits in the left humerus and skull.

diopharmaceuticals will give positive uptake in benign conditions such as fracture, infection, and the arthritides.

Cavalieri and Scott (1968) initially reported on the use of sodium selenite labeled with ^{75}Se to allow differentiation between malignant and benign osseous disease. In our experience to date, we have not had as much success as the original reporters, but nonetheless we believe this is the best agent available when the question of benign-versus-malignant cause arises concerning a lesion demonstrated by scanning techniques (O'Mara and Hall, unpublished data). If a repeat scan performed with selenite is positive, one can be assured of a neoplastic nature to the underlying disease process. However, if the scan is normal or negative, neoplasm cannot be excluded. One of the major reasons for this is in the handling of selenite, which oxidizes quite readily to sodium selenate. Tumor localization of this compound is quite poor. At present, I believe this represents the best secondary scanning agent available when this bothersome question is raised.

Summary

Bone scanning techniques are a sensitive, although nonspecific, method of detecting neoplastic involvement of the skeletal system. This procedure has been shown to be superior to evaluation via clinical symptomatology, alkaline phosphatase levels, and skeletal radiographs in the detection of early or occult metastatic lesions. Positive areas identified by scanning techniques should be correlated with radiographic changes because of the nonspecific nature of the scan. Besides assisting in the detection of neoplastic involvement, scanning techniques are useful in the evaluation of therapeutic regimens and in delineating areas for biopsy purposes.

Acknowledgment

This work has been supported in part by Grant No. CI-10 from the American Cancer Society.

REFERENCES

Abrams, H. L., Spiro, R., and Goldstein, N.: Metastases in carcinoma: Analysis of 1000 autopsied cases. *Cancer*, 3:74–85, January 1950.

Bachman, A. L., and Sproul, E. E.: Correlation of radiographic and autopsy findings in suspected metastases in the spine. *Bulletin of the New York Academy of Medicine*, 31:146–148, 1955.

Bauer, G. C. H., and Wendeberg, B.: External counting of ^{47}Ca and ^{85}Sr in studies of localised skeletal lesions in man. *Journal of Bone and Joint Surgery*, 41B: 558–580, August 1959.

Borak, J.: Relationship between the clinical and roentgenological findings in bone metastases. *Surgery, Gynecology and Obstetrics*, 75:599–604, November 1942.

Cavalieri, R. R., and Scott, K. G.: Sodium selenite ^{75}Se. A more specific agent for scanning tumors. *The Journal of the American Medical Association*, 206:591–595, October 14, 1968.

DeNardo, G. L., and Volpe, J. A.: Detection of bone lesions with the Strontium-85 scintiscan, *Journal of Nuclear Medicine*, 7:219–236, March 1966a.

_____: The [85]Sr scintiscan in bone disease. *Annals of Internal Medicine*, 65:44–53, July 1966b.

Edelstyn, G. A. Gillespie, P. J., and Grebbell, F. S.: The radiological demonstration of osseous metastasis: Experimental observations. *Clinical Radiology*, 18:158–162, April 1967.

Greenberg, E. J., Weber, D. A., Pochaczevsky, R., Kenny, P. J., Myers, W. P. L., and Laughlin, J. S.: Detection of neoplastic bone lesions by quantitative scanning and radiography. *Journal of Nuclear Medicine*, 9:613–620, December 1968.

Harmer, C. L., Burns, J. E., Sams, A., and Spittle, M.: The value of [18]Fluorine for scanning bone tumours. *Clinical Radiology*, 20:204–212, April 1969.

Jaffe, H. L.: Tumors metastatic to skeleton. In Jaffe, H. L., Ed.: *Tumors and Tumorous Conditions of the Bone and Joints*. 1st edition. Philadelphia, Pennsylvania, Lea and Febiger, 1958, pp. 589–617.

Legge, D. A., Tauxe, W. N., Pugh, D. G., and Utz, D. C.: Radioisotope scanning of metastatic lesions of bone. *Mayo Clinic Proceedings*, 45:755–761, November–December 1970.

O'Mara, R. E.: Unpublished data.

O'Mara, R. E., and Baker, V. H.: The use of radiography and radionuclides in metastatic skeletal disease. *Applied Radiology*, 2:17–20, 1973.

O'Mara, R. E., Brettner, A., Danigelis, J. A., and Gould, L. V.: [18]F uptake within metastatic osteosarcoma of the liver. *Radiology*, 100:113–114, July 1971.

O'Mara, R. E., and Hall, J. N.: Unpublished data.

Samuels, L. D.: Lung scanning with [87m]Sr in metastatic osteosarcoma. *The American Journal of Roentgenology, Radium Therapy and Nuclear Medicine*, 104:766–769, December, 1968.

Sauerbrunn, B. J. L., Hansen, H., and Napoli, L.: Strontium bone scans in carcinoma of the lung, a comparative prospective study. (Abstract) *Journal of Nuclear Medicine*, 13:465–466, June 1972.

Sharma, S. M., and Quinn, J. L.: Sensitivity of ^{18}F bone scans in the search for metastases. *Surgery, Gynecology and Obstetrics*, 135:536–540, October 1972.

Shirazi, S. P. H., Rayudu, G. V. S., and Fordham, E. W.: Review of solitary ^{18}F bone scan lesions. (Abstract) Presented at Radiological Society of North America Meeting, Chicago, Illinois, 1972. (In press.)

Silberstein, E. B., Saenger, E. L., Tofe, A. J., Alexander, G. W., and Park, H.: Imaging of bone metastases with ^{99m}Tc-Sn-EHDP (Diphosphonate), ^{18}F, and skeletal radiography. *Radiology*, 107:551–555, June 1973.

Sklaroff, D. M., and Charkes, N. D.: Diagnosis of bone metastasis by photoscanning with [85]Strontium. *The Journal of the American Medical Association*, 188:1–4, April 6, 1964.

_____: Bone metastases from breast cancer at the time of radical mastectomy. *Surgery, Gynecology and Obstetrics*, 127:763–768, October 1968.

Spencer, R., Herbert, R., Rish, M. W., and Little, W. A.: Bone scanning with

[85]Sr, [87m]Sr and [18]F. *British Journal of Radiology*, 40:641–654, September 1967.

Subramanian, G., McAfee, J. G., Bell, E. G., Blair, R., O'Mara, R. E., and Ralston, P.: ^{99m}Tc-labelled polyphosphate as a skeletal imaging agent. *Radiology*, 102:701–704, March, 1972.

Subramanian, G. McAfee, J. G., O'Mara, R. E., Rosenstreick, M., and Mehter, A.: [99m]Tc polyphosphate pp 46; A new radiopharmaceutical for skeletal imaging. (Abstract) *Journal of Nuclear Medicine* 12:399–400, June 1971.

Willis, R. A.: Metastasis. In Willis, R. A., Ed.: *Pathology of Tumors*. 4th edition. London, England, Butterworth and Company, Ltd., 1967, pp. 163–190.

Woodbury, D. H., and Beierwaltes. W. H.: Fluorine-18 uptake and localization in soft tissue deposits of osteogenic sarcoma in rat and man. *Journal of Nuclear Medicine*, 8:646–651, September 1967.

Yano, Y., McRae, J., VanDyke, D. C., and Anger, H. O.: ^{99m}Tc-labelled tin (11)-diphosphonate: A bone scanning agent. (Abstract) *Journal of Nuclear Medicine*, 13:480–481, June 1972.

Thermography in Malignant Diseases of the Bone

JOHN DOYLE WALLACE, B.A.

Department of Radiology, Thomas Jefferson University,
Philadelphia, Pennsylvania

AS IS THE CASE with every new technique, thermography has been tried in a myriad of clinical situations by the enterprising investigator. Some of these trials have met with success, some have produced equivocal results, and some were downright failures. However, it is only by such a process that any new technique finds its rightful place, if a place at all, in the armory of clinical medicine.

That the early detection of bone tumors is of prime importance to prognosis is axiomatic. Once the detection is accomplished, the differential diagnosis also has a great influence on the subsequent course of the disease. In the instance of bone lesions, radiologic procedures are probably the technique of choice in the initial diagnosis; this is not to suggest that the techniques of nuclear medicine do not have an important role to play in bringing about a differential diagnosis.

The development of the use of thermography in the detection of breast lesions has led, not unreasonably, to the investigation of its capabilities in detecting bone lesions. Lawson (1956) based his original work on the premise that in malignant processes, there was "accelerated local metabolism which could be detected by estimating the change in temperature caused by the tumor in its immediate environment." This premise would seem, at first glance, to apply to bone lesions.

The initial or first reported use of thermography in the investigation of a bone lesion seems to be the citing of a single case by Gershon-Cohen and Haberman (1964). They published a thermogram of the left shoulder of a 55-year-old male who had had a subtotal thyroidectomy for "cancer" 3 years previously. The left shoulder area was obviously hot, and the X-ray examination done at the same time suggested "metastatic thyroid cancer of the scapula and left fifth rib." Three months later, after a course of ^{131}I therapy, thermography was repeated and there was a substantial reduction in the elevated temperature of the shoulder. These researchers reported again in 1965 on single case of metastatic carcinoma of the lumbar vertebrae from a primary tumor of the prostate (Gershon-Cohen and Haberman, 1965). There was a diffuse area of excessive heat centered over the lumbar spine, where the abnormal temperature elevation was about 2°C. Two years later, single examples of vertebral metastatic disease from thyroid and pancreatic primaries were published (Gros, Keiling, and Vrousos, 1967). The following year brought the last of the publications citing single examples—a lumbar spine metastasis from a primary breast tumor (Farrell, Mansfield, and Wallace, 1968).

Osteosarcoma

A study of 19 patients with osteosarcoma was reported in 1968 by Farrell, Wallace, and Edeiken. Their interest stemmed from a thermographic study of the breasts of a 23-year-old female who complained of a "warm feeling" in her left breast. While the thermogram (Fig. 1) detected an abnormally hot vein in the left breast, it also showed a bizzare pattern of abnormal heat from the left arm. The subsequent radiograph suggested osteosarcoma. In following cases, we found that the thermographic pattern caused by the primary tumor was so striking that it was easily recognizable in all 14 patients who retained their primary lesions at the initial examination. The patterns were of 2 basic types: (1) hot areas over the diseased member and (2) venous signs which radiated from the hot areas. Figure 2 is a lateral thermogram of the knee which demonstrates the abnormally hot area over the involved member. The small warm areas over the proximal femur may have been the result of so-called "skip areas." Figure 3 is a clear example of venous signs in conjunction with the primary hot area. This 17-year-old female presented with pain in the left knee of 5 weeks duration following minor trauma. A recent paper reported in part on a series of 9 patients with primary osteosar-

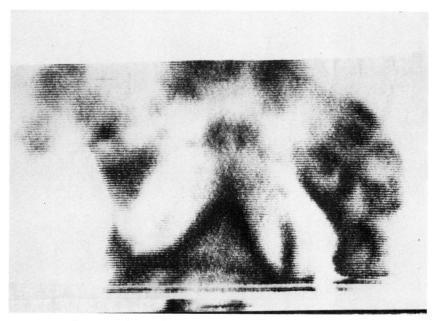

FIG. 1.—Thermographic study of a 23-year-old female with a subsequent diagnosis of osteosarcoma of the left humerus.

coma (Zweymuller and Strassl, 1973). The researchers found the thermograms "uniformly positive" in all 9 cases. Figure 4 is an example from their series, in this instance an osteosarcoma of the proximal tibia. It is of interest that Zweymuller and Strassl found in 2 cases of periosteal osteosarcoma and 1 case of osteosarcoma of the talus that the angiograms showed vessel displacement but there was no dye in either the tumor or the pathologic vessels.

With the exception of the 3 cases cited by Zweymuller and Strassl, there has been no indication that thermography can be relied upon for early detection; there has not been sufficient experience in this area. What may prove to be of clinical importance was the suggestion made by Farrell and associates (1968) that a thermographic finding of radiating veins may be an "ominous prognostic sign." They found that the presence of the venous sign in several patients was shortly thereafter followed by the discovery of pulmonary metastases.

Because of the few cases reported, there is little point, at this stage, in trying to derive any performance characteristics. Suffice it to state that primary osteosarcomas produce readily readable thermographic signs.

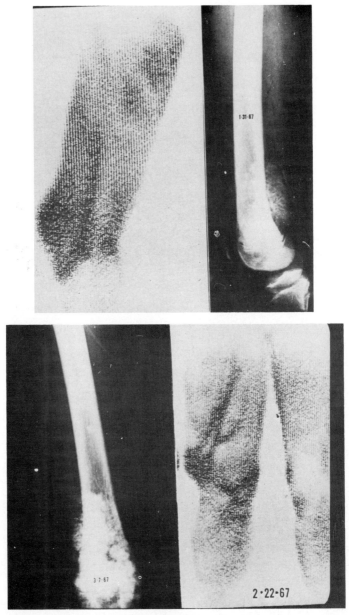

FIG. 2 *(top).*—Lateral thermogram of knee of patient with osteosarcoma.
FIG. 3 *(bottom).*—AP thermogram of legs of 17-year-old female with osteosarcoma.

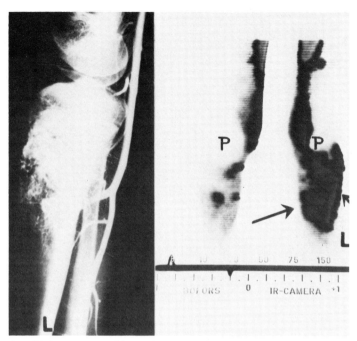

FIG. 4.—AP thermogram of legs of patient with osteosarcoma. (Courtesy of Zwey-muller and Strassl, 1973.)

Metastatic Disease

A second area of clinical interest where the use of thermography has been investigated is in detecting the presence of metastatic disease. The literature contains the reports on 3 series of patients who have been subjected to thermography.

The first report was of a total-body thermographic study of 126 patients with known carcinoma of the breast (Farrell, Wallace, and Mansfield, 1971). The thermographic findings were compared with the medical and radiation therapy records, roentgenograms, nuclear medicine studies, and pathological findings. While no breakdown was given to permit segregation of the bone involvements, a number of the findings pertained to metastatic bone disease. The authors reported that 87 per cent of the blind-read thermographic findings for the presence or absence of metastatic disease were confirmed, 10 per cent of the findings were falsely suspicious at the time of the examination, and 3 per cent of the findings were negative in the presence of positive findings by the other modalities. Of the 72 instances of initial readings classified as false-positive, 7 findings were confirmed as positive in 3 to 6 months, based on roentgen studies.

The second report included 20 patients with primary bone tumors, 95 patients with primary tumors of the breast, and 6 patients with other primary tumors (Nicholson, Rogers, and Tosh, 1971). In the thermography study of the 121 patients, the results were judged to be false-negative in 5 instances (4 per cent) and seemingly false-positive in 15 instances (12 per cent).

A third study consisted of 80 patients with confirmed cancer who had 110 bone involvements (Amalric, Spitalier, Seigle, and Altschuler, 1972). In the 90 instances of metastatic disease as confirmed by radiological or clinical examination, 76 (85 per cent) of the cases were thermographically suspicious. The 14 metastatic sites missed included 2 metastases from primary tumors of the prostate which previously had been treated with estrogens. It is of interest that these researchers cited 13 cases in which the thermography was suspicious and the standard roentgen films were inconclusive. In these

FIG. 5 *(left).*—Lumbar spinal thermogram of premenopausal female with confirmed carcinoma of the breast.

FIG. 6 *(right).*—Lumbar spinal thermogram of postmenopausal female with confirmed carcinoma of the breast.

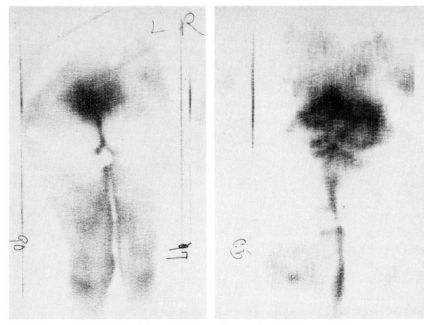

instances, the presence of bone metastases was finally confirmed by tomography.

Figures 5 and 6 are anteroposterior (AP) thermograms of the lumbar spinal areas of a premenopausal and a postmenopausal female with confirmed cancer of the breast. The principal complaint of both patients was low back pain. Figure 7 is again the (AP) view of a pa-

FIG. 7 *(top).* — Thermography (isothermal) of lumbar spine of patient with low back pain and carcinoma of the breast. (Courtesy of Amalric, Spitalier, Seigle, and Altschuler, 1972.)

FIG. 8 *(bottom).* — Thermogram (isothermal) of patient with metastatic disease of right humerus from a bronchial primary tumor. (Courtesy of Amalric, Spitalier, Seigle, and Altschuler, 1972.)

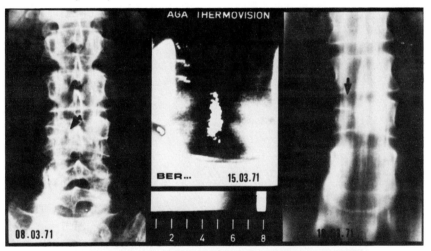

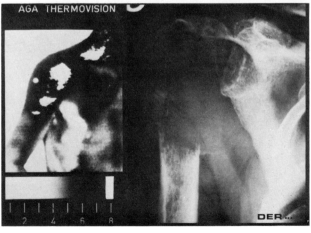

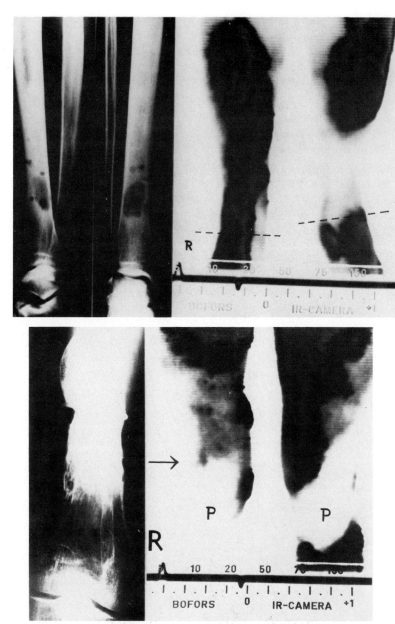

FIG. 9 *(top).*—Thermogram of 26-year-old male with acute osteomyelitis of right distal tibia. (Courtesy of Zweymuller and Strassl, 1973.)

FIG. 10 *(bottom).*—Thermogram of 25-year-old male with chronic osteitis. (Courtesy of Zweymuller and Strassl, 1973.)

tient with low back pain and a primary breast tumor which had been treated for the previous 5 years. The thermography technique used was that of isothermals. The white pattern over the lumbar spine is the isothermal area at the high temperature range of the thermographic thermal window. Tomography of the spine confirmed a metastatic lesion at L-3.

Amalric and his associates (Amalric, Spitalier, Seigle, and Altschuler, 1972) also demonstrated a case of bronchial carcinoma with a right humeral metastasis (Fig. 8).

Benign Lesions

Implied in the achievement of a differential diagnosis is a recognizably different characteristic of the benign lesion as compared with the malignant one. Zweymuller and Strassl (1973) sought to learn whether it was possible to make differential diagnoses based upon thermography alone. While, as stated previously, they found obviously positive thermograms in all the osteosarcoma cases, for instance, they also made a similar finding in all of the 5 instances of acute osteomyelitis (Fig. 9). Conversely, chronic osteitis cases resulted in thermograms which had little or no excess abnormal heat (Fig. 10). It was their conclusion, based on the few cases in their study, that differential diagnosis based upon thermography alone was not possible in the case of bone problems.

Summary

There is no doubt that malignant lesions of the bone, in a high percentage of the cases, produce highly abnormal thermograms. Some investigators have suggested an early detection capability, but experience is extremely limited both in numbers and pathology.

As has been the experience with other primary tumors, thermography has little or no differential diagnosis capability.

REFERENCES

Amalric, R., Spitalier, J. M., Seigle, J., and Altschuler, C.: Diagnostic precoce des metastases osseuses et thermovision. *Corse Mediterranee Medicale*, 216:32–35, 1972.
Farrell, C. B., Mansfield, C. M., and Wallace, J. D.: Thermography as an investigative method. *Pennsylvania Medicine*, 71:38–40, December 1968.
Farrell, C. B., Wallace, J. D., and Edeiken, J.: Thermography in osteosarcoma. *Radiology*, 90:792–793, April 1968.

Farrell, C. B., Wallace, J. D., and Mansfield, C. M.: The use of thermography in detection of metastatic breast cancer. *The American Journal of Roentgenology, Radium Therapy and Nuclear Medicine*, 111:148–152, January 1971.

Gershon-Cohen, J., and Haberman, J. D.: Thermography. *Radiology*, 82: 280–285, February 1964.

_____: Medical thermography. *The American Journal of Roentgenology, Radium Therapy and Nuclear Medicine*, 94:735–740, July 1965.

Gros, C., Keiling, R., and Vrousos, C.: Apport de la thermographie dans le diagnostic de localization et d'extension dans les affections malignes. *Journal de Radiologie*, 48:89–92, January–February 1967.

Lawson, R. N.: Implications of surface temperatures in the diagnosis of breast cancer. *Canadian Medical Association Journal*, 75:309–310, August 15, 1956.

Nicholson, J. P., Rogers, R. T., and Tosh, D. C.: The relative merits of thermoscanning and gamma scanning in the detection of metastatic bone disease. *British Journal of Radiology*, 44:898, November 1971.

Zweymuller, K., and Strassl, R.: Erfahrungen mit der Thermographie bei Knochentumoren. *Zeitschrift fur Orthopaedie und ihre Grenzgebiete*, 111: 41–47, 1973.

Skeletal Complications of Radiation Therapy

THOMAS S. HARLE, M.D.,* and
J. BARNETT FINKELSTEIN, M.D.†
*Department of Radiology, *The University of Texas
Medical School at Houston, and †Department of
Diagnostic Radiology, The University of Texas System
Cancer Center M. D. Anderson Hospital and Tumor
Institute, Houston, Texas

WHILE THE COMPLICATIONS of radiation therapy are few compared to the benefits, skeletal abnormalities following irradiation have been documented for many decades (Ewing, 1926).

Pathophysiology

Radiation produces a variety of osseous abnormalities, although the pathologic features are more consistent (Dalinka, Edeiken, and Finkelstein, in press). Radiation may cause immediate or delayed cell death, arrest of cellular division, vascular disturbances, injury with recovery, abnormal repair, and neoplasia (Vaughan, 1968; Pappas, 1969).

Similar skeletal changes occur whether the inciting radiation is in the form of alpha, beta, gamma, or roentgen rays (Rubin, Andrews, Swarm, and Gump, 1959; Rubin, Duthie, and Young, 1962; Frantz, 1950; Fabrikant and Smith, 1964; Arkin, Pack, Ranshoff, and Simon, 1950; Arkin and Simon, 1950; Barr, Lingley, and Gall, 1943; Engel, 1939; Hinkel, 1943).

The primary factors determining skeletal sequelae following radiation therapy concern the intensity of radiation, the area exposed, and the age of the patient (Rutherford and Dodd, in press; Rubin, Andrews, Swarm, and Gump, 1959; Neuhauser, Wittenborg, Berman, and Cohen, 1952; Vaeth, Levitt, Jones, and Holtfreter, 1962; Whitehouse and Lampe, 1953). Resultant disorders may be categorized as developmental abnormalities, osteroradionecrosis, and neoplasia.

Developmental Abnormalities

Rubin and co-workers demonstrated the effects of radiation on the 3 divisions of a growing tubular bone (Rubin, Andrews, Swarm, and Gump, 1959). Irradiation of these zones produces the following: (a) epiphysis, arrest of chondrogenesis and therefore growth; (b) metaphysis, failure of absorptive processes of calcified cartilage and bone; and (c) diaphysis, alterations in periosteal activity which result in modeling errors.

Since the most common indication for radiation therapy in chil-

FIG. 1.—*A, B*, growth arrest lines as well as demineralization and flattening are seen in the lumbar vertebral bodies of a 7-year-old girl who received radiation therapy at 5 weeks of age for Wilms' tumor. The left ilium is hypoplastic.

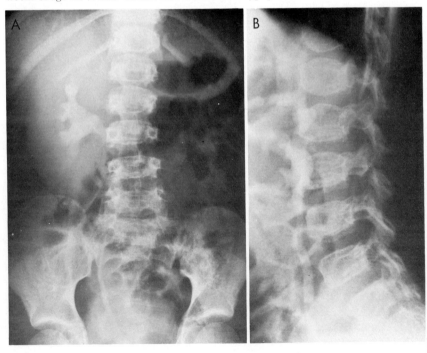

dren is an abdominal tumor, the most common skeletal sequelae involve the lumbar spine, adjacent ribs, and pelvis. The sequelae usually involve alterations of normal growth resulting in hypoplasia. Experimental and clinical studies document the effect of radiation on the growing spine (Neuhauser, Wittenborg, Berman, and Cohen, 1952; Arkin, Pack, Ranshoff, and Simon, 1950; Arkin and Simon, 1950). Initial changes in the vertebral body usually occur 9 to 12 months following irradiation and consist of subcortical lucent zones

FIG. 2.—A, B, notable flattening of multiple vertebral bodies and anterior central beaking of T10–12 is present in a 13-year-old child who received radiation of Wilms' tumor at age 16 months. C, D, associated hypoplasia of the lower portion of the right hemithorax and right ilium.

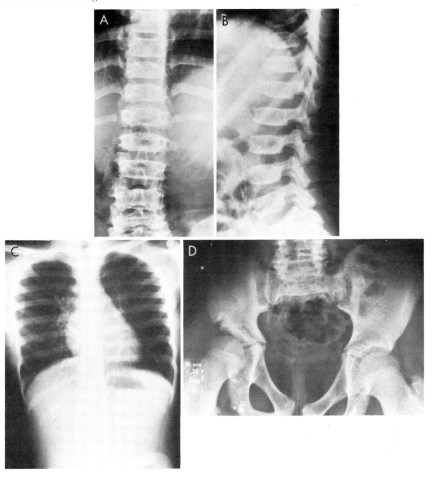

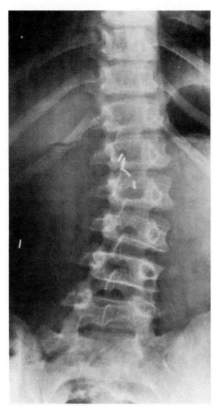

FIG. 3 *(left)*.—Rotoscoliosis in an 11-year-old child, 7 years after surgery and radiation therapy for Wilms' tumor of the right kidney. Note the hypoplasia of the right side of the vertebral bodies and posterior elements of L1–3.

FIG. 4 *(below)*.—Hypoplasia of the right orbit and maxillary sinus in a 13-year-old girl 10 years following enucleation of the right eye and radiation therapy for retinoblastoma.

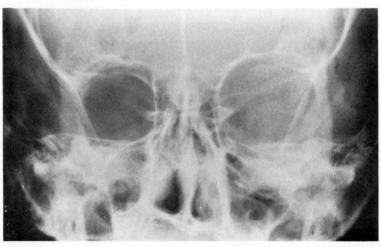

which progress to growth arrest lines that parallel the epiphyses (Rutherford and Dodd, in press) (Fig. 1). It is believed that 1,000 to 2,000 rads are necessary to produce this change. Katzman, Waugh, and Berdon (1969) noted that vertebral bodies have a more bulbous contour in the early period following irradiation. Gross irregularity or scalloping of vertebral epiphyseal plates occurs only in the field of irradiation and requires exposures of 2,000 to 3,000 rads. Vertebral bodies with central beaking, resembling those found in osteochondrodystrophy, require 2,500 rads or more and result in a greater retardation of axial growth (Fig. 2, *A* and *B*). Asymmetrical distribution of radiation to the spine decreases growth on the irradiated side producing scoliosis (Fig. 3). Both lateral flexion curve with concavity on the treated side and rotary scoliosis may be present as a result of changes not only in the vertebral bodies but also in the laminae and pedicles (Greenfield, 1969). Scoliosis is usually of moderate degree and increases minimally with growth (Katzman, Waugh, and Berdon, 1969; Neuhauser, Wittenborg, Berman, and Cohen, 1952). Narrowing of the interpedicular distance, similar to that found in achondroplasia, has been observed (Rubin, Duthie, and Young, 1962).

Since treatment portals for abdominal masses in children often include the lower ribs and upper pelvis, hypoplasia of these structures occurs (Fig. 2, *C* and *D*). Hypoplasia of the orbit, associated with varying degrees of growth arrest of the adjacent maxilla, nasal bones, and temporal bones, may develop following therapy for occular lesions (Fig. 4).

Radiation of an entire tubular bone results in cessation of growth within a few days (Rubin, Andrews, Swarm, and Gump, 1959). These bones are overtubulated and fragile. When radiation is restricted to the epiphysis, tubulation is normal but metaphyseal flaring occurs, with dwarfing similar to that in the hypoplastic form of achondropla-

FIG. 5.—Film made 6 years after radiation therapy for a neurofibrosarcoma of the soft tissues of the forearm in a 9-year-old girl. There is thinning of the radius and ulna, bowing of the radius, and shortening of the ulna with distal dislocation.

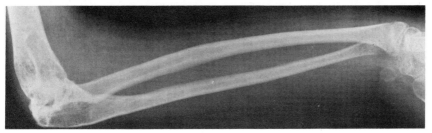

sia. Decrease in length and bowing result from metaphyseal irradiation primarily as a result of a failure of absorptive processes of calcified cartilage and bone. Diaphyseal irradiation results in narrowing of the shaft caused by interference with periosteal new bone formation. Clinically, the degree of shortening, bowing, or deformity is related to the intensity and distribution of the radiation (Fig. 5).

Osteoradionecrosis

Necrosis of bone results primarily from the direct effect of radiation on osteocytes with vascular changes aggravating and prolonging the radiation effects (Pappas, 1969). Unopposed osteoclastic activity leads to demineralization and osteoporosis. Notable thickening of the walls of arteries and arterials follows radiation, while veins and capillaries are unaffected. Cutright and Brady (1971) demonstrated that with exposures above 4,000 roentgens, approximately 70 per cent of the vasculature is destroyed while the other 30 per cent remains up

FIG. 6.—*A*, film of a gold grain implant for recurrent pelvic mass in a 34-year-old woman who was treated initially 5 years ago with external radiation and radium for carcinoma of the cervix (Stage II). *B*, 10 years later, extensive destructive changes are present about the right hip, with a pathologic fracture. Changes are consistent with osteoradionecrosis.

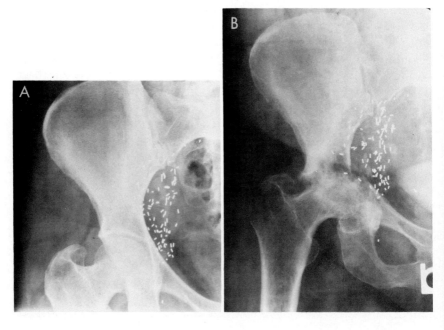

to 10,000 roentgens. There was no recovery of vascular damage, which they believe supports the impression that irradiated bone is irreparably damaged.

The following conditions predispose to the development of radiation osteitis: (a) superficial position of bone, (b) presence of infection in or around the bone, (c) high intensity of radiation, and (d) poor blood supply (Schuknecht and Karmody, 1966).

Common sites of involvement are the mandible, chest wall, shoulder girdle, pelvis, and hips. The roentgenographic appearance of radionecrosis is well described by Dalinka and Bragg and their co-workers (Dalinka, Edeiken, and Finkelstein, in press; Bragg, Shindinia, Chu, and Higinbotham, 1970). Demineralization is the most frequent radiographic finding. The trabecular pattern is coarsened and

FIG. 7.—Film of a 66-year-old woman who was treated with x-ray therapy and radium applications for carcinoma of the cervix 7 years previously. Note the sclerotic areas in the ilia and sacrum similar to those of osteitis condensans ilii. A pathological fracture has occurred in the right femoral neck secondary to osteonecrosis. No tumor is present.

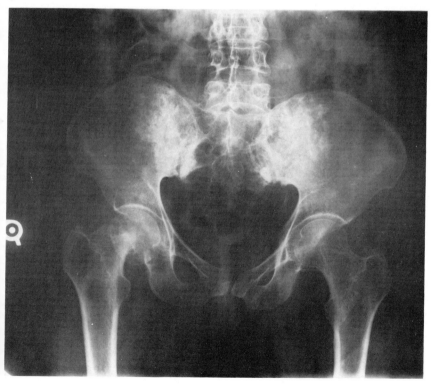

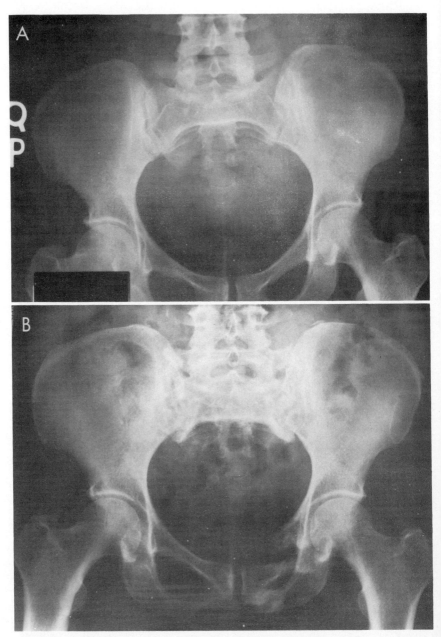

FIG. 8.—Film of a 55-year-old woman treated with 1 intrauterine radium application and supervoltage external beam therapy for Stage IIIA carcinoma of the cervix: *A*, normal-appearing pelvis at time of treatment. *B*, sclerotic sacrum and sacroiliac joints as well as pathological fractures of left pubis 5 years after therapy.

disorganized with a "Pagetoid appearance." Ill-defined areas of destruction may be present, often with a loss of cortical bone (Fig. 6). In most bones, there is no associated sclerosis, although within the pelvis changes resembling osteitis condensans ilii may be seen (Fig. 7). The sacroiliac joints may be widened, irregular, and sclerotic (Fig. 8). Pathological fractures occur and while these may heal, they do so more slowly than normal. The appearance of the osteonecrosis is determined, in part, by the status of the involved area. If the structure already is demineralized from the disuse osteoporosis, the additional necrotic changes may cause complete loss of radiodensity simulating neoplasia.

Superimposed infection which frequently is present may result in rapid progression of the previously described osseous changes. This probably is the result of lack of the normal defense mechanisms of bone. Sequestrum formation is rare.

Neoplasia

Tumors developing within the treatment field are more often malignant than benign (Rutherford and Dodd, in press). Benign exostoses have been reported developing in long bones and in flat bones such as ribs, ilium, scapula, and clavicle, as well as in the spine (Rutherford and Dodd, in press; Katzman, Waugh, and Berdon, 1969; Neuhauser, Wittenborg, Berman, and Cohen, 1952; Simpson and Hempelmann, 1957; Murphy and Blount, 1962). Radiation-induced sarcoma most frequently occurs following treatment of a benign osseous lesion, but also has been noted following successful therapy for a malignant tumor or in previously normal bone included in the treatment field of an unrelated problem (Finkelstein, 1970; Arlen *et al.*, 1971; Sagerman, Cassady, Tretter, and Ellsworth, 1969; Forrest, 1961). Cahan's criteria for classification of radiation-induced sarcomas stipulate that: (a) the original condition must be microscopically or roentgenographically normal or nonmalignant, (b) sarcomas must arise within portals of irradiation, (c) a long, asymptomatic, latent period must exist before sarcoma appears, and (d) all sarcomas must be histologically proven (Cahan *et al.*, 1948). Complaints of pain or swelling within the irradiated area in a patient who has received treatment several years previously should alert the physician to the possible diagnosis of radiation-induced sarcoma (Figs. 9 and 10). Osteosarcoma and fibrosarcoma are the most common cellular types, with chondrosarcoma occurring less often. Although as little as 1,200

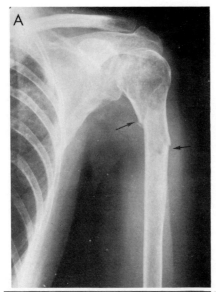

FIG. 9.—*A*, pathological fracture in a 58-year-old woman 6 years after radiation therapy for carcinoma of the breast. *B*, ununited fractures with increased demineralization of the humerus and scapula. *C*, the patient continued to have pain which prompted amputation of her arm. Undifferentiated sarcoma involving bone and soft tissues was present.

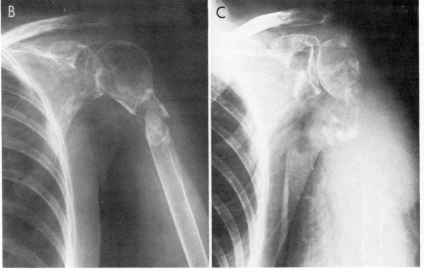

rads in 2 weeks has resulted in sarcomatous change, usually the higher the exposure the greater the incidence of malignant change (Arlen *et al.*, 1971; Rutherford and Dodd, in press).

The following points help to differentiate radiation-induced sar-

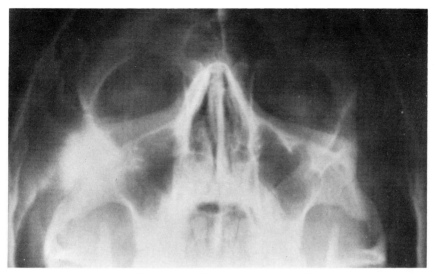

FIG. 10.—Osteosarcoma below the right orbit in a 14-year-old girl who was irradiated at age 6 months for retinoblastoma.

coma from radiation osteitis: (a) development of pain, (b) presence of a mass, (c) change in the radiographic appearance after a previously stable latent period of up to 5 years, and (d) identification of mineralized tumor matrix within soft tissues.

Comment

In general, the younger the patient, the higher the radiation exposure, and the higher the growth potential of the bone, the greater the probability and extent of skeletal damage (Rutherford and Dodd, in press; Berdon, Baker, and Boyer, 1965). Whenever possible, epiphyses of rapidly growing bone should be protected or excluded from the treatment field. With symmetrical epiphyses, unilateral deformities are prevented most effectively by utilization of a uniform exposure of the epiphyses. Skeletal abnormalities continue to occur even in the age of supervoltage therapy.

Fortunately, few patients require orthopedic or other methods of treatment for abnormalities or disabilities following radiation therapy. The cure or control of malignant disease by radiation therapy outweighs the undesirable side effects that occasionally occur.

REFERENCES

Arkin, A. M., Pack, G. T., Ranshoff, N. S., and Simon, N.: Radiation-induced scoliosis, a case report. *The Journal of Bone and Joint Surgery*, 32 – A:401 – 404, April 1950.

Arkin, A. M., and Simon, N.: Radiation scoliosis: An experimental study. *The Journal of Bone and Joint Surgery*, 32-A:396 – 401, April 1950.

Arlen, M., Higinbotham, N. L., Huvos, A. G., Marcove, R. C., Miller, T., and Shah, I. C.: Radiation-induced sarcoma of bone. *Cancer*, 28:1087 – 1099, November 1971.

Barr, J. S., Lingley, J. R., and Gall, A. E.: The effect of roentgen irradiation on epiphyses growth. I. Experimental studies upon the albino rat. *The American Journal of Roentgenology, Radium Therapy and Nuclear Medicine*, 49: 104 – 115, January 1943.

Berdon, W. E., Baker, D. H., and Boyer, J.: Unusual benign and malignant sequelae to childhood radiation therapy. *The American Journal of Roentgenology, Radium Therapy and Nuclear Medicine*, 93:545 – 556, March 1965.

Bragg, D. G., Shindinia, H., Chu, F. C. H., and Higinbotham, N. L.: The clinical and radiographic aspects of radiation osteitis. *Radiology*, 97:103 – 111, October 1970.

Cahan, W. G., Woodard, H. Q., Higinbotham, N. L., Stewart, F. W., and Coley, B. L.: Sarcoma arising in irradiated bone, report of eleven cases. *Cancer*, 1:3 – 29, May 1948.

Cutright, D. E., and Brady, J. M.: Clinical long-term effects of radiation on the vascularity of rat bone-quantitative measurements with a new technique. *Radiation Research*, 48:402 – 408, November 1971.

Dalinka, M. K., Edeiken, J., and Finkelstein, J. B.: Radiation changes in bone. *Seminars in Radiology*. (In press.)

Engel, D.: Experiments on the production of spinal deformities by radium, part I. *The American Journal of Roentgenology, Radium Therapy and Nuclear Medicine*, 42:217 – 234, August 1939.

Ewing, J.: Radiation osteitis. *Acta Radiologica*, 6:399 – 412, 1926.

Fabrikant, J. I., and Smith, C. L. D.: Radiographic changes following the administration of bone seeking radionuclides. *British Journal of Radiology*, 37:53 – 62, January 1964.

Finkelstein, J. B.: Osteosarcoma of the jaw bones. *Radiologic Clinics of North America*, 8:425 – 443, December 1970.

Forrest, A. W.: Tumors following radiation about the eye. *Transactions of the American Academy of Ophthalmology and Otolaryngology*, 65:694 – 717 September – October 1961.

Frantz, C. H.: Extreme retardation of epiphyseal growth from roentgen irradiation, a case study. *Radiology*, 55:720 – 724, November 1950.

Greenfield, G. B.: *Radiology of Bone Diseases*. Philadelphia, Pennsylvania, J. B. Lippincott Company, 1969, 200 pp.

Hinkel, C. L.: The effect of roentgen rays upon the growing long bones of albino rats. II. Histological changes involving endochondral growth centers. *The American Journal of Roentgenology, Radium Therapy and Nuclear Medicine*, 49:321 – 348, March 1943.

Katzman, H., Waugh, T., and Berdon, W.: Skeletal changes following irradiation of childhood tumors. *The Journal of Bone and Joint Surgery*, 51-A: 825–842, July 1969.

Murphy, F. D., Jr., and Blount, W. P.: Cartilaginous exostoses following irradiation. *The Journal of Bone and Joint Surgery*, 44-A:662–668, June 1962.

Neuhauser, E. B. D., Wittenborg, M. H., Berman, C. Z., and Cohen, J.: Irradiation effects of roentgen therapy on the growing spine. *Radiology*, 59: 637–650, November 1952.

Pappas, G. C.: Bone changes in osteoradionecrosis. *Oral Surgery, Oral Medicine, and Oral Pathology*, 27:622–630, May 1969.

Rubin, P., Andrews, J. R., Swarm, R., and Gump, H.: Radiation induced dysplasias of bone. *The American Journal of Roentgenology, Radium Therapy and Nuclear Medicine*, 82:206–216, August 1959.

Rubin, P., Duthie, R. B., and Young, L. W.: The significance of scoliosis in post-irradiated Wilms' tumor and neuroblastoma. *Radiology*, 79:539–559, October 1962.

Rutherford, H., and Dodd, G. D.: Radiation injuries to the treated bone. *Seminars in Radiology*. (In press.)

Sagerman, P. H., Cassady, J. R., Tretter, R., and Ellsworth, R. M.: Radiation induced neoplasia following external beam therapy for children with retinoblastoma. *The American Journal of Roentgenology, Radium Therapy and Nuclear Medicine*, 105:529–535, March 1969.

Schuknecht, H. F., and Karmody, C. S.: Radionecrosis of the temporal bone. *Laryngoscope*, 76:1416–1428, August 1966.

Simpson, C. L., and Hempelmann, L. H.: The association of tumors and roentgen ray treatment of the thorax in infancy. *Cancer*, 10:42–56, January–February 1957.

Vaeth, J. M., Levitt, S. H., Jones, M. D., and Holtfreter, C.: Effects of radiation therapy in survivors of Wilms' tumor. *Radiology*, 79:560–568, October 1962.

Vaughan, J.: The effects of skeletal irradiation. *Clinical Orthopedics*, 56: 283–303, January–February 1968.

Whitehouse, W. M., and Lampe, I.: Osseous damage in irradiation of renal tumors in infancy and childhood. *The American Journal of Roentgenology, Radium Therapy and Nuclear Medicine*, 70:721–729, November 1953.

Pulmonary Angiography, Azygography, and Mediastinoscopy in the Diagnosis and Staging of Bronchogenic Carcinoma

CLIFTON F. MOUNTAIN, M.D., and
HECTOR MEDELLIN-LASTRA, M.D.
*Departments of Surgery and Diagnostic Radiology, The
University of Texas System Cancer Center M. D.
Anderson Hospital and Tumor Institute,
Houston, Texas*

SURVIVAL IN BRONCHOGENIC CARCINOMA is largely dependent upon the ability to successfully implement definitive surgical resection. There is ample evidence which indicates that objective assessment of mediastinal involvement, in lung cancer, is of crucial importance in judging resectability and in estimating prognosis. The question posed is: "What constitutes a reliable, valid, and rational method for such objective assessment?" Our personal experience with pulmonary arteriography and azygography, and our observations in more than 300 mediastinoscopies have convinced us of the independent value of such studies both in the diagnostic and the evaluative process. These conclusions are widely supported in a host of studies reported in the international literature (Ikeda, *et al.*, 1968; Bernardi, *et al.*, 1970; Petrikova, Polak, and Mottl, 1971; Sharov and Sumnaia, 1969; Willa, *et al.*, 1971; Delarue and Strasberg, 1966; Dux, Bucheler, and Sobbe, 1970). The most recent studies, by Delarue and his co-workers and by Greenough, reporting on the complementary value of mediastinoscopy and angiography have led us to examine our own experience in this regard (Delarue and Starr, 1967; Greenough, 1972). In reporting our results, we will comment briefly upon the techniques utilized and demonstrate several cases which typify various situations encountered where the studies were complementary to mediastinoscopy.

Pulmonary Angiography

Pulmonary angiography has been employed in evaluating patients suspected of having lung cancer since the late 1930's (Steinberg and Robb, 1938). Continuous refinement in techniques has improved its reliability and validity in indicating the relationship of lesions to major vessels and therefore its value in judging resectability. Malignant tumors of the lung or mediastinum are the most numerous causes of failure of the pulmonary artery to fill, and although this has been described as a cardinal sign of cancer, it is not specifically diagnostic. In the case of a patient with known bronchogenic cancer, this finding contributes significantly to the evaluative picture (Greenspan and Capps, 1963). While some investigators define a relationship between histologic type and the degree of bronchial vascularization of pulmonary tumors, the procedure does not give evidence as to the histologic pattern of disease, and therefore it must be regarded as evaluative rather than diagnostic per se (Ikeda, *et al.*, 1968). In a study by Steinberg and Finby (1959) of vascular changes revealed by angiocardiography in 250 patients with primary lung cancer, involvement of the superior vena cava system or the major pulmonary artery was present in 30 per cent of the cases. Although a high correlation between angiographic interpretation and operative findings has been reported, a normal angiogram does not exclude intrathoracic extension remote from the heart and great vessels. Therefore, the procedure does not replace the need for other examinations.

The procedure is performed routinely via basilic vein puncture and catheterization utilizing the Seldinger technique. For lesions of the right upper lobe, the right brachycephalic vein and superior vena cava are first visualized, and if the vena cava is normal, the pulmonary arteries are examined subsequently. The left brachycephalic vein is utilized for left-sided lesions with particular attention directed toward the innominate vein. Injection of the pulmonary artery trunk is preferred to selective bilateral injection in order to determine any differences in perfusion between the 2 lungs. These procedures are done under local anesthesia on an outpatient basis with continuous electrocardiographic monitoring. The attendant morbidity and mortality of the procedure are extremely low while the instances of critically important positive findings are relatively high. We now regard this procedure as routinely justified in the evaluation of all centrally placed lesions.

The information obtained from azygography is supplementary and distinct from that provided by other methods of study, but is clearly complementary to pulmonary arteriography. The abnormal azygogram has proved a reliable index of inoperability. In the evaluation of 86 cases of primary lung cancer at the University of Maryland Hospital, Wolfel and his co-workers report 4 false-negative and 1 false-positive azygograms among 35 surgical patients. In the nonsurgical group, 28 patients had an abnormal azygogram and all 28 had clinical and/or roentgenographic evidence of nonresectability (Wolfel, Lindberg, and Light, 1966). In a report of 63 cases of suspected lung cancer, Rinker found that in 14 cases, both examinations were abnormal. One patient had a false-positive examination of the azygos system. In 6 cases, only the azygogram was abnormal and in 4 cases, only the vena cava was involved (Rinker *et al.*, 1967). In a study of inoperable patients, Skinner reported 77 per cent to have a positive azygogram (Skinner, 1962).

Our criteria of inoperability by angiography include: (1) involvement of a main pulmonary artery within 1.5 centimeters of its origin for the left artery and from the triforcation for the right, (2) involvement of the main pulmonary veins at the pericardial reflection, (3) invasion or compromise of the innominate vein or superior vena cava, (4) clear-cut evidence of involvement in the azygos system, and (5) evidence indicating direct invasion of the heart. It should be noted here that our 1 case of false-positive angiography involved a highly suggestive compromise of the azygos system in the absence of any other index of nonresectability. In retrospect, it was felt that this resulted from a positive valsalva maneuver by the patient during examination. Every effort should be made to instruct the patient before examination so as to prevent this occurrence. If it is observed to occur, considerable weight should be given to this in the evaluation of the study.

Mediastinoscopy

Transcervical mediastinoscopy, introduced by Carlens in 1959, permits direct surgical exploration and biopsy of the middle and posterior portions of the superior mediastinum (Carlens, 1959; Carlens and Hambraeus, 1967). It is important to appreciate the anatomic relationships as they bear upon the extent of the examination (Mountain, 1970). The scope lies directly anterior to the trachea and beneath the pretracheal fascia. Because the instrument is posterior to the innominate artery and vein and to the arch of the aorta, the contents of the anterior mediastinum are not accessible. The procedure does, however, permit biopsy and examination of both peritracheal regions and the subcarinal space as well as the first 3 to 4 centimeters of each main stem bronchus. More than 4,500 cases now have been reported in the world literature, with a remarkably low index of morbidity and mortality (Ashbaugh, 1970). In our own experience, we have had no deaths and only 1 case of serious bleeding in over 300 procedures. Between 35 and 50 per cent of all patients with bronchogenic carcinoma will have evidence of mediastinal metastatic adenopathy or of direct mediastinal invasion depending upon cell type (Sarin and Nohl-Oser, 1969; Goldberg, Glicksman, Khan, and Nickson, 1970). We now routinely employ this procedure in all patients suspected of having lung cancer in which the question of diagnosis or resectability remains unsolved. Our specific contraindications to resection, based upon the findings at mediastinoscopy, are as follows: (1) any evidence of undifferentiated small cell (oat cell) carcinoma, (2) contralateral peritracheal lymph node involvement, (3) ipsilateral peritracheal lymph node involvement in the upper half of the intrathoracic trachea, (4) any evidence of direct tumor invasion of the mediastinal structures, and (5) any evidence of lymph node involvement with adenocarcinoma. We continue to resect the tumors of patients with squamous cell carcinoma and undifferentiated large cell carcinoma having nodal metastasis at the tracheobronchial angle or in the subcarinal space if there is no other evidence of inoperability. This is based on our recent observations that 14 per cent of patients with Stage III squamous cell carcinoma and 11 per cent of those with undifferentiated large cell carcinoma will survive more than 5 years following definitive resection under these circumstances.

Case Presentations

The following cases are illustrative of the types of defects encountered. In the first case, a left hilar mass is clearly demonstrated in the PA view of the chest, as shown in Figure 1A. The pulmonary arteriogram showed narrowing and deformity of the left pulmonary artery starting at its origin from the main trunk (Fig. 1B). The oblique view showed this to an even better extent (Fig. 1C). The azygogram dem-

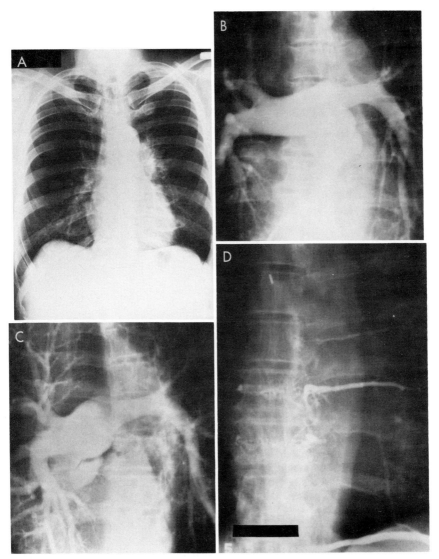

FIG. 1.—*A*, posterior-anterior view of chest demonstrating left hilar mass. *B*, pulmonary arteriogram demonstrating narrowing and deformity of the left pulmonary artery at its origin from the main trunk. *C*, oblique view of arteriogram clarifying extent of arterial involvement. *D*, azygogram demonstrating prominent intercostal veins draining into the hemiazygos system. There is notable irregularity of the azygos vein in its first portion and occlusion superiorly.

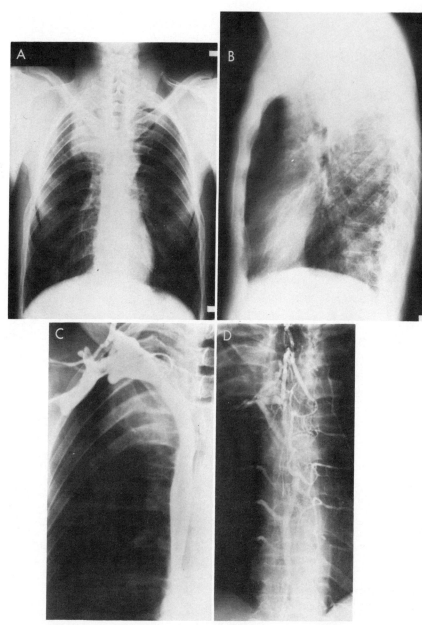

FIG. 2.—*A*, posterior-anterior view of chest demonstrating a right upper lobe mass. *B*, lateral view of chest showing posterior location of tumor. *C*, visualization of innominate vein and superior vena cava suggesting extrinsic compression of vena cava without invasion. *D*, azygogram demonstrating obstruction of the vein with filling of multiple collaterals.

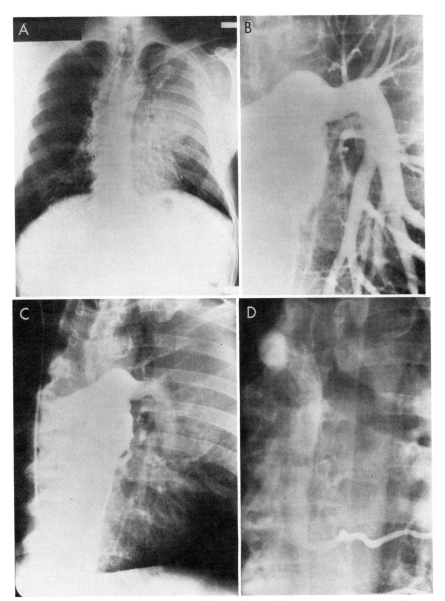

FIG. 3.—*A*, posterior-anterior view of chest showing large left hilar mass with complete atelectasis of the upper lobe and anterior herniation of the right lung. *B*, pulmonary arteriogram demonstrating narrowing of the left artery at its origin. *C*, oblique view confirming involvement. *D*, azygogram demonstrating normal vein.

onstrates prominent intercostal veins draining into the hemiazygos system. There is notable irregularity in the first portion of the azygos vein and then frank interruption superiorly (Fig. 1*D*). The patient had a negative sputum test for exfoliated cells, a negative bronchoscopy, and a negative mediastinoscopy. Exploratory thoracotomy was undertaken for diagnostic purposes, and nonresectability was confirmed.

The second case represents our 1 false-positive interpretation. On the PA and lateral views of the chest, a large right upper lobe lesion was seen posteriorly (Figs. 2*A* and *B*). Except for some extrinsic compression, the pulmonary arteriogram was judged normal as were the right innominate vein and superior vena cava (Fig. 2*C*). The azygogram was interpreted as showing obstruction with collateral vessels filling (Fig. 2*D*). All other examinations revealed no contraindication to resection. An exploratory thoracotomy was undertaken to confirm nonresectability. At exploration, the tumor was found to compress but not to invade the innominate vein and superior vena cava. It was adherent to the azygos vein, but it was possible to resect the lesion en bloc by pneumonectomy. Of 23 mediastinal lymph nodes examined, none contained metastasis.

In the third case, the chest films revealed a large left hilar mass with atelectasis of the complete left upper lobe and anterior herniation of the right lung (Fig. 3*A*). The pulmonary arteriogram revealed narrowing of the left pulmonary artery at its origin (Fig. 3*B*), and this was confirmed in subsequent views (Fig. 3*C*). The azygogram was negative, and again the mediastinoscopy was negative (Fig. 3*D*). Diagnosis was proven at bronchoscopy.

Results

All diagnostic and evaluative studies of 60 patients who had both mediastinoscopy and angiography were reviewed. The results are demonstrated in the table. In approximately 47 per cent of the cases, no evidence suggesting nonresectability was found preoperatively and thoracotomy was carried out. Of these patients, 3 were found to have nonresectable tumors for a resectability rate of 89.3 per cent. In carefully examining these 3 cases, we found 1 which we subsequently judged as incompletely studied since no azygogram had been performed. One other patient had a borderline pulmonary arteriogram. If we consider, then, only those patients in whom all studies were completed and in whom there was no suggestion of nonresectability, the resectability rate is 96 per cent for the series. In 6 patients, both

Table

Correlation of Resectability Criteria and Resectability Rates

Resectability Criteria						
Medias-tinoscopy	Angi-ography	Other Contrain-dications	No. Cases (N=60)	Per cent Total	Per cent Resected	Number not Explored
Neg.	Neg.	Neg.	28	46.7	89.3°	0
Neg.	Neg.	Pos.	6	10.0	0.0	3‡
Neg.	Pos.	+/−	7	11.6	14.2†	2
Pos.	Neg.	+/−	4	6.7	0.0	4
Pos.	Pos.	+/−	15	25.0	0.0	13

°One patient incompletely studied, one patient with borderline angiogram: resectability rate with all studies complete and negative = 96%
†False-positive azygogram
‡Two patients medically inoperable, one refused surgery

the mediastinoscopy and angiography studies were negative, but there was some other evidence of nonresectability. Of these patients, 3 were subsequently explored and all were found to have nonresectable tumors. In approximately 12 per cent of this series, the mediastinoscopy was negative while the angiography was positive, and of 5 such patients explored, only 1 was found to have a resectable tumor. This was the case illustrative of the false-positive azygogram. In 4 patients, the mediastinoscopy was positive while the angiography was negative; these cases were all judged nonresectable and none was explored. In the final category, constituting 25 per cent of the series, both the mediastinoscopy and angiography were positive. Of these patients, 2 were explored to confirm nonresectability or to establish a tissue diagnosis and neither was found to have a resectable tumor. Thus, 43.3 per cent of the total series had positive mediastinoscopy and/or angiography findings, with a resectability rate in this group of 3.9 per cent. This compares very closely with the reports of Delarue (Delarue, Sanders, and Silverberg, 1970) and his associates who cited 46.8 per cent with a positive finding at mediastinoscopy and/or angiography, for a resectability rate of 5.8 per cent for the group. For our total series of completed studies, we observed a false-negative rate of 8.3 per cent and an absolute false-positive rate of 1.6 per cent.

Conclusions

On the basis of these observations, we are persuaded that there is substantial value in both mediastinoscopy and angiography for the staging and determination of resectability in lung cancer. Further, the finding that the examinations were complementary to each other in more than 43 per cent of all patients with positive tests indicates the value of complete examination. As a result, we currently believe that mediastinoscopy and angiography, with visualization of the pulmonary arteries, the azygos system, the innominate vessels, and the superior vena cava, are indicated in all patients suspected of having lung cancer in which the lesions are centrally or posteriorly placed and in which there are no other obvious contraindications to surgical exploration as determined by conventional evaluative procedures.

REFERENCES

Ashbaugh, D. G.: Mediastinoscopy. *Archives of Surgery*, 100:568–573, May 1970.

Benfield, J. R., Gonney, H., Crummy, A. B., and Cleveland, R. J.: Azygograms and pulmonary arteriograms in bronchogenic carcinoma. *Archives of Surgery*, 99:406–409, September 1969.

Bernardi, R., Frasson, F., Dsellafore, D., Peracchia, A., and Pistolesi, G. F.: Place of selective retrograde azygography in angiographic study of lung cancer: 70 randomly chosen patients. *Journal de Radiologie et d'Electrologie*, 51:229–236, May 1970.

Carlens, E.: Mediastinoscopy. *Diseases of the Chest*, 36:343–352, October 1959.

Carlens, E., and Hambraeus, G. M.: Mediastinoscopy. Indications and limitations. *Scandinavian Journal of Respiratory Diseases*, 48:1–10, 1967.

Delarue, N. C., Sanders, E. D., and Silverberg, S. A.: Complementary value of pulmonary angiography and mediastinoscopy in individualizing treatment for patients with lung cancer. *Cancer*, 26:1370–1378, December 1970.

Delarue, N. C., and Starr, J.: A review of some important problems concerning lung cancer: Part II. *Journal of the Canadian Medical Association*, 96: 8–20, January 1967.

Delarue, N. C., and Strasberg, S. M.: The rationale of intensive preoperative investigation in bronchogenic carcinoma. *Journal of Thoracic and Cardiovascular Surgery*, 51:391–411, March 1966.

Dux, A., Bucheler, E., and Sobbe, A.: Die klinische bedeutung der direkten azygographie. *Der Radiologe*, 10:192–201, May 1970.

Goldberg, E. M., Glicksman, A. S., Khan, F. R., and Nickson, J. J.: Mediastinoscopy for assessing mediastinal spread of carcinoma of the lung. *Cancer*, 25:347–353, February 1970.

Greenough, W. G.: Role of pulmonary angiography in carcinoma of the lung. *Chest*, 62:206–210, August 1972.

Greenspan, R. H., and Capps, J. H.: Pulmonary angiography: Its use in diagnosis and as a guide to therapy in lesions of the chest. *Radiologic Clinics of North America*, 1:315–330, August 1963.

Ikeda, M., Neyazaki, T., Chiba, S., Yoneti, M., and Suzuki, C.: Bronchial vascular pattern of various pulmonary diseases with particular emphasis on its diagnostic value in pulmonary cancer. *Journal of Thoracic and Cardiovascular Surgery,* 55:642–652, May 1968.

Janower, M. L., Dreyfuss, J. R., and Skinner, D. B.: Azygography and lung cancer. *The New England Journal of Medicine,* 275:803–808, October 1966.

Mountain, C. F.: The role of mediastinoscopy in the management of lung cancer. In *Sixth National Cancer Conference Proceedings.* Philadelphia, Pennsylvania, J. B. Lippincott Company, 1970, pp. 829–834.

_____: Unpublished data.

_____: Surgical therapy in lung cancer: Biologic, physiologic, and technical determinants. *Seminars in Oncology.* (In press.)

Petrikova, J., Polak, J., and Mottl, V.: Comparative study of angiography and lung scanning in the preoperative diagnosis of bronchogenic carcinoma. *International Surgery,* 55:335–342, May 1971.

Rinker, C. T., Templeton, A. W., MacKenzie, J., Ridings, G. R., Almong, C. H., and Kephart, R.: Combined superior vena cavagraphy and azygography in patients with suspected lung cancer. *Radiology,* 88:441–445, March 1967.

Sander, E. D., Delarue, N. C., and Lou, G.: Angiography as a means of determining resectability of primary lung cancer. *The American Journal of Roentgenology, Radium Therapy and Nuclear Medicine,* 85:884–891, May 1962.

Sanders, E. D., Delarue, N. C., and Silverberg, S. A.: Combined angiography and mediastinoscopy in bronchogenic carcinoma. *Radiology,* 97:331–339, November 1970.

Sarin, C. L., and Nohl-Oser, H. C.: Mediastinoscopy: A clinical evaluation of 400 consecutive cases. *Thorax,* 24:585–588, September 1969.

Sharov, B. K., and Sumnaia, E. M.: On pneumomediastinography and azygography in pulmonary cancer. *Voprosy Onkol.,* 15:24–30, 1969.

Skinner, D. B., Dreyfuss, J. R., and Nordi, G. L.: Azygography in the evaluation of operability of pulmonary carcinoma. *The New England Journal of Medicine,* 267:232–237, August 1962.

Steinberg, I., and Finby, N.: Great vessel involvement in lung cancer: Angiocardiographic report on 250 consecutive proved cases. *The American Journal of Roentgenology, Radium Therapy and Nuclear Medicine,* 81:807–818, May 1959.

Steinberg, I., and Robb, G. P.: Mediastinal and hilar angiography in pulmonary disease. *American Review of Tuberculosis,* 38:557–569, November 1938.

Tucker, J. A.: Mediastinoscopy: 300 cases reported and literature reviewed. *Laryngoscope,* 82:2226–2248, December 1972.

Willa, C., Favex, G., Essinger, A., Hessler, C., and Nour, T.: Apport de l'angiographie pulmonaire au diagnostic pneumologique. *Schweizerische Medizinsche Wochenschrift,* 101:207–213, February 1971.

Wolfel, D. A., Lindberg, E. J., and Light, J. P.: The abnormal azygogram–an index of inoperability. *The American Journal of Roentgenology, Radium Therapy and Nuclear Medicine,* 97:933–938, August 1966.

133-Xenon Studies in the Preoperative Evaluation of Bronchogenic Carcinoma

M. KHALIL ALI, M.D.
*Department of Medicine, The University of Texas
System Cancer Center M. D. Anderson Hospital and
Tumor Institute, Houston, Texas*

IN NO SITUATION is the time-honored surgical fact that a patient must survive an operation before he can be considered cured more applicable than in the treatment of bronchogenic carcinoma. This is a result of the unfortunate situation that most patients with bronchogenic carcinoma are cigarette smokers and chronic obstructive lung disease coexists in varying degrees of severity.

The subject of this communication is, therefore, twofold: first, to present data concerning the pulmonary function evaluation both over-all and regional, using ^{133}Xe gas in lung cancer patients; and, second, to analyze the results of these tests in the patients who underwent pneumonectomy in an effort to predict the postoperative pulmonary status.

Material and Methods

Fifty consecutive lung cancer patients referred to us for preoperative evaluation were studied. Tests were repeated after pneumonectomy in 27 patients, 1 to 47 months following operation. In 12 patients, more than one serial follow-up postpneumonectomy study was obtained over that period of time.

SPIROMETRY AND ARTERIAL BLOOD GASES

The simplest tests for assessing over-all pulmonary function are the determination of the forced vital capacity (FVC) and the volume expired in the first second ($FEV_{1.0}$). We use the FVC and the $FEV_{1.0}$/FVC percentage to classify the impairment as either restrictive or obstructive, or both. Recently it has been recognized that $FEV_{1.0}$, expressed in liters or as a percentage of the predicted value, is the most reliable parameter of the routine pulmonary function studies (Boushy *et al.*, 1971). We utilize this index to classify our lung cancer patients into 4 functional groups: Group I includes patients with an $FEV_{1.0}$ of 2½ liters or more, corresponding to a minimum of 85 per cent of the predicted value; Group IV consists of patients with an $FEV_{1.0}$ of less than 1.2 liters, or 40 per cent of their predicted value. Groups II and III have values of 2 to 2.5 and 1.2 to 2 liters, respectively. While Group I patients are considered essentially normal, Groups II, III, and IV have mild, moderate, and severe ventilatory impairment, respectively. Arterial oxygen (PaO_2) and carbon dioxide ($PaCO_2$) tensions are routinely measured in all patients.

REGIONAL PULMONARY FUNCTION STUDIES

Regional distribution of pulmonary blood flow and ventilation were studied with ^{133}Xe gas. The studies were done during normal breathing at rest. The technique used is similar to that reported by Ball, Bates, Newsham, and Stewart (1962), and the basic methodology has been reported previously (Miller, Ali, and Howe, 1970).

Eight scintillation detectors, 4 for each lung, were positioned behind the chest. The apical pair of counters was placed at the level of the fourth thoracic spine and the other 3, directly below in a fixed arrangement. An intravenous injection of 1 to 2 mc. was used for the perfusion study. ^{133}Xe in a concentration of 1 to 1.5 mc. per liter of air was used for the study of zonal ventilation and zonal volume. Ventilation was measured from a single breath of the ^{133}Xe-air mixture of 500 to 700 ml. and from the wash-in and wash-out curves obtained during closed-circuit equilibration for volume determination.

The mean normal values and range for 14 healthy subjects are given in Figure 1. These values indicate that both perfusion and ventilation per unit lung volume—$\dot{Q}/V$ and $\dot{V}/V$, respectively—rises gradually from apex to base in the healthy lung, studied in the upright position. A zonal defect in perfusion or ventilation was detected

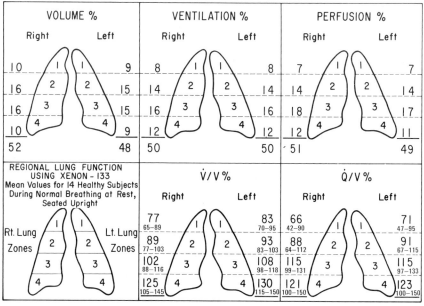

FIG. 1.—Distribution of ventilation and perfusion in the healthy adult lung during normal breathing at rest as determined by studies using ^{133}Xe gas.

when the absolute value fell below the normal range for the zone or when the value was less than that of the zone above.

Results

LUNG CANCER SERIES (50 PATIENTS)

Biometric data and the mean values for simple ventilatory tests and arterial blood gases are given in Table 1. The mean age and smoking habits were similar in all groups. The severity of airways obstruction, as detected by the $FEV_{1.0}/FVC$ percentage, increased steadily from Group I to Group IV. The arterial oxygen tension decreased from 83 mmHg in Group I to 66 mmHg in Group IV, while the CO_2 tension was within normal limits. ^{133}Xe studies revealed zonal function defects in the tumor-bearing lung in 47 of 50 patients. Zonal reductions of ventilation were more frequent than zonal perfusion defects, and the extent of reduction varied from mild to severe. Most of these defects were in the vicinity of, and hence related to, the tumor mass.

Table 1
Mean Spirometry and Arterial Blood Gas Values in Lung Cancer—50 Patients

Functional Group	No. of Patients	Age (Yrs.)	Smoking (Pkg.-Yrs.)	FEV$_{1.0}$ (L)	FVC (L)	FEV$_{1.0}$/FVC × 100	PaO$_2$ (mmHg)	PaCO$_2$ (mmHg)
I	8	57	63	3.2	4.4	72	83	43
II	18	63	64	2.3	3.7	63	79	42
III	19	61	61	1.7	2.8	58	70	40
IV	5	62	64	1.0	2.6	37	66	45

Abbreviations: FEV$_{1.0}$, forced expiratory volume in 1 second; L, liters; FVC, forced expiratory vital capacity; Pkg.-Yrs., package years, the number of daily packs of cigarettes × the number of years person has been smoking.

One of our patients presented with repeated hemoptysis and nega-tive results for chest X-ray study, bronchoscopy, and sputum cytolo-gy. The regional pulmonary function studies revealed perfusion and ventilation defects in the left upper lung zones. On bronchography, the contrast medium failed to fill the left upper lobe. Left upper lo-bectomy was performed and squamous cell carcinoma was reported in the resected specimen.

The findings in the contralateral lung were of more clinical significance, since this lung will support the life of the patient if pneumonectomy is contemplated. Of the 50 patients studied, 25 had zonal
function defects in the nontumor-bearing lung. The incidence of
defects increased as the $FEV_{1.0}$ decreased, so that all 5 patients in
Group IV had severe zonal abnormalities of function, and pulmonary
resection was considered to carry an increased funtional risk (Fig. 2).

FIG. 2. — Incidence of ventilatory defects in the nontumor-bearing lung of 50 patients
with lung cancer. A shift to the right downward (high $FEV_{1.0}/FVC$ percentage) indicates that the reduction in $FEV_{1.0}$ is mainly restrictive in nature. The 5 patients whose
study results were of this type had almost total obstruction of the tumor-bearing lung,
with a healthy contralateral lung. A shift to the left downward is compatible with significant airway disease. The high incidence of major ventilatory defects for test results
of this type strongly substantiates the conclusion that these defects are the result of
emphysema and/or chronic bronchitis.

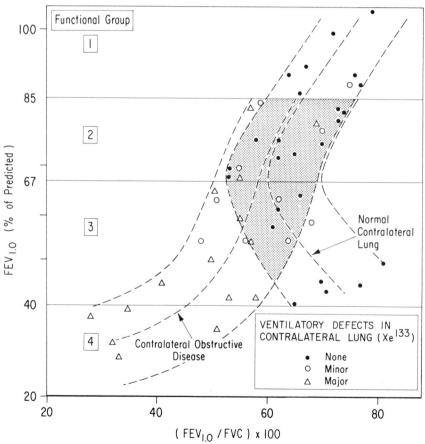

Only 1 patient of the 8 in Group I had localized perfusion defect; ventilation was normal in all 8, making pneumonectomy functionally tolerable. The majority of our patients were in Groups II and III, with an intermediate degree of over-all functional impairment. Figure 2 illustrates the fact that the incidence and severity of zonal function defects increased as the degree of airway obstruction increased (shift to the left downward). Conversely, patients with similar $FEV_{1.0}$ who had normal values for $FEV_{1.0}/FVC$ percentage had normal contralateral lungs (shift to the right downward); Figure 3 illustrates the findings in one of the patients in the latter group. The near loss of ventilation to the tumor-bearing lung was responsible for the pure, restrictive functional impairment.

FIG. 3 — Regional pulmonary function distribution in a patient with a right main stem bronchus carcinoma and total atelectasis of the right lung. Twenty-two per cent of the pulmonary blood flow perfuses the tumorous lung, which acts as a right-to-left shunt. Distribution of ventilation and perfusion within the right lung are considered normal, with progressively rising values for both indices from apex to base.

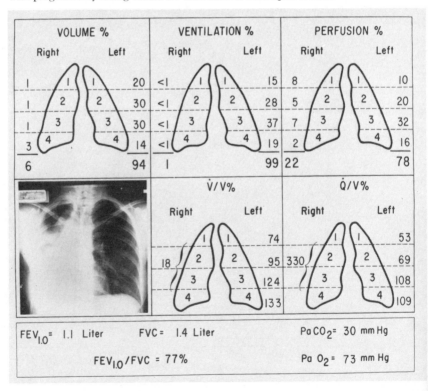

PNEUMONECTOMY SERIES (27 PATIENTS)

The classification and over-all pulmonary function data of these patients are shown in Table 2. This series does not represent the whole spectrum of lung cancer because of the obvious rejection of the bad-risk patients. However, as in the lung cancer series, most of the patients were in Groups II and III (22 of the 27). Group I patients had the approximate values we would expect for a healthy, nontumor-bearing lung after pneumonectomy. Of these 4, 3 are living and well, 1 to 4½ years following pneumonectomy. The fourth patient died of brain metastasis 2½ years after his operation. The only borderline patient who had 39 per cent of his predicted $FEV_{1.0}$ had a totally airless tumor-bearing lung, called medical pneumonectomy, and his spirometry values were unchanged following its removal. However, the $FEV_{1.0}/FVC$ percentage indicated a mild degree of airway obstruction. He died in respiratory failure 6 months after pneumonectomy. It is worth mentioning that both the $FEV_{1.0}/FVC$ percentage and the arterial oxygenation improved after pneumonectomy in nearly all these patients.

By comparing the pre- and postpneumonectomy ^{133}Xe studies in the 27 patients, we found that the distribution of regional ventilation was identical before and after pneumonectomy when the remaining lung was healthy (Fig. 4, Group A). Similarly, regional pulmonary blood was unaltered (Fig. 5, Group A). However, preoperative defects in ventilation persisted following pneumonectomy (Fig. 5, Group B). The apical blood flow was slightly increased at the expense of the basal zones in this group after pneumonectomy (Fig. 5). This loss of gravity effect on the blood flow distribution following pneumonectomy is indirect evidence of mild pulmonary hypertension developing in patients with preoperative regional function defects. Among the nonpulmonary conditions contributing to abnormal distribution of regional pulmonary perfusion in our patients were liver cirrhosis and old myocardial infarction.

Some of the resected lungs were inflated and fixed by formaline fumes. Pathological examination of the 2-cm. slices of the whole lung revealed structural disruption comparable in location to defects in regional function detected by the preoperative studies (Fig. 6).

Plots of the percentage of ventilation carried out by the tumor-bearing lung versus the percentage of loss of $FEV_{1.0}$ following pneumonectomy showed that most of the patients fell on, or in close proximity to, the 45° ideal regression line (Fig. 7). The line graphed in

Table 2
Mean Spirometry and Arterial Blood Gas Values Before and After Pneumonectomy — 27 Patients

Functional Group	No. of Patients	Age (Yrs.)	Smoking (Pkg-Yrs.)	$FEV_{1.0}(L)$		FVC(L)		$FEV_{1.0}/FVC \cdot 100$		PaO_2(mmHg)		$PaCO_2$(mmHg)	
				Pre	Post	Pre	Post	Pre	Post	Pre	Post	Pre	Post
I	4	54	53	3.1	1.6	4.1	2.1	75	77	82	85	38	36
II	16	62	54	2.3	1.3	3.7	1.9	65	68	81	84	41	39
III	6	63	70	1.9	1.4	3.5	2.2	56	65	76	83	36	40
IV	1	72	78	1.2	1.2	1.8	1.8	65	65	63	78	43	45

Abbreviations: Pre, preoperative; Post, postoperative; $FEV_{1.0}(L)$ = forced expiratory volume in liters in one second; FVC(L) = forced expiratory vital capacity in liters.

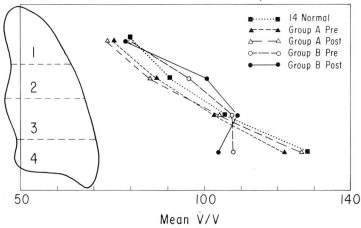

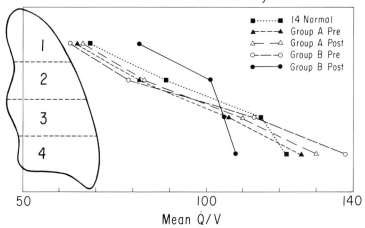

FIG. 4 *(top).*—Ventilation distribution before and after pneumonectomy in patients with healthy contralateral lung (Group A) and those with ventilatory defects (Group B).

FIG. 5 *(bottom).*—Pulmonary blood flow distribution before and after pneumonectomy in patients with a healthy contralateral lung (Group A) and those with ventilatory defects (Group B). Notice the increased apical blood flow (Zones 1 and 2) after pneumonectomy in Group B patients.

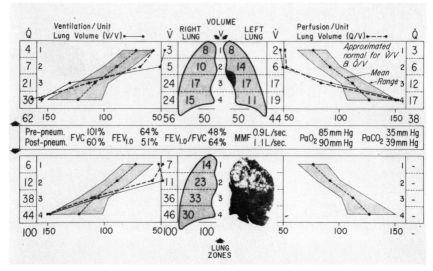

FIG. 6.—Regional pulmonary function distribution before (upper panels) and after (lower right panel) left pneumonectomy in a patient with bronchogenic carcinoma and bilateral, apical bullae. A 2-cm. slice of the inflated, fixed left lung showed the emphysematous cystic formations in the left upper zones, corresponding to the defective function of those areas in the preoperative study.

FIG. 7.—Percentage ventilation to the tumor-bearing lung, plotted against the percentage loss in FEV$_{1.0}$ following pneumonectomy.

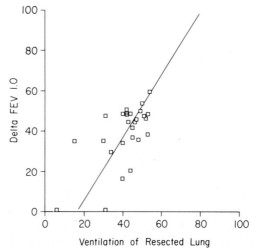

this figure, however, is the regression line for our data. Using this line and the preoperative $FEV_{1.0}$, the following regression equation was constructed for predicting the postpneumonectomy $FEV_{1.0}$:

$$\text{Predicted } FEV_{1.0} \text{ after pneumonectomy} = (1.25 - 0.0155\text{V})$$
$$\text{x Preoperative } FEV_{1.0}.$$
$$\dot{V} = \text{Ventilation of the tumor-bearing lung.}$$

Discussion

The widespread use today of pneumonectomy in treating patients with primary carcinoma of the lung, as well as the frequent perform- ance of extensive bilateral pulmonary resection for metastatic nod- ules, created the necessity for knowing the share of function per- formed by each lung and preferably by the individual zones within the lungs. Spirometry is occasionally of help in deliberations con- cerning operability or the choice of operation in individual patients, especially if the results are normal (Group I) or very poor (Group IV). Another situation in which it is useful is when the tumor-bearing lung is totally airless, a conditon we refer to as medical pneumonec- tomy (Fig. 3). While arterial oxygenation is usually of little help in this respect, carbon dioxide retention is an ominous sign and warns against sacrificing functioning lung tissue. However, the value of these over-all pulmonary function tests in the preoperative evalua- tion of the majority of lung cancer patients (Groups II and III) is lim- ited because of their distortion by the disease for which surgery is contemplated, as well as by the concomitant emphysema and chronic bronchitis. The shaded area in Figure 2 illustrates the value of the regional function studies in categorizing patients with identical mechanical function into those with healthy contralateral lung and those who are bad-risk patients who have major ventilatory defects in the nontumor-bearing lung. In addition, the regression equation de- rived from Figure 6 enables us to predict the postoperative $FEV_{1.0}$ with a great deal of accuracy.

Some investigators believe that if the relative perfusion to the tu- morous lung is less than one third of the total pulmonary blood flow, the tumor is unresectable (Jackson, Provan, and Walker, 1971). Our pneumonectomy studies proved that this philosophy is not uniformly true, since involvement of the major pulmonary vessels is only one of several mechanisms responsible for hypoperfusion. Four of our pa- tients had successful pneumonectomies with a relative pulmonary blood flow of 9, 15, 27, and 30 per cent to the tumorous lung; 3 of these patients are living and well, 1 to 4½ years postoperatively.

The effect of the increased blood flow through the remaining capillary bed over the course of the years was also of interest to us. Serial follow-up studies were performed on 12 patients. The repeat studies were very similar when the remaining lung was healthy, indicating the remarkable degree to which the capillary bed can be enlarged to accommodate the doubled blood flow (Fig. 8). However, preoperative abnormalities became progressively worse. In one patient, there was evidence that pulmonary hypertension in the remaining lung produced vascular changes that resulted in pathological disruption of the lung parenchyma. This was suggested by the gradual develop-

FIG. 8.—Serial, follow-up postpneumonectomy regional studies showing the persistence of the normal pattern of blood flow and ventilation over a period of 38 months.

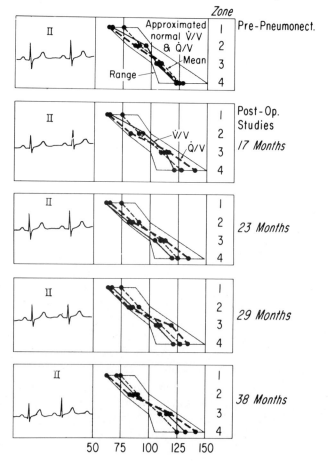

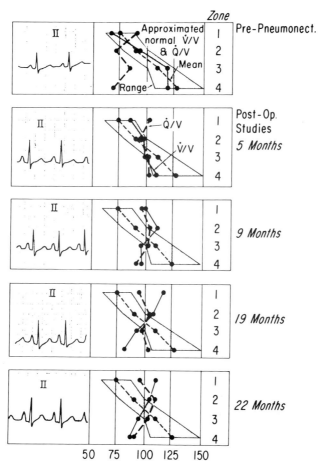

FIG. 9.—Serial, follow-up postpneumonectomy regional studies in a patient with abnormal distribution of blood flow. Abnormalities in ventilation distribution evolved and gradually became worse. Tall, peaked P-waves indicated the development of cor pulmonale.

ment of abnormalities in regional ventilation which were not evident in earlier studies (Fig. 9).

Conclusion

These data show that ^{133}Xe regional studies provide a safe, noninvasive substitute for other tedious and unpleasant methods of determining differential pulmonary function. We believe that pneumonectomy should be functionally tolerated if the distribution of ventilation and pulmonary blood flow within the nontumor-bearing lung is normal, and if the calculated postpneumonectomy $FEV_{1.0}$, using the regression equation, is more than 1 liter.

Acknowledgments

The technical assistance of Mr. R. L. Burdett is greatly appreciated. Parts of this work were presented before the combined meeting of the Central Society and the Mid-Western Section of the American Federation for Clinical Research, Nov. 1, 1969, in Chicago, Illinois, and at the National meeting of the American Federation for Clinical Research, May 2, 1970, at Atlantic City, New Jersey.

The work reported in this paper was partially supported by Grant No. ACS-IN-43-N from the American Cancer Society.

REFERENCES

Ball, W. C., Jr., Bates, D. V., Newsham, L. G. S., and Stewart, P. B.: Regional pulmonary function studied with xenon[133]. *Journal of Clinical Investigation*, 41:519–531, March 1962.

Boushy, S. F., Billig, D. M., North, L. B., and Helgason, A. H.: Clinical course related to preoperative and postoperative pulmonary function in patients with bronchogenic carcinoma. *Chest*, 59:383–391, April 1971.

Jackson, J. A., Provan, J. L., and Walker, R. H. S.: Lung scanning in carcinoma of the bronchus. *Thorax*, 26:23–32, January 1971.

Miller, J. M., Ali, M. K., and Howe, C. D.: Clinical determination of regional pulmonary function during normal breathing using xenon[133]. *American Review of Respiratory Disease*, 101:218–229, February 1970.

Iatrogenic Pulmonary Disease in the Cancer Patient

ARNOLD M. GOLDMAN, M. D.
Department of Diagnostic Radiology, The University of
Texas System Cancer Center M. D. Anderson Hospital
and Tumor Institute, Houston, Texas

DISEASES OF THE LUNG seen in the cancer patient which can be attributed to medical intervention begin with the infections and infestations associated with altered immunity. This usually is the result of chemotherapy, and virtually every effective chemotherapeutic agent causes a profound effect in the patient's immune mechanism. The only possible exception is bleomycin, and that drug causes a direct effect on the lung itself. The cancer patient, especially the one with leukemia or lymphoma, may have a faulty immune mechanism resulting from the primary disease, or deficient immunity may accompany the inanition which can be seen with any advanced neoplasm.

The usual problem that we face is a patient with fever or dyspnea and an abnormal chest X-ray film. The problem of fever in the cancer patient, especially the one with leukemia or lymphoma, is considerable. Most of these patients will be febrile at some point in their disease, and in the great majority of leukemia patients and at least half of the lymphoma patients, this fever is caused by an infection. The infection involved is often septicemia, but the single organ most commonly involved is the lung.

In the severely neutropenic patient, pneumonia may not be visible radiologically because of the failure to pour out the fluid and cells into the alveolae on which we depend for the radiologic diagnosis.

Only careful clinical evaluation for the presence of rales in a febrile patient will bring about that diagnosis.

NEOPLASTIC CHANGES

Figure 1 shows examples of changes in the lung which are caused by the neoplasm itself rather than by an infection. Figure 1A is the only identified case of leukemic involvement of the lung which was visible radiologically in the past 7 years at M. D. Anderson Hospital. This is not to say that the pathologist does not see leukemic infiltration of the lung very commonly, but for all intents and purposes, that diagnosis should not be considered in the leukemia patient with an abnormal chest X-ray film. The cause of such pulmonary abnormality is almost always infection, although occasionally an alveolar hemorrhage may occur.

Hodgkin's disease and lymphoma show neoplastic involvement of

FIG. 1.—A, cords of leukemic deposits manifested as linear densities superimposed on the right pleural effusion in a patient with chronic myelogenous leukemia. Pneumonia at the left base. B, recurrent Hodgkin's disease showing a combination of interstitial, nodular, and alveolar change in the lungs. C, Hodgkin's disease with a cavitated nodule. D, section of a lung showing diffuse interstitial spread of Hodgkin's disease at the time of initial presentation of the patient with peripheral adenopathy. E and F, recurrent hilar mass and density over the right upper lobe resulting from a plaque of tumor over the anterior pleura.

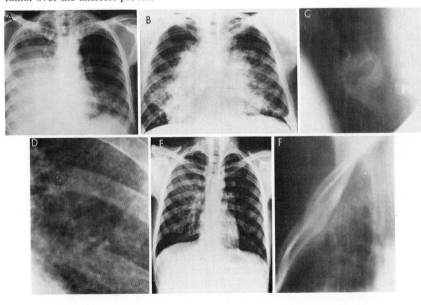

the lung much more commonly than leukemia does. It has been estimated that 30 per cent of patients with Hodgkin's disease eventually have pulmonary deposits. Most of these show interstitial deposits evidenced by a streaky change in the region of the hila and sometimes associated with recurrent disease or a new mass in the hila
(Fig. 1*B*). In our experience, most of these patients have received
previous radiation therapy to the hila and mediastinum. Nodular disease is the next most common manifestation, while alveolar spread of
tumor is least common.

In Figure 1*B* there are also multiple nodules, and in Figure 1*C* we
see a thick irregular cavity which represents an excavated Hodgkin's
nodule. These may sometimes be thin-walled and multiple.

A diffuse interstitial pattern in Hodgkin's disease, such as is seen
in Fig. 1*D* is very rare. Lymphangitic spread is not rare in other cancers and may be confused with interstitial pneumonias.

One additional type of spread of neoplasm which could be confused with infection is seen in Figure 1*E* in which a uniform density
which does not correspond to any lobe or segment is seen over the
right upper lung field and is not identified in the lung in the lateral
projection. On the oblique tomogram (Fig. 1*F*) of that area, it can be
seen that we are dealing with a plaque of tumor.

Infections

Although the ordinary infectious agents usch as diplococcus pneu-
moniae and mycoplasma occur in the immunologically incompetent
patient, it is more common to find ourselves dealing with unusual
and sometimes exotic organisms which have been termed opportunistic because of their uncommon appearance in the otherwise
healthy patient and their relative frequence in the group we are considering. In our hospital, the most common organisms identified in
these patients are *Klebsiella, E. coli,* and *Candida.* Figure 2 shows a
patient with *Klebsiella* pneumonia, and it is apparent that a differentiation of this from staphylococcal or fungal pneumonia with necrotiz-
zation usually is not possible. When the *Klebsiella* infection results
in an increase in volume of a lobe, the specific etiology may be suggested, but still is not certain.

THE COMMON GRANULOMATOUS INFECTIONS

The common granulomatous infections are surprisingly uncommon
in these immunologically incompetent patients. When one considers

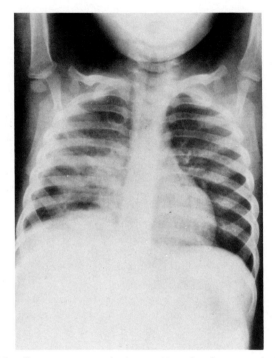

FIG. 2.—*Klebsiella* pneumonia in leukemia. Note the abscess in the lower lobe and the pneumatocele in the upper lobe.

the number of patients who must have old tuberculous, Histoplasma, or coccidioidal foci, it is surprising that these organisms are not a common problem, and yet that is the case. Figure 3 shows a patient with widespread tuberculosis including massive mediastinal nodes. We have also seen acute tuberculous pneumonia as well as an occasional case of breakdown of an old lesion in a patient receiving chemotherapy or in an area of radiation therapy.

Viral infections include a fairly high incidence of unusual organisms. The patient illustrated in Figure 4 had giant cell pneumonia without clinical evidence of measles. The organism, which is thought to be the same in these diseases, often does not cause a rash in the patient with altered immune response. The finding of spontaneous pneumomediastinum seems to be an almost specific finding, among the infections, for giant cell pneumonia and is seen in perhaps 30 to 40 per cent of the patients with that disease (Gilmartin, 1971).

Rounded, nodular-appearing densities approximately 1 centimeter

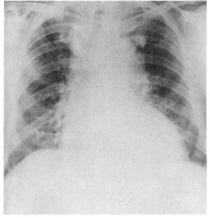

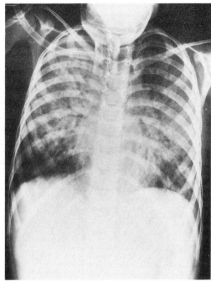

FIG. 3 *(above).* — Massive mediastinal adenopathy caused by diffuse tuberculosis, with virtually clear lungs in a patient with leukemia.

FIG. 4 *(right).* — Giant cell pneumonia with interstitial emphysema and pneumomediastinum.

in diameter and showing fluffy edges are fairly common in chickenpox pneumonia. This finding in the upper lung fields is supposed to suggest the presence of cytomegalic inclusion disease but in our experience that is not a helpful sign. The patients in whom that diagnosis has been established usually show areas of patchy pneumonia or occasionally an appearance almost like that of diffuse pulmonary edema. Additional information may be obtained by examining the urine or saliva for cells containing the characteristic findings of the cytomegalovirus syndrome, but it should be pointed out that only a minority of patients do show recognizable changes; furthermore, the presence of the abnormal cells does not always indicate the presence of active disease.

PROTOZOANS

The only protozoan which is a common problem is *Pneumocystis carinii,* although *Toxoplasma gondii* is seen on rare occasions.

Pneumocystosis is usually believed to be an interstitial disease, but the radiologic appearance is more often that of an alveolar process or a mixture of alveolar and interstitial findings. The usual descriptions state that the early radiologic findings are perihilar streaky density, but in our experience, this is an unusual appearance. More commonly, the sequence of events will include an area or areas of small linear nodular densities which tend to enlarge and become confluent, resulting in diffuse alveolar filling (Fig. 5). The most

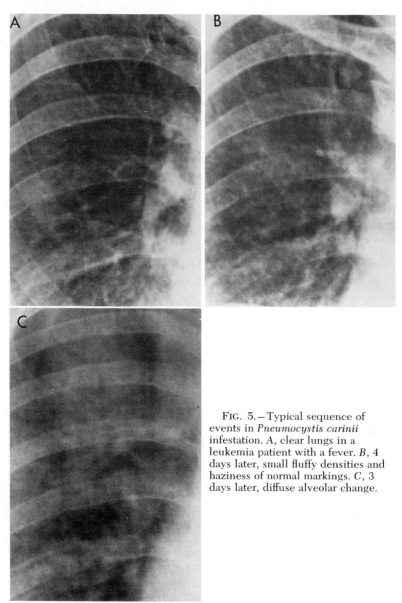

FIG. 5.—Typical sequence of events in *Pneumocystis carinii* infestation. *A*, clear lungs in a leukemia patient with a fever. *B*, 4 days later, small fluffy densities and haziness of normal markings. *C*, 3 days later, diffuse alveolar change.

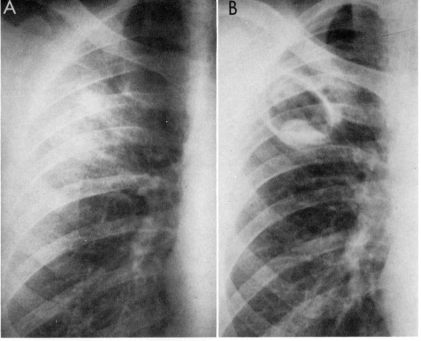

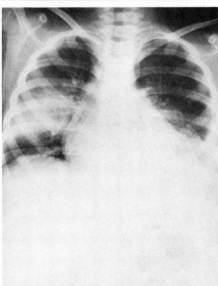

FIG. 6 *(above).*—*A,* an area of pneumonia which cavitated in the next few days and shows a large cavity containing debris or a fungus ball as well as a small amount of fluid. *B,* 3 weeks later. This may have been the result of a *Candida* infection.

FIG. 7 *(left).*—Mucormycosis with disseminated intravascular coagulation resulting in areas of pulmonary as well as splenic infarction.

unusual manifestation of pneumocystosis is that of lobar consolidation. Pleural effusion is very uncommon and we have not seen hilar adenopathy.

The incidence of pneumocystosis of the lungs seems to have decreased at M. D. Anderson Hospital in the past 2 or 3 years, but it is still an important disease to identify because of the possibility of specific treatment being given.

FUNGAL INFECTIONS

The fungi are most important in the consideration of opportunistic pulmonary infection. The organism that we see most frequently is *Candida*. It is often difficult to establish the presence of invasive *Candida* pneumonia beyond a doubt, but Figure 6 shows a case in which the pneumonia was found at the same time that there was a *Candida* fungemia. The pneumonia broke down into a cavity which contained either a fungus ball or necrotic debris. This appearance of a cavity with solid contents also may be seen in multiple areas in which case the presence of septic embolization is suspected.

Aspergillus and *Nocardia* are, in some institutions, the most common fungi seen in the group of patients with immunologic defects, but that has not been our experience at M. D. Anderson Hospital. Unusual fungal diseases such as mucormycosis (Fig. 7) are occasionally seen.

As was mentioned previously, histoplasmosis and coccidioidomycosis, although fairly common granulomatous diseases of the general population, do not often cause difficulty in these patients. We have seen 1 or 2 Histoplasma pneumonias but have not identified a case in which a known lesion has broken down. Figure 8 shows an interesting sequence of films in which the patient had an acute coccidioidomycosis pneumonia with hilar adenopathy followed by granuloma formation. Several years later, he developed leukemia and while being treated these areas did break down and an acute coccidioidal pneumonia was diagnosed at that time.

Direct Effect of Chemotherapeutic Agents on the Lungs

Myleran (busulfan) (Fig. 9) and perhaps Cytoxan (cyclophosphamide) can cause extensive interstitial and alveolar changes in the lungs. Following withdrawal of the drug, partial clearing can occur, but considerable residual fibrosis may be seen.

Methotrexate therapy has been reported as causing diffuse areas of

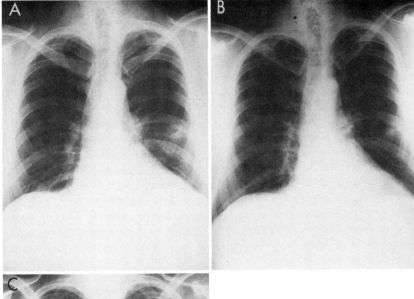

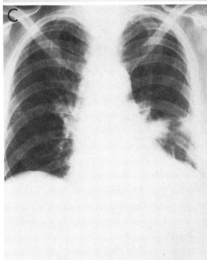

FIG. 8. — Coccidioidomycosis. *A*, small area of acute pneumonia with left hilar adenopathy. *B*, 2 months later, granulomata seen in lung and hilum. *C*, breakdown with acute coccidioidomycosis pneumonia during chemotherapy for leukemia 2 years later.

pneumonia and a number of patients also have hilar adenopathy, a finding which may help in suspecting that diagnosis. We have had no cases that could be definitely attributed to methotrexate although the diagnosis has been suspected several times.

From time to time, cases of diffuse lung disease in which no organism or other cause can be definitely identified are suspected as being the result of chemotherapeutic agents other than the ones men-

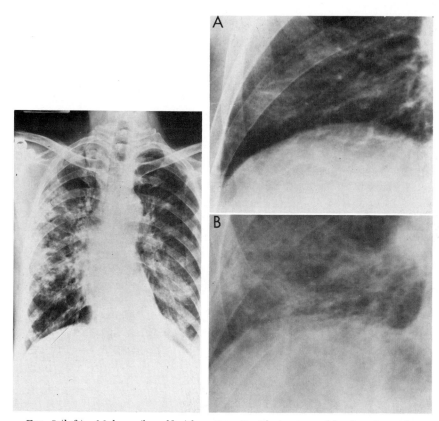

FIG. 9 *(left)*. — Myleran (busulfan) lung in patient being treated for chronic myelogenous leukemia. The chest cleared considerably after medication was stopped. Residual fibrosis did remain.

FIG. 10 *(right)*. —A, typical early changes in bleomycin lung toxicity showing interstitial markings and fuzziness with some confluence. B, progression with considerable interstitial fibrosis as well as confluent alveolar density. There were changes in the other costophrenic angle and slight changes in the upper portions of the lung at this time.

tioned above, but the exact relationship thus far has been questionable (Dohner, Wart, and Standor, 1972).

One other drug which definitely does cause pulmonary disease is bleomycin. The typical sequence can be seen in Figure 10. It should be emphasized that the majority of our patients who have had bleomycin lung disease show an almost identical evolution; that is, radiologically visible changes begin in the lower portions of the lung, especially near the costophrenic angles. The disease may of course become diffuse.

The Radiologist's Place in the Definitive Diagnosis of Pulmonary Disease

It must be perfectly understood that, although an occasional specific diagnosis can be made with a fairly high degree of confidence and accuracy, the usual situation requires histologic or microbiologic proof. The radiologist, using the techniques of percutaneous needle biopsy (either aspiration or core) and bronchial brushing, can contribute materially to rapid, accurate diagnosis. Although the application of these methods must be well thought out in each case, procrastination can result in the patient becoming a poor candidate if the disease is permitted to progress too far.

Summary

Iatrogenic pulmonary disease in the cancer patient usually is a result of an induced immunologic deficiency which permits infection, often by unusual organisms. The radiologist's role includes differentiation of such disease from neoplastic disease, usually by both the appreciation of the varied radiologic findings in both of these types of diseases and an evaluation of the clinical situation. The radiologist may further aid in specific diagnosis by the use of needle biopsy or bronchial brushing.

REFERENCES

Dohner, V. A., Wart, H. P., and Standor, R. E.: Alveolitis during procarbazine, vincristine, and cyclophosphamide therapy. *Chest*, 62:636–639, November 1972.

Gilmartin, D.: Mediastinal emphysema in Melbourne children. *Australasian Radiology*, 15:27–31, February 1971.

Rosenow, E. C.: The spectrum of drug-induced pulmonary disease. *Annals of Internal Medicine*, 77:977–991, December 1972.

Differentiation of Renal Masses: A Systematized Approach

HOWARD M. POLLACK, M.D., BARRY B.
GOLDBERG, M.D., JOSÉ O. MORALES, M.D., and
MORTON BOGASH, M.D.

Departments of Radiology, Nuclear Medicine, and
Urology, Episcopal Hospital and Temple University
Health Sciences Center, Philadelphia, Pennsylvania

DIFFERENTIATION OF RENAL MASSES constitutes one of the most vexing problems facing radiologists and urologists. The reasons for this are: First, renal masses are common and seem to be encountered more frequently now than in years gone by. This is no doubt the result of recent improvements in urography whereby masses are more readily detected. Second, many masses have a gross radiographic similarity, and special examinations are required to differentiate them. Most of these special procedures are complex, time consuming, and expensive. It would be helpful, therefore, if a method of selecting the most appropriate examinations could be devised whereby cases could be so individualized that only those procedures considered essential to the diagnosis in a particular patient would be employed, thus eliminating all extraneous studies. The "correct" set of studies would vary from case to case, of course, but would proceed in general according to a flow diagram or decision-making tree constructed according to previous experiences. Such a method is outlined in this paper.

Numerous types of renal masses are encountered in clinical practice. Of these, cysts are by far the most common (Lang *et al.*, 1972). In an asymptomatic population, cysts outnumber the combined total of all other renal masses by approximately 2 to 1. Since, generally speaking, they require less aggressive management than other masses, they provide our major task; namely, how to separate them from other renal masses in a simple and reliable way, thus allowing attention to be concentrated on the more significant entities. Tumors, of course, are our main concern. Inflammatory masses occur rather infrequently, but from time to time one encounters pyogenic abscesses, tuberculous abscesses, xanthogranulomatous inflammatory masses, and nodular hypertrophy of the kidney occurring as a result of chronic pyelonephritis. Intrarenal hematomas may easily simulate any other type of renal mass, although they usually occur in patients who are on anticoagulant therapy or otherwise predisposed to spontaneous bleeding. Hydronephroses usually are not a problem unless they present as a localized hydrocalyx or a duplicated collecting system, in which case they may have a masslike appearance. Retroperitoneal masses including adrenal lesions may either invade the kidney or become so intimately involved with it that differentiation from primary renal masses may be accomplished only with difficulty. Finally, the group known as "pseudotumors," including enlarged columns of Bertin and the numerous lumps and bumps which occur as normal variants, may produce very real problems in their differentiation from pathological entities (Felson and Moskowitz, 1969). We believe, however, that these spurious masses can be readily sorted out from the significant ones by means of the protocol which will be described.

Procedures available for the discrimination of renal masses include urography, nephrotomography, angiography, ultrasound, radionuclide imaging, and cyst aspiration. By using them in various combinations, one may readily determine which are likely to provide the information necessary to arrive at a correct diagnosis in any given case.

Excretory urography, while a very sensitive indicator of a renal mass, is a very poor discriminator of masses. It cannot differentiate cysts from tumor except in rare cases. There are 2 findings, however, which, if seen on urography, are extremely suggestive, if not conclusive, proof of the nature of the mass in question. The presence of amorphous calcification within the central or the nonperipheral portion of the mass almost invariably indicates renal cell carcinoma (Daniel, Hartman, and Witten, 1972). All other distributions of calcification in or around a renal mass may be seen in either cyst or tumor or, indeed, in other masses. The other finding in question is the presence of fat within the mass as visualized on a plain film of the abdomen. If present, this indicates the presence of either a lipoma or, more likely, an angiomyolipoma (hamartoma) (Adelman, 1965).

We believe that the primary function of nephrotomography is the demonstration that a given lesion is a cyst. Such an inference, however, may be reliably drawn only when all of the typical findings of renal cyst are present; namely, (a) a pencil-line thin, smooth wall; (b) notable radiolucency when compared with the opacified adjacent renal parenchyma, and (c) a sharp, smooth margination of the mass at its interface with the normal renal parenchyma. If all of these findings are present, then it is extremely likely that such a renal mass is a simple cyst (Evans and Bosniak, 1971). A mass lacking all of the typical findings may also represent a renal cyst, but to render such a diagnosis under any but the conditions outlined above incurs the hazard of misdiagnosing a tumor as a cyst. The usual cause for such a false-negative examination lies in a deficiency in the technical performance of the procedure. Nephrotomography is an examination which must be performed meticulously, employing sufficient contrast medium, dependable equipment, and close monitoring (Pfister and Shea, 1971). Usually, multiple projections are required. This type of tomography cannot be performed during screening urography. The addition of "cuts" to a urographic study, while often helpful, does not in our opinion constitute the type of nephrotomography required to produce reliable discrimination of masses. When the procedure is performed with the requisite attentiveness, however, its accuracy is probably between 90 and 95 per cent (Evans, 1968). Other findings which may aid in diagnosis include the so-called spur or beak sign which occurs at the junction of the extrarenal portion of the cyst wall with the adjacent renal parenchyma (Dautrebande, Duckett, and Roy, 1967). This is usually a sign of renal cyst as opposed to tumor, but exceptions have been recorded. Occasionally, the existence of collateral veins may be seen around the mass when no other sign of tumor is apparent. This has been of help on several occasions in our experience (Genereux, 1968). The so-called "Swiss cheese nephrogram" is also very helpful when it occurs, and indicates the presence of polycystic disease (Evans and Bosniak, 1971). This is usually not a consideration in the differential diagnosis of a solitary renal mass although occasionally it may be. Finally, it should be pointed out that the demonstration of a thick wall (more than a millimeter in diameter) is a very alarming sign which, when present, should suggest that a mass is probably not a simple, uncomplicated renal cyst (Bosniak and Faegenburg, 1965). We have been able to demonstrate the wall of a renal cyst in almost all cases unless the cyst was entirely intrarenal. Tumors, however, may or may not have a readily demonstrable wall. At times, a wall may be more apparent on nephrotomography than at angiography.

Arteriography has long been a dominant factor in the discrimination of renal masses. Its accuracy is quite high, being at the same level of reliability, or perhaps slightly higher, than nephrotomography (Watson, Fleming, and Evans, 1968). Unquestionably, however, a significant percentage of renal parenchymal tumors escape detection by selective renal arteriography (Meaney, 1969) in spite of the addition of pharmacoangiography and magnification studies to the armamentarium. There are a number of neoplasms which may, at times, be hypovascular and some which are characteristically so, particularly the papillary cystadenocarcinoma, a cellular variant of renal cell carcinoma. In fact, any renal cell carcinoma, regardless of cell type, may undergo sufficient necrosis or hemorrhage to render the demonstration of neovasculature within the tumor impossible. Wilms' tumors are another variety which are noted for their scanty neovasculature. Their unique clinical setting, however, makes them rather easy to recognize, and angiography usually is not necessary for their diagnosis. Renal sarcomas, lymphomas, and metastatic deposits are further examples of tumors which may be confusing in diagnosis because of a lack of vascularity. One must be aware, therefore, that a renal arteriogram must be scrutinized for the presence of even 1 small vessel abnormal in location or in appearance, since this may be the only evidence that a mass is not innocuous. Conversely, such subtle areas of neovasculature are not necessarily pathognomonic of renal neoplasms but may be seen as well in inflammatory processes, especially abscesses. The major drawback of renal angiography is not the occasional misleading appearances it may present, 5 to 10 per cent of cases (Meaney, 1969), but rather the fact that it is an incommodious procedure with a significant morbidity rate (Reiss, Bookstein, and Bleifer, 1972). Whereas the other procedures employed in renal mass evaluation all may be performed on an outpatient basis, angiography usually requires overnight hospitalization. In addition, it is time-consuming, expensive, and requires more technical expertise than the other studies. None of these criticisms, however, mitigate its indispensable nature in the evaluation of solid lesions of the kidney, and we have come more and more to employ it selectively in this regard, once the cystic lesions and pseudotumors have been excluded.

The next procedure to be considered is that of radionuclide imaging. It is well known that the diuretic, chlormerodrin, is localized to the cells of the proximal renal tubules. Uptake of this substance labeled with [197]Hg, therefore, occurs only in areas of functioning renal cortex. Since no pathological renal mass contains such functioning tissue, a renal scan will demonstrate a defect in the image when a tumor, cyst, or other mass is present, but will not demonstrate such a defect when an irregularity of renal configuration is attributable to a normal variant (Rosenthall, 1971). Therefore, such pseudotumors as columns of Bertin and nodular compensatory hypertrophy will be associated with intact renal scans, devoid of "cold spots." This observation holds true only in the case of renal masses larger than 2.5 cm. in diameter. Lesions smaller than this are beyond the limits of resolution of current imaging systems and may well escape detection (Pollack, Edell, and Morales, 1974). However, since such small masses usually are not detected on the urogram (Cope, Hackett, and Raphael, 1965), a significant clinical problem does not occur. Satisfactory imaging may be obtained by the use of either a rectilinear scanner or an Anger camera. In view of the frequency with which pseudotumors are seen, especially those involving the left kidney, renal imaging has assumed greater importance in separating real from spurious masses. In our experience, it is now rarely necessary to resort to angiography to make this distinction. Nephrotomography may be of help, but only if the mass proves to be a renal cyst, since tomographic appearances of solid renal lesions may be extremely deceptive and may resemble normal renal parenchyma. [99m]Technetium iron ascorbate complex also accumulates in the renal tubules and may be used instead of chlormerodrin for renal imaging. Once the presence of a bona fide renal mass has been confirmed by renal scanning, it may be desirable, while the patient is still within the nuclear medicine department, to perform a renal flow study. This procedure, of course, requires the use of an Anger camera, but will allow the detection of vascularity within certain renal neoplasms. But, as in the case of renal arteriography, there are a significant number of false-negative flow studies in renal tumors, and failure to demonstrate vascularity within the mass by this method is no assurance that a tumor does not exist. This procedure is helpful, therefore, only if positive, for if so, the diagnostic possibilities are reduced to 2 — tumor or arteriovenous abnormality.

The newest diagnostic tool to be employed in the study of renal masses is ultrasound (Goldberg and Pollack, 1971). Both the A-mode and the B-scan modalities are utilized, the latter for a 2-dimensional anatomical perspective of the relationship of the mass in question to its surrounding environment and the former for a more definitive and critical assessment of the nature of the echoes arising from and around the mass (Pollack and Goldberg, 1973). With solid masses, numerous acoustical interfaces exist, all of which provide sound reflection, represented on the A-mode format as vertical peaks from the baseline, or echoes, A fluid-filled mass, however, is acoustically homogeneous and no echoes will be reflected from within it. Such a transonic or sonolucent zone almost invariably indicates the presence of a fluid-containing structure, usually a cyst (Goldberg and Pollack, 1971). A localized hydronephrosis may produce a similar picture and on several occasions, we have detected a transonic zone emanating from a hematoma. An occasional tumor may appear at first to be transonic but with circumspection, it will be noted to have absorbed more sound that would be expected from a cyst of comparable dimensions. This is manifested by a notable diminution in the number and intensity of the far wall echoes. Apparent exceptions to this rule are usually attributable to technical lapses which, when recognized and corrected, provide a strong measure of reliability to the ultrasonic differentiation of solid from cystic masses. Small renal masses, of approximately 2.5 cm. in diameter or less, may be overlooked with ultrasound just as they have been a source of false or misleading results with radionuclide imaging. One further advantage of ultrasound is its ability to provide accurate dimensions of the mass. Not only may the diameter of the lesion be measured but its depth below the skin surface may also be readily ascertained by direct measurement from the A-mode or B-scan readouts.

We have separated the A-mode patterns in renal masses into 3 varieties: the cystic, the solid, and the complex or mixed (Goldberg and Pollack, 1971). Cystic patterns, as stated above, are seen in cysts, hydronephroses, and hematomas. Solid patterns are seen only in the presence of parenchymal masses. Since normal renal tissue is in a sense a parenchymal mass, one must be certain that a pathological mass is present before attributing significance to a solid ultrasound pattern. If this is not done, it is possible to misinterpret a normal variant, such as a dromedary hump, as a neoplasm. This type of catastrophe can be avoided by preliminary radionuclide scanning in uncertain or ambiguous cases. Complex patterns are seen when there is a mixture of fluid and solid components such as in cystic or necrotic tumors. We have also encountered this pattern in infected cysts, polycystic disease, multilocular cysts, abscesses, and certain Wilms' tumors. Here again, the interdependence of ultrasound and radiology is apparent for although a polycystic kidney may be indistinguishable from a necrotic tumor to the ultrasonic beam, these entities are readily separable radiographically. Ultrasound cannot stand alone as a diagnostic modality but must be integrated with other information, both clinical and roentgenographic, if it is to have maximum effectiveness and reliability.

We consider aspiration, with the instillation of both air and opaque media for double contrast cystography, to be the definitive examination in the diagnosis of renal cysts. When combined with cytology and chemical analysis of the aspirate, especially for fat content, it becomes a modality which we believe is of absolute reliability when performed in a technically satisfactory fashion. We utilize the examination for confirmation once a strong suspicion of renal cyst has been established. We have not needled, either knowingly or unknowingly, any renal neoplasms, but were this to occur there is no valid reason to believe that any great harm would be done. We are more concerned with the possibility of inadvertently needling a renal abscess or large arteriovenous malformation and for this reason, we do not employ needle aspiration as a primary study as has been advocated by others (Lalli, 1973). Although initially we performed aspiration with fluoroscopic guidance, the development of a special ultrasonic transducer, designed to permit needle aspiration and biopsy through its core, has dramatically changed our approach (Goldberg and Pollack, 1973). All renal cyst aspirations are now performed under ultrasonic guidance with a resultant increase in accuracy and efficiency. This procedure, which requires only an A-mode ultrasound unit rather than the more expensive B-scanner, is easily performed on outpatients. No complications attributable to its performance have occurred in our experience. Water-soluble contrast media are employed, since in our experience, the instillation of oily opaques generally has been ineffective in permanently decreasing the size of cysts. Routine filming includes the obtaining of multiple radiographs in various projections including prone, supine, and both lateral decubitus views. A smooth inner lining to the cyst wall in association with normal cytology and a lack of fat in the aspirate all point to a diagnosis of benignity. In a 5-year period, we have not seen a single case of a mass diagnosed as a benign cyst by this method which later proved to be a tumor.

Figures 1 to 5 demonstrate a series of flow diagrams showing how we attempt to integrate, in a logical or algorithmic fashion, the various diagnostic modalities available for the discrimination of renal masses. The facts determining the selection of the next most appropriate examination are depicted in the form of a decision-making tree. To illustrate: After the intravenous urogram, a decision must be reached regarding the presence or absence of a renal mass (Fig. 1). If

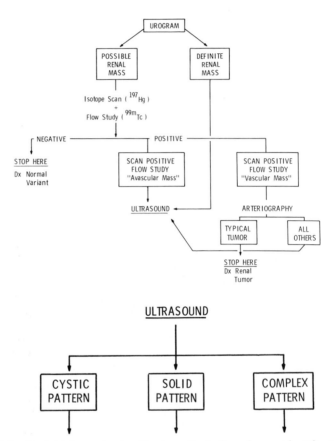

FIG. 1 *(top)*. — Initial step in algorithmic method of renal mass identification. Used only when the presence of a mass is equivocal on urography.

FIG. 2 *(bottom)*. — Ultrasound provides excellent method of initial "triage" of masses. Of those demonstrating cystic pattern, 90 per cent will prove to be simple renal cysts, and these are immediately sequestered from the remaining more significant lesions.

such a mass is questionable, then the next examination performed is a renal scan using, preferably, ^{197}Hg chlormerodrin. If this examination proves negative, then the investigation is halted at this point and it is presumed that a normal variant in the contour of the kidney exists. We have seen no false results in 33 cases evaluated in this way. A positive examination at this stage indicates the presence of a definite renal mass, and the procedure from that point on is similar to that followed for any renal mass with the following exception: If the patient is still in the nuclear medicine department and a flow study is elected (which we consider to be an optional procedure), the demonstration of a vascular mass will allow the patient to go directly to arteriography with the elimination of all intermediate steps. A negative flow study is of little help, as pointed out previously.

After the intravenous urogram has demonstrated the presence of a definite renal mass, we perform ultrasound as the next examination (Fig. 2). In our experience, ultrasound has proved an extremely effective "triage" agent since it allows immediate separation of fluid-filled from solid and mixed masses. This examination is noninvasive, painless, rapid, relatively inexpensive, and has an initial accuracy rate of between 90 and 95 per cent. It, too, like the other studies previously described, may be performed easily on outpatients. The subsequent method of evaluation following ultrasound depends upon the type of sonic pattern disclosed.

If a cystic pattern is demonstrated, nephrotomography is the next procedure of choice (Fig. 3). If the findings of a typical renal cyst are revealed, this diagnosis is probable with a 95 per cent confidence

FIG. 3.—Renal masses showing a cystic pattern on ultrasound are studied next by nephrotomography. If typical cyst findings are disclosed by this method also, diagnosis of simple cyst is extremely likely. Aspiration with double contrast cystography is desirable as a confirmatory study, but is not mandatory. If the tomographic findings are not classical, however, aspiration is imperative.

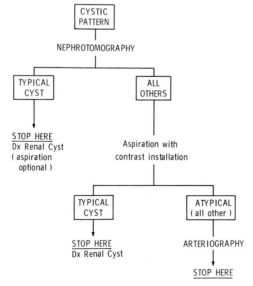

level. Although there are those who recommend discontinuing the
diagnostic protocol at this point, we prefer to go on to renal cyst aspiration wherever practicable in an attempt to raise the diagnostic accuracy rate as close to 100 per cent as possible. If, however, even 1 of
the typical features of renal cyst is lacking by nephrotomography,
then aspiration with contrast instillation becomes mandatory. Although most such cases will prove to be renal cysts which, for technical or other reasons, did not result in typical nephrotomograms, an
occasional inflammatory cyst or even a cystic neoplasm may be overlooked if further study is not done. These unusual lesions will be
disclosed following renal cyst aspiration and double contrast cystography. If the findings on double contrast cystography are equivocal
or in any way suggest the presence of abnormality of the inner wall,
arteriography is recommended to rule out the presence of a cystic
type of tumor. This is an unusual combination of findings which also
may be seen in some hematomas or multilocular cysts.

If a complex pattern is disclosed by nephrosonography, then once
again nephrotomography is the procedure of next choice (Fig. 4). It is
difficult to predict what the examination will reveal in this group.
Many possibilities exist. A cyst for example, if loculated or infected,

FIG. 4.—Flow diagram for renal masses having a complex ultrasonic pattern. Some
of these cases will be renal cysts, in which case the nephrotomogram will provide pre-
sumptive evidence of such a diagnosis. Many, however, will represent more formidable
lesions such as necrotic tumors or abscesses. Here again, nephrotomography will prove
invaluable in pointing out the direction of the necessary ancillary studies.

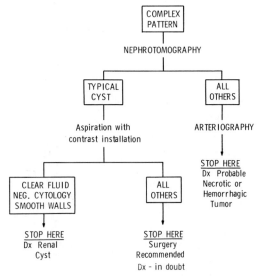

could easily account for these findings. Therefore, aspiration is done if typical cyst findings are present. If the cytology is negative and the walls are smooth, the investigation is concluded. In all other circumstances, that is, if the cytologic examination is abnormal or if there is irregularity, surgery is recommended. The presence of bloody fluid or calcification in the wall of the presumed cyst also may be an acceptable indication for surgical exploration, although it must be realized that numerous examples of calcification and bloody fluid are recorded with benign cysts. If nephrotomography is not typical for a benign renal cyst, we believe that arteriography should be performed next because of the appreciable number of necrotic and cystic renal tumors which can produce complex patterns. At times, there may be valid indications to deviate from this general approach. For example, the nephrotomogram may clearly demonstrate the presence of previously unsuspected polycystic disease. If this is so, then further studies usually are unnecessary. Each case must be individualized. Under certain circumstances, it is conceivable that aspiration might be the next recommended procedure. This, of course, depends on the integration of all available information – tomographic, ultrasonic, and clinical. At this point in the evaluation of masses, the number of cases in which a definite diganosis cannot be rendered should be less than 15 per cent and the accuracy rate in the remaining cases should approximate 100 per cent.

The disclosure of a solid pattern by ultrasound indicates that a renal mass is almost certainly a neoplasm. The only exceptions to

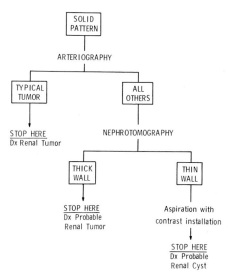

FIG. 5. – Flow diagram for renal masses having solid ultrasonic pattern is geared toward arteriography. Almost all such masses will be tumors, but occasional confusion may be produced by small cysts or hypovascular neoplasms. Nephrotomography may serve to distinguish between the two.

this which we have seen have been those cysts measuring less than 2.5 cm. in diameter which have been confused with adjacent normal renal parenchyma. Arteriography should be the procedure employed next (Fig. 5). If the renal arteriogram confirms the suspicion of tumor, the evaluation is then complete from the diagnostic standpoint. If, however, angiography does not conclusively demonstrate the presence of a tumor, other studies should be employed since there is still a possibility, albeit small, that a renal cyst exists. The disclosure of a thick wall by nephrotomography will sometimes confirm the suspicion of an avascular tumor which was not demonstrable at arteriography. The demonstration of a thin wall, however, either alone or in combination with other cyst characteristics, will suggest the desirability of attempted renal cyst aspiration. It should be pointed out that we have successfully aspirated renal cysts as small as 2 cm. in diameter without difficulty using the ultrasonic approach. Under certain conditions, however, especially with an obese patient, a high lying kidney, or an upper pole lesion, it may not be possible to aspirate such a small lesion and exploratory surgery may be necessary to establish the identity of the mass.

We have studied 196 real and potential renal masses by the diagnostic protocol outlined (Table 1). In only 20 cases was the diagnosis still indefinite after all of the recommended studies had been performed. Surgery was necessary in these cases since a tumor could not be conclusively ruled out. In only 1 of these 20 cases was a neoplasm discovered. The other 12 tumors in this group of patients were detected early in the work-up. By strongly urging surgery when results are indeterminate, we feel that the likelihood of overlooking an atypical renal tumor is removed. In all cases, a final diagnosis was available based either on surgical or autopsy proof, a follow-up period of not less than 3 years in the nonoperated cases, or cyst aspiration

Table 1

Distribution of Masses Evaluated by Systematized Approach

Cyst	130
Pseudotumor	33
Tumor	13
Hydronephrosis	6
Polycystic disease	5
Abscess	4
Hematoma	4
Perirenal pseudocyst	1
Total	196

Table 2
Types and Accuracy of Diagnostic Studies in Renal Masses

	Urog-raphy	Renal Scan	Ultra-sound	Nephro-tomog-raphy	Needle Punct.	Arteriog-raphy	No. of Cases	Definitive Diagnosis Rendered	Number Rendered Correctly	Diagnosis Indefinite	
Preliminary	Yes	Yes	No	No	No	No	33	31(95%)	31(100%)	2(5%)	9 scans positive
Step I	Yes	No	Yes	No	No	No	163	139(85%)	130(93%)	24(15%)	22 scans negative
Step II a	Yes	No	Yes	Yes	No	No	140	125(90%)	119(95%)	15(10%)	
Step II b	Yes	No	Yes	No	No	Yes	5	5(100%)	5(100%)	—	All 5 were carcinomas
Step III a	Yes	No	Yes	Yes	Yes	No	66	61(92%)	61(100%)	5(8%)	5 cases technically unsatisfactory
Step III b	Yes	No	Yes	Yes	No	Yes	16	10(60%)	8(80%)	6(40%)	
Step IV	Yes	No	Yes	Yes	Yes	Yes	5	3(60%)	3(100%)	2(40%)	
Total							196	176(90%)	176(100%)*	20(10%)	

*Incorrect diagnosis assigned only if patient with life-threatening lesion was treated for clinically less-significant lesion.

studies, the results of which we accept as conclusive. The choice of 3 years as an adequate follow-up period is of course arbitrary, but we believe that most false-negative studies will come to light within that time. Although a few minor mistakes in diagnosis were made, such as diagnosing an infected renal cyst as an abscess, in no instance was a potential life-threatening lesion such as a tumor falsely diagnosed as a less significant lesion such as a cyst. Since the basic purpose of the protocol was to separate benign lesions from the potentially more serious ones, a diagnosis was considered correct insofar as this was accomplished satisfactorily. Equally important is the fact that most masses were completely evaluated on an outpatient basis, often in a single afternoon. As a result, great savings in economy as well as in utilization of medical resources were realized, not the least of which derived from the avoidance of unnecessary exploratory surgery. Table 2 summarizes, step by step, the diagnostic accuracy which was realized at each level of the systematized method of renal mass evaluation.

Analysis of the distribution of masses included in this study indicates that cysts and pseudotumors predominate by far. Significantly, these are the 2 entities which can most simply and expediently be separated from the remaining lesions, thus allowing more time and energy to be directed toward those masses most likely to be of the greatest clinical significance.

Summary

By use of a flow diagram or logic chart, a sequence of the most appropriate studies necessary for determining the nature of a given renal mass is developed. By following this schema, developed during the evaluation of approximately 200 renal masses, duplication of studies is avoided, hospitalization and cost are minimized, complications are lessened, radiation exposure is reduced, and conservative treatment for benign lesions is encouraged. The expeditious identification of innocuous lesions allows medical resources to be concentrated on the potentially more serious masses. An accuracy rate approaching 100 per cent may be anticipated in the ability to separate life-threatening renal masses from all others.

REFERENCES

Adelman, B. P.: Angiomyolipoma of the kidney. *The American Journal of Roentgenology, Radium Therapy and Nuclear Medicine*, 95:403–405, October 1965.

Bosniak, M. A., and Faegenburg, D.: The thick-wall sign: An important finding in nephrotomography. *Radiology*, 84:692–698, April 1965.

Cope, V., Hackett, M., and Raphael, M. J.: Some observations on the value of excretion urography in the detection of renal tumors. *British Journal of Urology*, 37:691–693, December 1965.

Daniel, W. W., Hartman, G. W., and Witten, D. M.: Calcified renal masses. *Radiology*, 103:503–508, June 1972.

Dautrebande, J., Duckett, C., and Roy, P.: Claw sign of cortical cysts in renal arteriography. *Journal of Canadian Association of Radiologists*, 18:240–250, March 1967.

Evans, J.: The accuracy of diagnostic radiology, arteriography and nephrotomography. *The Journal of the American Medical Association*, 204:223–226, April 15, 1968.

Evans, J. A., and Bosniak, M.A.: *The Kidney*. 1st edition. Chicago, Illinois, Year Book Medical Publishers, Inc., 1971, 382 pp.

Felson, B., and Moskowitz, M.: Renal pseudotumors: The regenerated nodule and other lumps, bumps and dromedary humps. *The American Journal of Roentgenology, Radium Therapy and Nuclear Medicine*, 107:720–729, December 1969.

Genereux, G. P.: The collateral vein sign in renal neoplasia. *Journal of Canadian Association of Radiologists*, 19:46–55, June 1968.

Goldberg, B. B., and Pollack, H. M.: Differentiation of renal masses using A-mode ultrasound. *Journal of Urology*, 105:765–771, June 1971.

————: Ultrasonically guided renal cyst aspiration. *Journal of Urology*, 109:5–7, January 1973.

Lalli, A.: *The Tailored Urogram*. 1st edition. Chicago, Illinois, Year Book Medical Publishers, Inc., 1973, 252 pp.

Lang, E. Johnson, B., Chance, H. L., Enright, J. R., Fontenot, R., Trichel, B. E., Wood, M., Brown, R., and St. Martin, E. C.: Assessment of avascular renal mass lesions. *Southern Medical Journal*, 65:1–10, January 1972.

Meaney, T. F.: Errors in angiographic diagnosis of renal masses. *Radiology*, 93:361–366, August 1969.

Pfister, R. E., and Shea, T. E.: Nephrotomography: Performance and interpretation. *Radiologic Clinics of North America*, 9:41–62, April 1971.

Pollack, H. M., Edell, S., and Morales, J. O.: Radionuclide imaging in renal pseudotumors. *Radiology*, 111:639–644, June 1974.

Pollack, H. M., and Goldberg, B. B.: Differentiating renal masses with ultrasound. *Medical World News*, pp. 31–32, 1973.

Reiss, M. D., Bookstein, J. J., and Bleifer, K. H.: Radiologic aspects of renovascular hypertension. Part 4: Arteriographic complications. *The Journal of the American Medical Association*, 221:374–378, July 24, 1972.

Rosenthall, L.: Static and dynamic renal imaging. *Current Problems in Radiology*, 1:3–50, May–June 1971.

Watson, R. C., Fleming, R. J., and Evans, J. A.: Arteriography in the diagnosis of renal carcinoma: Review of 100 cases. *Radiology*, 91:886–887, November, 1968.

Radiologic Diagnosis of Early Gastric Cancer

HIDETAKA DOI, M.D.
*Department of Diagnostic Radiology, National Cancer
Center, Tokyo, Japan*

GASTRIC CANCER is one of the 3 major causes of mortality in adults in Japan. This compelled us to look for advanced diagnostic technology in order to detect gastric cancer at an early stage.

At present, the most important method of improving the survival rate of gastric cancer patients is the detection of the disease at an early stage when there is minimal invasion and no metastasis. Our statistics clearly indicate that there is a distinct relationship between the survival rate and the depth of cancerous invasion in the gastric wall. Table 1 and Figure 1 indicate this relationship.

Table 1
Five-year Survival Rate in Relation to the Depth of Cancerous Invasion

	Invasion	Deaths	Survivors	Survival Rate (%)
Early Cancer	Mucosa	7	113	94.2
	Submucosa	21	99	82.5
	Muscularis propria	42	56	57.1
Advanced Cancer	Subserosa	109	96	46.8
	Serosa	532	157	22.8
Totals		711	521	42.2

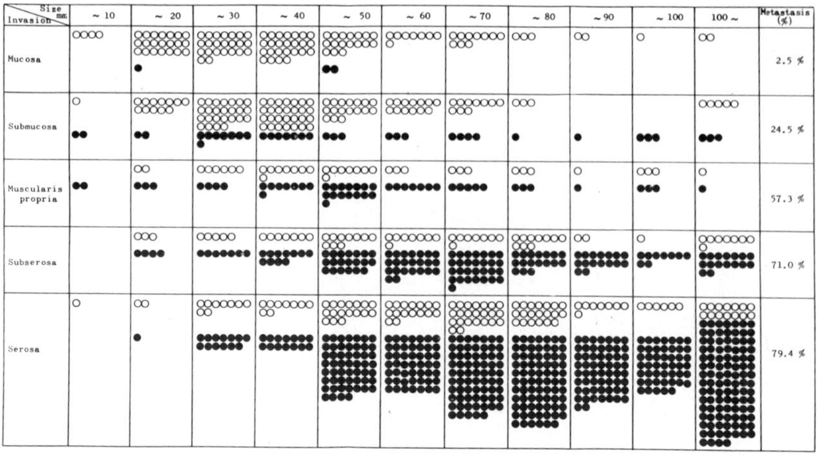

FIG. 1.—Size and invasion of gastric cancer. Open circles, metastases (−); closed circles, metastasis (+).

Definition and Classification of Early Gastric Cancer

According to the Japanese Endoscopic Society, early gastric cancer is defined as that in which the cancerous invasion is limited to the mucosa only, or to the mucosal and submucosal layers, regardless of whether there is regional lymph node metastasis. The reason is that preoperative diagnosis cannot determine lymph node metastasis.

Our statistical study indicates that the 5-year survival rate in patients with early gastric cancer is as high as 92 per cent. In patients who have deeper invasion such as into the muscle layer, the rate is 57 per cent. In patients with deep invasion into the serosa, the rate decreases to 28 per cent, which corresponds to the rate for patients with regional lymph node metastasis.

Early gastric cancer is classified according to the characteristic appearance of the mucosal surface. When the lesion is obviously prominent on the mucosa, it is classified as Type I or the protruded

FIG. 2.—Macroscopic classification of early gastric cancer.

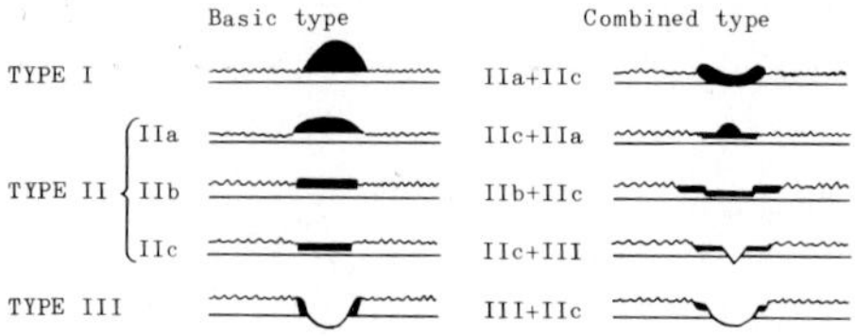

Table 2
Lesions by Type

Type I	Protruded Type. Protrusion into the gastric lumen is very obvious.
Type II	Superficial Type. Unevenness of the surface is relatively inconspicuous. In this category, the following 3 types are included:
Type IIa	Elevated Type. The surface is slightly elevated.
Type IIb	Flat Type. There is no recognizable elevation or depression from the surrounding mucosal surface.
Type IIc	Depressed Type. The surface is slightly depressed.
Type III	Excavated Type. An excavation in the gastric wall is prominent.

type. When the lesion is almost flat, it is classified as Type II, or the superficial type. This type is further divided into 3 subtypes. When the lesion is only slightly elevated from the mucosa when compared with Type I, it is classified as the superficial elevated type (Type IIa). When the level of the lesion is almost the same as the mucosal layer, this is the flat type (Type IIb). When the lesion is slightly depressed under visual observation, we classify this as the superficial depressed type (Type IIc). When the lesion shows a fairly deep excavation, it is classified as the excavated type (Type III). This classification is founded on the macroscopic appearance of the lesion. In practice, we often encounter cases which show a mixed pattern. These lesions may be described by combined classifications such as IIc+IIa (Fig. 2, Table 2).

Clinical Material

The age distribution of early gastric cancer patients at operation is about 10 years younger than the age at death from gastric cancer (Fig. 3). This may suggest that it takes about 10 years for the cancer to be fatal. The sex ratio for early cases does not differ from that for advanced cases (Table 3).

From 1962 to 1972, 2,463 patients with gastric cancer underwent operation in our hospital. Of these, 535 are classified as early cancer (approximately 22 per cent) (Table 4). Since our hospital specializes in cancer, our detection rate of early cases is not high. By mass survey, early gastric cancer accounts for 40 per cent of detected cases (Table 5).

Since almost half of the cases of early gastric cancer are combined with ulcerative lesions, 46.5 per cent of these patients complain of epigastralgia. However, in 23.2 per cent of cases, there are no symptoms (cf. Tables 6 and 7).

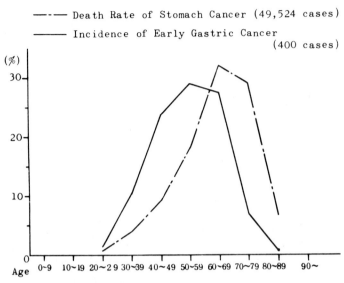

——·—— Death Rate of Stomach Cancer (49,524 cases)

——— Incidence of Early Gastric Cancer
(400 cases)

FIG. 3.—Age distribution of 400 early gastric cancer cases in comparison with death rate from stomach cancer in Japan in 1969.

In our hospital, fluoroscopic television examination is the initial survey, with a gastrocamera examination 1 week later. Of these 535 cases of early gastric cancer, 68 per cent were examined for some abnormality discovered by the mass survey or were referred by other clinics. Table 8 describes the means of detection in our patients. Of the cases, 8.7 per cent escaped detection by radiologic examination,

Table 3
Sex Ratio of 400 Cases of Early Gastric Cancer

Male:	251 cases (62.75%)
Female:	149 cases (37.25%)

Table 4
Incidence of Early Gastric Cancer (1962–1972)*

Early gastric cancer	535 Cases
Resectable cases of gastric cancer	2,463 Cases
Detection rate of early gastric cancer	21.7%

*National Cancer Center, Tokyo, Japan.

Table 5
Annual Statistics in Mass Survey of the Stomach (1969)*

Total Number Examined		1,539,521
Detected Disease:		
	Gastric Cancer	3,931 cases (0.26%)
	Gastric Polyp	6,835 cases (0.44%)
	Gastric Ulcer	41,686 cases (2.71%)
	Duodenal Ulcer	25,155 cases (1.63%)
	Gastric and	
	Duodenal Ulcer	2,709 cases (0.18%)
Early Gastric Cancer		
	40.5% of Gastric Cancer	

°Japanese Society of Gastric Mass Survey.

Table 6
Incidence of 499 Cases by Type

	Type	No. Cases	%
I	Protruded Type	69	(13.8)
IIa	Elevated Type	38	(7.6)
IIa + IIc		46	(9.2)
IIb	Flat Type	12	(2.4)
	(7 cases with ulcer)		
IIc	Depressed Type	223	(44.7)
IIc + III	(197 cases with ulcer)	65	(13.1)
III	Excavated Type	11	(2.2)
III + IIc		35	(7.0)
Total		499	(100.0)

Table 7.
Initial Symptom of 535 Cases of Early Gastric Cancer

Symptom	No. Cases	%
No Complaint	124	(23.2)
Epigastralgia or Hunger Pain	249	(46.5)
Discomfort or Nausea	99	(18.5)
Weight Loss	4	(0.8)
Anorexia	17	(3.2)
Others	42	(7.8)
Total	535	(100.0)

and 6.1 per cent could not be found using both radiologic and gastro-camera examinations. However, cases overlooked with our routine examinations were found by the follow-up studies. Only 2 cases among 535 were not detected in the early stage.

Table 8.
Means of Detection in 535 Cases of Early Gastric Cancer

Source	No. Cases	%
Mass Survey or Referred by Other Clinics	364	(68.0)
Routine Radiologic Study	125	(23.3)
Additional Routine Gastrocamera Study	14	(2.6)
Follow-Up Study	30	(5.7)
Other	2	(0.4)
Total	535	(100.0)

Radiographic Technique

The positioning of the patient and the technique of our routine radiographic examination is conducted in the following sequence:

1. Mucosal study with about 30 cc. of barium with the patient in a prone position.

2. PA and right anterior oblique projections of the esophagus with the patient in an upright position.

3. PA view of the barium-filled stomach with the patient in an upright position.

4. Right anterior oblique projection of the barium-filled stomach with the patient in an upright position.

4'. Swallowing of the vesicant to produce approximately 300 cc. of gas.

5. Barium-filled stomach studied with the patient in a prone position.

6. Double contrast study of the gastric angle with the patient in a supine position.

7. Double contrast study of the antrum with the patient in a 45° right-side-up position.

8. Double contrast study of the gastric body with the patient in a 45° left-side-up and head-down position.

9. Double contrast study of the cardiac region with the patient in a 45° semierect position in the left anterior oblique projection.

10. PA view with the patient in an upright position.

SPECIAL NOTES ON THE DOUBLE CONTRAST TECHNIQUE

In radiographic diagnosis of early gastric cancer, the double contrast technique is essential for a clear demonstration of superficial pathologic changes. For example, a barium-filled stomach may show a marginal pathologic lesion, as a niche or filling defect. In addition, it may present deformity of the viscus caused by an underlying lesion which is reflected by rigidity of the wall or shortening of the curvature. The advantage of the double contrast X-ray study over the barium-filled stomach examination is that it simultaneously demonstrates both the primary and secondary evidences of tumor.

Two important aspects of the double contrast study are first, the stomach should be adequately expanded with additional air through a stomach tube or by a vesicant if necessary; second, the gastric mucosa should be thinly and evenly coated with barium so that the network pattern of the mucosa appears clearly.

We recommend that a fairly large amount of viscous barium (about 300 cc. of 100 per cent barium suspension) be used for each patient. About 200 cc. of additional air is normally sufficient, but the amount is adjusted according to the fluoroscopic findings to meet individual requirements. In order to demonstrate the fine network pattern of the posterior wall clearly, the barium suspension must be made to adhere to the mucosa by repeated rotation of the patient. For double contrast study of the anterior wall, the patient is placed in the prone position. The amount of barium used is about 100 cc., of the same thickness as is used for examining the posterior wall, and the amount of additional air increases to about 400 cc. It is still necessary to rotate the patient in order to have barium adhere evenly to the mucosa.

When the lesion is located in the upper stomach, the patient is positioned about 30° semierect; for lower lesions, the patient is placed in approximately a 15° head-down position.

Radiographic Findings

Except for functional disorders, radiologic diagnosis of the gastrointestinal tract is dependent upon morphologic demonstration of mucosal abnormalities. Therefore, the degree to which findings can by analyzed depends upon the capability of demonstrating the lesion radiographically.

Type I (Protruded Type)

This type may be categorized roughly into 2 different histological origins: one is a so-called polypoid carcinoma which resembles a pedunculated adenoma, and the second has a rounded shape but no stalk.

According to our statistics, when the head of a pedunculated polyp was less than 2 cm. in diameter, none of 54 lesions studied was malignant. When the diameter was larger than 2 cm., 4 of 11 cases showed malignant change of early carcinoma. For the rounded, sessile mass, when the diameter of protrusion was less than 2 cm., 14 of 82 cases (17.1 per cent) had early stage malignant disease. When larger than 2 cm. in diameter, we found 28 early gastric cancer lesions and 18 advanced lesions among 53 cases. This rate of malignancy is 86.7 per cent. Malignant lesions generally show a rough irregular mucosa which occasionally has shallow erosion.

Important considerations in radiographic diagnosis of the protruded type are shape, size, and surface appearance.

Type IIa (Superficial Elevated Type)

Since Type IIa has a lesser degree of elevation when compared to Type I, radiographic findings are characterized by a small, flat filling defect without a stalk. They are generally irregularly shaped with an uneven surface reflecting shallow erosion. To differentiate this from a submucosal tumor, a bridging fold should be demonstrated.

Type IIb (Superficial Flat Type)

Because the Type IIb lesion has no difference in elevation from the surrounding mucosa, it is extremely difficult to detect by radiographic examination or endoscopy. Characteristic findings of this lesion are unevenness of size and shape of the area gastrica and space occupation in the mucosa. Radiographically, this lesion shows an unmatched rough mucosal pattern with barium adherence. Discoloration and loss of the normal glossy appearance may be seen by endoscopy.

Type IIc (Superficial Depressed Type)

This type had the highest incidence of about 58 per cent. Since 71 per cent of this type are associated with ulceration, detection of the lesion is relatively easy. Type IIc has a shallow depression with various-sized nodules in the depressed area. Mucosal folds are abruptly interrupted at the periphery of the depression. The tips of the interrupted folds are slightly enlarged with a bulging shape and concavity toward the center. The depressed area is usually surrounded by the steplike shelf. Conversely, a benign ulcer has smooth folds radiating from the center with no evidence of interruption, indentation, or notching.

TYPE III (EXCAVATED TYPE)

This type is rather difficult to differentiate from a benign peptic ulcer since often there is no cancerous change at the bottom of the ulcer while only the ulcer margin presents a bandlike, shallow cancerous depression. This finding corresponds to the irregular narrow space between the end of the mucosal folds and the ulcer margin seen radiographically. With close observation, interruption of converging mucosal folds with concave ends should be noted. Potential confusion with healing stages of benign ulcers is easily understandable.

DIFFERENTIAL DIAGNOSIS

Recently, "atypical epithelium" which resembles Type IIa or IIc lesions has presented a problem for us. This is not classified histologically as cancer because the structural atypia is not suficiently disordered. For these cases, the diagnosis may be confirmed only by biopsy.

Another problem is "reactive lymphoid hyperplasia" which may be confused with Type IIc lesions, as both have a shallow mucosal depression. The major points of difference from Type IIc are that the mucosal depression does not have a sharp demarcation, and it is associated with multiple ulcers within the shallow depression. Radiographic diagnosis may be possible but, usually, biopsy is required. Histologically, these lesions show focal hyperplasia of the lymphoid tissue in the submucosa with no cancerous invasion.

Summary

At present, the most promising means of improving the 5-year survival rate of patients with gastric cancer is to detect the lesion at the earliest possible stage. Our statistics clearly indicate that the double contrast radiologic technique is essential in the detection of early gastric cancer, especially Type IIc.

It is my opinion that the radiographic diagnosis of early gastric cancer is not overly difficult when an adequate radiologic study is obtained. In addition, endoscopy with biopsy or cytologic techniques are valuable in diagnosis. However, atypical epithelium and reactive lymphoid hyperplasia have recently presented a problem because they are difficult to differentiate radiographically from early gastric cancer.

REFERENCES

Ichikawa, H.: Differential diagnosis between benign and malignant ulcers of the stomach. In *Clinics in Gastroenterology*. London, England, W. B. Saunders, Co., Ltd., 1973, pp. 329–343.

Ichikawa, H., Yamada, T., and Doi, H.: *Practice of X-ray Diagnosis of the Stomach—Particularly for the Detection of Early Cancer*. Tokyo, Japan, Bunkodo Co., Ltd., 1964.

Kuru, M., Editor: *Atlas of Early Carcinoma of the Stomach*. Tokyo, Japan, Nakayama Shoten Co., Ltd., 1967, 240 pp.

Murakami, T., Editor: *Early Gastric Cancer*. Tokyo, Japan, Tokyo University Press, 1971, pp. 27–44, 93–142.

Shirakabe, H., Editor: *Atlas of X-ray Diagnosis of Early Gastric Cancer*. Tokyo, Japan, Igaku-Shoin Co., Ltd., 1966, 244 pp.

————: *Double Contrast Studies of the Stomach*. Tokyo, Japan, Bunkodo Co., Ltd., 1971, pp. 11–52, 209–218.

Gastroscopic and Radiologic Patterns in Gastric Lymphoma

ROBERT S. NELSON, M.D., and
FRANK L. LANZA, M.D.
*Department of Medicine, The University of Texas
System Cancer Center M. D. Anderson Hospital and
Tumor Institute, Houston, Texas and Hillcroft Clinic,
Houston, Texas*

THE RADIOLOGIC AND GASTROSCOPIC CHARACTERISTICS of gastric lymphoma have seldom been compared or correlated. There are many roentgenologic studies, but few include a significant number of patients in whom gastroscopy was also used in diagnosis (Culver, Bean, and Berens, 1955; Dixon and Shonyo, 1949; Favis and Saltzstein, 1964; Ferris, 1964; Frazer, 1959; Friedman, 1959; Garvie, 1965, Guest, 1961; Jacobs, 1963; Jensen, 1967; Joseph and Lattes, 1966; Marshall and Meissner, 1950; Masley, 1959; McNeer and Berg, 1959; Ochsner and Ochsner, 1955; Ruffin, 1950, Snoddy, 1952; Swain, 1961; Taylor, 1939; Tesler, 1959; Thorbjarnarson, Beal, and Pearce, 1956; Thorbjarnarson, Pearce, and Beal, 1959; Welborn, Ponka, and Rebuck, 1965; Worferth, Brady, Enterline, and Blakemore, 1959). In the largest previous series in which both methods were employed, neither procedure was particularly accurate in differentiating the gross appearances of these lesions from other gastric pathologic abnormalities, malignant or benign. Gastroscopic color photography was used for the first time with the purpose of determining whether further prospective study might be helpful in comparison and correlation (Nelson and Lanza, 1968). The present report deals with a

255

somewhat larger group of patients with gastric lymphoma in whom both gastroscopy and roentgenoscopy were used comparatively. Gastroscopic color photographs as well as the conventional roentgenograms were obtained in each patient.

Patient Material and Methods

All patients with gastric lymphoma admitted to The University of Texas System Cancer Center M. D. Anderson Hospital and Tumor Institute during the period July, 1967, to October, 1973, who had both radiologic and gastroscopic examinations, were included. There were 32 patients, 15 with primary and 17 with generalized disease. Of these, 25 had reticulum cell sarcoma, 5 lymphocytic sarcoma, and 2 were listed as unclassified. Roentgenoscopic examinations were for the most part performed in the Department of Diagnostic Radiology, although a few had records from other hospitals. Gastroscopy was performed in all these patients at M. D. Anderson Hospital with the Olympus GFBK and GIF fiberoptic instruments. Gastroscopic color photographs of each patient were obtained with the Olympus external camera, and biopsies were taken in all patients. Gastroscopic follow-up studies were carried out in a few individuals at varying intervals. Retrospective comparisons of the radiographic and gastroscopic findings were carefully made in each case.

Results

Diagnoses were judged correct if the firm opinion of "lymphoma" or "probable lymphoma" was given, regardless of the differential considered by either gastroscopy or roentgenoscopy. By these standards, there were 19 tumors correctly diagnosed by radiological examination and 24 by gastroscopy. Of the incorrect results, roentgenoscopy yielded 3 negative, 6 diagnosed as carcinoma, and 4 diagnosed as gastritis or benign ulcer; gastroscopic errors included 7 evaluated as carcinoma and 1 as gastritis.

Classification of Gross Findings

LARGE FOLDS. — These occurred in the majority of patients and appeared to be the major means of differentiation by roentgenoscopy. They were also noted on gastroscopy. The characteristics of the folds, such as rigidity, nodularity, or ulceration, were prime considerations of the latter method, although they were mentioned in a number of cases in radiologic descriptions as well. The direct feel of a large fold when biopsied afforded a gastroscopic clue in some cases.

LARGE INFILTRATIVE MASSES. —Lymphomatous masses were hard to distinguish from carcinoma in most patients, although they tended to take more bizarre shapes and, unlike carcinoma, were polypoid in very few instances. In lymphoma, major distortions appeared with relatively smooth overlying mucosa more often than in carcinoma.

ULCERATIONS. — In a few patients, ulcer was the most prominent finding although in most, abnormal folds predominated. Ulcers occurred in a few instances as large, deep, and surrounded by rolled, heaped-up edges. In others, superficial necrosis of the tops of heavy folds predominated. In general, they did not resemble benign ulcers, mainly because of the heavy submucosal infiltrate produced by the lymphoma.

VOLCANO-LIKE CRATER ULCERS. —This peculiar lesion was noted only in reticulum cell sarcoma, appeared in approximately 30 per cent of those seen, and was associated with massive involvement of the stomach. The ulcerations were round, for the most part, and seemed to develop initially at the level of the mucosa and to gradually rise, giving the final appearance of a smoothly tapered volcano with the ulcer at the top. In several such patients serially evaluated, it became clear with time that these lesions represented only the "tip of the iceberg," and that massive submucosal infiltrate also was present. "Volcano" ulcers often were associated with small polypoid or more conventional-appearing ulcerative lesions. They appear to be pathognomonic, when found, for reticulum cell sarcoma, and one of the few reliable gross clues in gastric lymphoma of any type. Small lesions of this type were not demonstrated roentgenographically.

ATYPICAL LESIONS. —Occasionally gastric lymphoma may be completely atypical by both gastroscopy and roentgenoscopy. Two such cases appeared to be gastritis and other multiple benign ulcerations; these occurred in patients with generalized disease. Biopsy was the only determining factor.

GASTROSCOPIC BIOPSY. —Suspicion of lymphoma may be confirmed at present in better than 80 per cent of all patients by gastroscopic biopsy. Despite the submucosally infiltrative nature of most lesions, adequate biopsy technique is highly successful.

Discussion

Comparison of the results obtained with a previous study (Nelson and Lanza, 1968) shows considerable improvement in diagnosis by both gastroscopy and roentgenography. In the primary gastric lymphoma group, gastroscopy was correct in 1 of 11 patients, and roentgenoscopy in 5 of 11 previously studied; in the present study, gastroscopy was correct in 10 of 15 and roentgenoscopy in 7 of 15. In the patients with generalized lymphoma and stomach involvement, radiologic examination diagnosed 7 of 12, and gastroscopy 11 of 12 in the earlier study, compared to 12 of 17 by roentgenoscopy, and 15 of 17 by gastroscopy in the present study. This improvement in accuracy appears to be the result of increased awareness of certain gross features of the disease as demonstrated by both methods, as well as the opportunity to compare roentgenograms and gastroscopic color photographs retrospectively. In general, gastroscopic characteristics seemed slightly more definite than radiologic ones, and many more smaller lesions were seen gastroscopically than radiologically. The X-ray examination will continue to be the main screening device, however, and the first signs of pathologic abnormality will usually be obtained in this manner. An alert department of radiology can help immeasurably in diagnosis by suggesting referral for endoscopy in suspicious cases. The most common source of error, about equally divided between the 2 methods, is the diagnosis of carcinoma rather than lymphoma. The "volcano crater ulcer," best seen by gastroscopy in 30 per cent of reticulum cell sarcoma patients (the most common type of gastric lymphoma noted in the majority of publications), is perhaps the most definitive clue, followed by the presence of large, nodular, and irregular folds. In generalized lymphoma, any gastric pathology should be evaluated by both methods, and particularly by gastric biopsy, bearing in mind the rare atypical findings resembling gastritis or benign ulcer in 3 of our patients, all of whom had positive biopsies.

The value of a nonoperative or preoperative diagnosis is considerable in the case of gastric lymphoma. Both radiology and gastroscopy can assist in determining the extent of involvement and the possibility of resection in primary disease, especially in aged or poor-risk patients. In generalized lymphoma, gastric lesions often produce severe morbidity and present a parameter for determination of effectiveness of treatment best assessed by these means. Gastroscopic biopsy, now readily available, is presently more than 80 per cent accurate in our experience, allowing histologic confirmation of atypical lesions. The routine employment of all these modalities has increased the accuracy of diagnosis considerably.

REFERENCES

Culver, G. J., Bean, B. C., and Berens, D. L.: Gastric lymphoma. *Radiology*, 65:518–528, October 1955.

Dixon, C. F., and Shonyo, E. S.: Differential diagnosis of sarcoma of the stomach. In *Sugical Clinics of North America*, Philadelphia, Pennsylvania, W. B. Saunders Co., 1949, pp. 1109–1113.

Favis, T. D., and Saltzstein, S. L.: Gastric lymphoid hyperplasia: A lesion confused with lymphosarcoma. *Cancer*, 17:207–212, February 1964.

Ferris, D. A.: *Gastric Sarcoma in Cancer of the Stomach.* Philadelphia, Pennsylvania, W. B. Saunders Co., 1964, pp. 158–162.

Frazer, J. W., Jr.: Malignant lymphomas of the gastrointestinal tract. *Surgery, Gynecology and Obstetrics*, 108:182–190, February 1959.

Friedman, A. I.: Primary lymphosarcoma of the stomach. A clinical study of seventy-five cases. *American Journal of Medicine*, 26:783–796, May 1959.

Garvie, W. H. H.: Leiomyosarcoma of the stomach. *British Journal of Surgery*, 52:32–38, January 1965.

Gastric lymphoma. *The Cancer Bulletin*, 14:49–51, May–June 1962.

Guest, J. L., Jr.: Lymphosarcoma of the stomach: A review and analysis of twenty-one cases. *Southern Medical Journal*, 54:175–179, February 1961.

Jacobs, D. S.: Primary gastric malignant lymphoma and pseudo-lymphoma. *American Journal of Clinical Pathology*, 40:379–394, October 1963.

Jensen, F. B.: Primary gastric sarcoma. *Acta Chirurgica Scandinavica*, 133:139–151, 1967.

Joseph, J. I., and Lattes, R.: Gastric lymphosarcoma. *American Journal of Clinical Pathology*, 45:653–669, June 1966.

Marshall, S. F., and Meissner, W. A.: Sarcoma of the stomach. *Annals of Surgery*, 131:824–837, June 1950.

Masley, P. M.: Leiomyosarcoma of the stomach. A review of ten cases. *American Journal of Digestive Diseases*, 4:792–811, October 1959.

McNeer, J., and Berg, J. W.: The clinical behavior and management of primary malignant lymphoma of the stomach. *Surgery*, 40:829–840, November 1959.

Nelson, R. S., and Lanza, F. L.: Endoscopy in the diagnosis of gastric lymphoma and sarcoma. *American Journal of Gastroenterology*, 50:37–46, July 1968.

Ochsner, S., and Ochsner, A.: Sarcoma of the stomach. Analysis of 17 cases. *Annals of Surgery*, 142:804–809, November 1955.

Ruffin, J.: Primary lymphosarcoma of the stomach with five-year survival after operation: Clinical, x-ray and gastroscopic features. *Gastroenterology*, 16:250–258, 1950.

Snoddy, W. T.: Primary lymphosarcoma of the stomach. *Gastroenterology*, 20:537–553, April 1952.

Swain, J.: Sarcoma of the stomach of lymphoid origin. *Medical Journal of Australia*, 48:479–481, September 16, 1961.

Taylor, E. S.: Primary lymphosarcoma of the stomach. *Annals of Surgery*, 110:200–221, August 1939.

Tesler, J.: Primary lymphosarcoma of the stomach. *American Journal of Gastroenterology*, 32:557–564, November 1959.

Thorbjarnarson, B., Beal, J. M., and Pearce, J. M.: Primary malignant lymphoid tumors of the stomach. *Cancer*, 9:712–717, July–August 1956.

Thorbjarnarson, B., Pearce, J. M., and Beal, J. M.: Sarcoma of the stomach. *American Journal of Surgery*, 97:36–42, January 1959.

Welborn, J. K., Ponka, J. L., and Rebuck, J. W.: Lymphoma of the stomach. A diagnostic and therapeutic problem. *Archives of Surgery*, 90:480–487, April 1965.

Wolferth, C. C., Jr., Brady, L. W., Enterline, H. T., and Blakemore, W. S.: Primary lymphosarcoma of the stomach. *Surgery, Gynecology and Obstetrics*, 109:755–761, December 1959.

CEA Antigen in the Management of Colonic and Rectal Carcinoma

RICHARD G. MARTIN, M.D.
*Department of Surgery, The University of Texas System
Cancer Center M. D. Anderson Hospital and Tumor
Institute, Houston, Texas*

In 1965, Doctors Phillip Gold and Samuel Freedman, at McGill University, isolated a substance believed to be an antigen from tumors arising from the entodermally derived digestive system epithelium. The same substance was also isolated from fetal colon tissue in the first 2 trimesters; because of this, the substance was called carcinoembryonic antigen (CEA). It was at this time considered to be tumor-specific, or at least organ-specific. This substance is obtained from plasma. The antigen is isolated using perchloric acid extraction, is dialyzed, and is precipitated with a gel solution and incubated with I^{125} and determined by using the gamma counter. This is a complicated radioimmune assay procedure that requires dialyzing for 18 hours. Each test takes approximately 2 working days to run.

Because of the belief that this substance was tumor-specific, the possibility of its use as a screening test immediately came to mind. However, like so many procedures, it could not be duplicated as to its specificity. The substance is a glucoprotein (glucosamine) with a molecular weight of 200,000, 45 per cent protein and 55 per cent carbohydrate. The antigen is measured in nanograms. One nanogram = 10 to the minus 9 grams. For the purpose of this study, any titer above 2.5 ng. has been considered significant.

The Hoffmann LaRoche Laboratories have studied specimens from over 10,000 patients during the past 3 years. They divided the studies into 3 protocols: (A) Cases with no previous history of carcinoma, (B) cases with no previous history of carcinoma and no evidence of any at the time of study, and (C) cases with obvious metastases. According to the group A protocol (Table 1), it can readily be seen that this is not a tumor- or organ-specific antigen. Carcinoma of the pancreas had the highest percentage of cases with a positive reading, with colon and rectum at approximately 72 per cent. Table 2 shows the results from studies of protocol B. Here again, it is obvious that benign lesions will show elevated titers. Of importance is the fact that patients with pancreatitis have elevated readings in 69.9 per cent of the cases; therefore, this prohibits CEA from being a good diagnostic tool in the differential diagnosis of carcinoma of the pancreas. The protocol C cases with obvious metastasis had almost 100 per cent positive readings. These studies led the Hoffman LaRoche Researchers to believe, as shown in Table 3, that those patients having titer between 2.6 and 5.1 are in a gray zone and really not too diagnostic. The majority of the benign lesions also fell in this range. Readings of 5.1 to 10 ng. showed a higher percentage to be positive for carcinoma so one could say this is beginning to be a strongly suggestive area, although, here again, many of the benign lesions

Table 1
Cases with No Previous History of Cancer

Site of Cancer	% Over 2.5 Ng.
Colon	72%
Lung	55%
Stomach	61%
Pancreas	90%
Breast	26%
Head and neck	19.5%
All others	20%

Table 2
Cases with No History of Previous Cancer and No Evidence of Any at Time of Study

Disease	% Over 2.5 Ng.
Pulmonary emphysema	40%
Alcoholic cirrhosis	29.2%
Ulcerative colitis	69.2%
Gastric ulcer	55%
Diverticulitis	70%
Pancreatitis	69.9%

also had titers in this range. Those cases with readings between 10 and 20 ng. became highly suspicious for cancer and anything over 20 ng. was almost invariably carcinoma. Also, those cases with titers of 20 or over frequently had liver metastases. In Table 4, the figures from the Hoffmann LaRoche study of CEA readings in patients who smoked are shown. It also shows that there is a definite increase in the number of positive titers among patients who smoke. This factor must be taken into consideration in interpreting CEA values. Table 5 shows the percentage of cases with positive readings when the carcinomas are broken down into the Dukes' A, B, or C classifications. It is disturbing to note that in the Dukes' groups A and B, only 40 per cent had a CEA value of 2.5 or above, whereas in group C, the more advanced cases, 90 per cent showed an elevated CEA reading. It is

Table 3

Significance of Titer Range

0.0– 2.5 ng.	Normal range
2.6– 5.1 ng.	Gray zone
5.1–10.0 ng.	Strongly suggestive
10.1–20.1 ng.	Highly suggestive
20.0 and over	Invariably has cancer

Table 4

Colonic and Rectal Carcinoma

Dukes' A and B	40% above 2.5 ng.
Dukes' C	90% above 2.5 ng.

Table 5

CEA and Smoking — Healthy Volunteers

	Titer Range	% Positive
Nonsmokers		
892 cases	0.0– 2.5 ng.	97%
	2.6– 5.0 ng.	3%
Former smokers		
235 cases	0.0– 2.5 ng.	93%
	2.6– 5.0 ng.	5%
	5.0–10.0 ng.	1%
	10.0 and over	1%
Active smokers		
620 cases	0.0– 2.5 ng.	81%
	2.6– 5.0 ng.	15%
	5.0–10.0 ng.	3%
	10.0 and over	1%

these early cases, groups A and B, that we are particularly interested in diagnosing before they develop into group C. As can be readily seen, these 2 groups show the poorest percentage of positive titers. Therefore, besides not being tumor-specific, the fact that early lesions often do not show positive titers makes the CEA antigen test a very poor screening device. How then can this test be of value in the management of carcinoma of the colon and rectum? We have at this institution been concentrating on following cases of known carcinoma of the colon and rectum over a long period of time with repeated CEA readings. We believe it is necessary to obtain readings before surgery, immediately after surgery, and at various intervals during the follow-up of the patient. If the patient has a high CEA reading which falls immediately after surgery to normal or near normal and remains at this level throughout the follow-up period, one is encouraged as to the prognosis in this case. If the CEA reading is moderately elevated in the so-called gray zone or under 10 ng. before surgery and remains so after surgery for a long period of time, one can possibly believe that factors other than the carcinoma may be contributing to the elevated CEA. This patient also probably will have a good prognosis. In those cases in which there is a significant drop in the titer following surgery, with a sharp rise during the follow-up period, one can almost invariably predict that the patient has recurrent or metastatic disease. This patient should be examined very carefully, to the extent that a second-look procedure possibly might be indicated. Those patients with an elevated CEA which falls only slightly and then continues to rise gradually most likely will have a poor prognosis with residual tumor present. CEA determinations are being obtained in our BCG and chemotherapy programs. It is too early to evaluate the use of this test in determining the effectiveness of the chemotherapy. To illustrate the value of following up patients with CEA titers, the following 5 cases are presented:

CASE 1. — The patient was a 66-year-old white male with carcinoma of the rectum proven by biopsy. An abdominoperineal resection was done in September 1972, at which time the lesion was classified as a Dukes' B lesion. It will be seen in Figure 1 that the preoperative CEA reading was 1.5 ng. It rose immediately following surgery to 2.9 ng. then fell back to 1.3 ng. Over the last year and 3 months it has remained below 1.0 ng. The patient's alkaline phosphatase, LDH, and SGOT levels have remained normal. He is not a smoker. Probably, this man has a good prognosis. The sharp rise in CEA titer immediately after surgery may indicate some liver damage resulting from the anesthetic agents. This phenomenon has been seen frequently in our series.

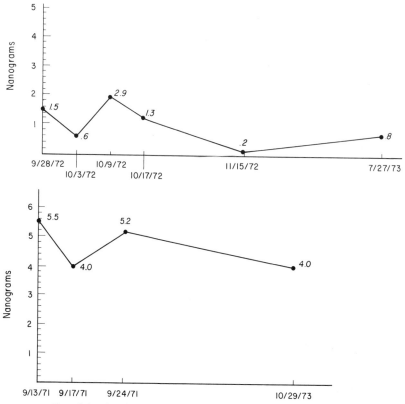

FIG. 1 *(top)*. — CEA readings, shown in nanograms, of Case 1.
FIG. 2 *(bottom)*. — CEA readings, shown in nanograms, of Case 2.

CASE 2. — This patient was another 66-year-old white male who in September 1971, had a right hemicolectomy for carcinoma of the cecum. The lesion extended through the serosa, but no lymph nodes or liver metastasis were noted. He had a 5.5 ng. reading before surgery (Fig. 2). It fell to 4.0 after surgery and then rose to 5.5. His last reading, approximately 2 years following surgery, was 4.0 ng. Clinically, there is no evidence of any recurrent disease. Liver function tests are still within normal limits. Although this man had an elevated CEA titer from the beginning, it has remained in the same approximate range. This man probably has a good prognosis, and the elevated CEA titer is caused by some factor other than the carcinoma of the colon.

CASE 3. — This 79-year-old man had 2 lesions, 1 a carcinoma of the rectum and 1 a carcinoma of the cecum. In March 1973, he had an AP resection and a right hemicolectomy. Two of 12 positive regional lymph nodes were found in the abdominoperineal specimen; no lymph nodes were noted in the cecal area. The liver showed no evidence of metastasis. Liver function tests were within normal limits. It is noted that this patient had an elevated CEA titer of 9.7 (Fig. 3). It fell after surgery to 5.4 ng. After falling to a low of 2.5 ng., it did rise in September 1973 to 4.4 ng. He has been asked to return in 4 months for repeat CEA reading. If this should continue upward, a second-look procedure might be indicated. If, however, it has dropped or remained the same with no clinical evidence of disease, only observation would be necessary.

CASE 4. — This 59-year-old man had a carcinoma of the right colon which extended through the serosa. At the time of surgery, no lymph nodes or liver metastasis were noted. In March 1973, he had a right hemicolectomy. At that time, the CEA reading was 7.8 (Fig. 4). It fell following surgery to 3.4, then 3.2. However, in July, 1973, he had had a notable rise to 8.0, although the liver functions were normal. The patient also had some clinical evidence of intestinal obstruction

FIG. 3. — CEA readings, shown in nanograms, of Case 3.

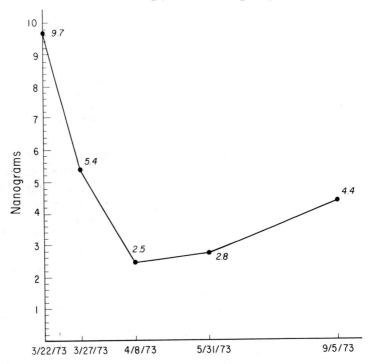

in the area of the ligament of Treitz; therefore, a second-look procedure was done and nonresectable nodes were noted in the area of the ligament of Treitz. The patient has been started on chemotherapy, but at the present, he is living in Mexico which makes follow-up rather difficult.

CASE 5. — This patient was a 76-year-old white male who, in March 1972, had an abdominoperineal resection for carcinoma of the rectum. The carcinoma extended through all layers into the surrounding tissue. No lymph nodes were noted however. At the time of surgery, his CEA reading was 1.4, dropping to 1.2 (Fig. 5). Two months following surgery it was 0.8 ng. At this time, his alkaline phosphatase, LDH, and SGOT levels were within normal limits. He was lost to follow-up from May 1972 until June 1973. At the time of his examination in June 1973, his CEA reading was well over 250. There was obvious metastatic disease involving the liver; he had an elevated alkaline phosphatase of 301, LDH 600, and SGOT 0.40. He was started on 5-fluorouracil, but there was no evidence of any decrease in CEA titer. He died in September 1973. This case stresses the necessity of frequent follow-up CEA studies. One should not wait a full

FIG. 4. — CEA readings, shown in nanograms, of Case 4.

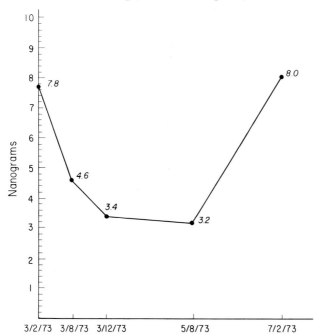

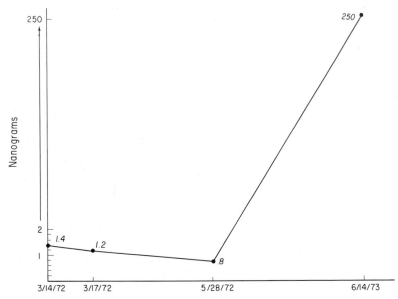

FIG. 5.—CEA readings, shown in nanograms, of Case 5.

year and probably, when possible, follow-up every 2 to 3 months would be more desirable.

In summary, the CEA test, although its exact nature or just what is being measured are not known, is an important test when serial readings are obtained. As a screening device it is not, unfortunately, specific enough to be of value. However, in following cases of carcinoma of the colon and rectum, it is a valuable aid because elevated CEA readings become important in the follow-up period if previous serial readings have been obtained.

Acknowledgment

The work in this report was supported in part by Hoffmann La-Roche Grant No. 168196.

REFERENCES

Dhar, P., Moore, T., Zamcheck, N., and Kupchik, H. Z.: Carcinoembryonic antigen (CEA) in colonic cancer. *The Journal of the American Medical Association*, 221:31–35, July 3, 1972.

Gold, P.: The role of immunology in human cancer research. *Canadian Medical Association Journal*, 103:1043–1051, Nov. 1, 1970.

_____: Tumor-specific antigen in GI cancer. *Hospital Practice,* 7(1):79–88, 1972.

Gold, P., and Freedman, S. O.: Specific carcinoembryonic antigens of the human digestive system. *The Journal of Experimental Medicine,* 122:467–481, September 1965.

Gold, P., Gold, M., and Freedman, S. O.: Cellular location of carcinoembryonic antigen of the human digestive system. *Cancer Research,* 28:1331–1334, July 1968.

Hansen, H. J., *et al.*: Carcinoembryonic Antigen (CEA) Assay: A Laboratory Adjunct in the Diagnosis and Management of Cancer. Hoffmann-LaRoche, Inc., New Jersey, 1973.

LeBel, S. J., Deodhar, S. D., and Brown, C. H.: Evaluation of a radioimmunossay for carcinoembryonic antigen of the human digestive system. *Cleveland Clinic Quarterly,* 39:25–31, Spring 1972.

_____: Newer concepts of cancer of the colon and rectum: Clinical evaluation of a radioimmunossay for CEA. *Diseases of the Colon and Rectum,* 15:111–115, March–April 1972.

Thompson, D. M. P., Krupey, J., Freedman, S. O., and Gold, P.: The radioimmunossay of circulating carcinoembryonic antigen of the human digestive system. *Medical Sciences,* 64:161–167, 1969.

Colonoscopy in the Detection of Colonic Cancer

NICHOLAS G. BOTTIGLIERI, M.D.

Department of Medicine, The University of Texas
System Cancer Center M. D. Anderson Hospital and
Tumor Institute, Houston, Texas; Present Address: The
American Cancer Society, Inc., 965 Hope Street,
Stanford, Connecticut

THE DEVELOPMENT OF THE AMAZINGLY EFFICIENT fibro-optic instrument has provided an additional method for examining the entire colon and rectum under direct vision as well as a means of biopsying lesions heretofore unreachable by standard proctosigmoidoscopy. Lesions seen through the colonoscope can be photographed in color easily, and some pedunculated colonic polyps can even be removed by the use of a cauterizing electrical current conducted by a wire snare which has been passed through a tubular lumen in the scope.

These instruments vary from about 86.5 to 186 cm. in length. The one we use has a functional length of 100 cm. and is a little over 1.4 cm. in diameter at its tip (Fig. 1). The illumination source is provided by a high-intensity xenon lamp; the light is carried through to the scope and through the entire length of the instrument via flexible bundles of very small glass strands (Fig. 2). The light source also contains a pump for the introduction of air or water through the instrument. Suction is provided by a simple connection to any standard vacuum apparatus. The tip of the scope can be flexed by remote manual controls to almost right angles in 4 directions. The biopsy forceps, the cytology brush, and polyp snare are all passed through a small channel built into the instrument (Fig. 3). The cautery source

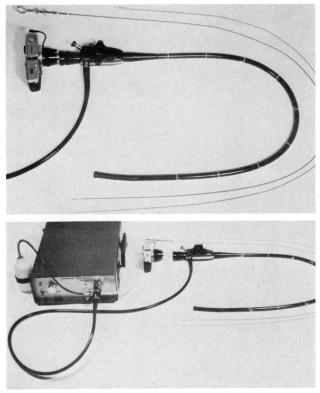

FIG. 1 *(top).*—Colonoscope, 100 cm. long with cytology brush and biopsy forceps. A 35-mm. camera may be attached to the head of the instrument as shown here.

FIG. 2 *(bottom).*—Colonoscope attached to light source which also contains a pump to be used for air insufflation or delivery of water through the instrument for use in cleaning the objective lens and the tip of the scope.

is small, easily portable, and includes a special cautery tipped suction tube for stopping postpolypectomy bleeding if necessary (Fig. 4).

It is not proposed that colonoscopy should replace radiographic studies of the large intestine because, indeed, there are cases where the colonoscope cannot be inserted properly because of problems such as a large redundant or sometimes a narrow serpiginous segment of the sigmoid colon in which the instrument will "curl" instead of advancing up the colon lumen normally; thus, the examination is incomplete.

However, because of technical difficulties, there are also instances when the radiologist's barium contrast study fails to demonstrate the cause of lower intestinal bleeding, such as a malignant tumor or a

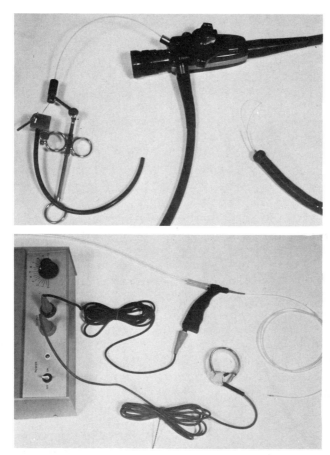

FIG. 3 *(top)*. — A polyp snare in position through a channel built into the shaft of the colonoscope.

FIG. 4 *(bottom)*. — Portable cautery source with cautery tipped suction tube.

bleeding benign polyp. In addition, it is sometimes difficult to differentiate radiographically between diverticulitis and carcinoma in the region of the lower portion of the descending colon, and biopsies obtained under direct vision at colonoscopy may, with relative ease, best provide the answer in these cases.

At our institution, we rely on our fine Radiology Department for the solution of day-to-day problems in the diagnosis of colonic disease, and we use colonoscopy primarily to obtain biopsies of "suspicious" lesions or to study further cases which cannot be clearly diagnosed by the usual contrast radiographic techniques. We do not perform colonoscopy in every case of colonic carcinoma which has already been demonstrated radiographically because of the resulting additional delay in definitive treatment and the added expense to the patient.

The procedure for colonoscopy may be very simple or very difficult depending upon anatomical and functional variations such as redundancy of the sigmoid, significant spasm of some colon segments, postsurgical adhesions, *etc*. With the patient in the left lateral decubitus position, the tip of the colonoscope is inserted up to the splenic flexure. If at that point there is any difficulty passing the scope farther, it may be necessary to turn the patient to the supine position; in most instances, however, the instrument can be inserted to its maximum extent with the patient lying on his left side. As the instrument is inserted, air or carbon dioxide may be used to insufflate the colon; the lumen of the bowel should always be kept in view before advancing farther. As the instrument is slowly withdrawn, a detailed examination of the colon and rectal mucosa is accomplished by appropriate insufflation of the bowel with air and by maneuvering the tip of the instrument so that all of the mucosa is seen. During recent examinations performed on approximately 100 patients by the staff of the gastroenterology service of our institution, the average distance from the anus that the 100-cm.-long instrument could be inserted into the colon was 76 cm., and the average time necessary to reach the point of maximum insertion was just less than 12 minutes. Most patients experienced mild-to-moderate discomfort from the procedure, but some had none. Most patients said that colonoscopy was not as uncomfortable as sigmoidoscopy.

When a lesion was identified, specimens for cytological examination were obtained by the brush technique and specimens for histological examination were obtained under direct vision with the biopsy forceps. Biopsy specimens have been taken from various lesions, including pedunculated polyps, sessile polyps, new large bowel adenocarcinomas, recurrent colonic carcinomas, lymphomas, and inflammatory disease of the colon. In some patients, the presence of small lower colon polyps was verified after being suspected on a barium enema radiograph; in other patients, polyps were found which had not been evident radiographically.

Colonoscopy is a relatively safe and simple diagnostic procedure which should be used as an adjunct to standard diagnostic techniques in selected cases of lower colon disease. It is imperative that colonoscopy be done in all patients who have blood in their stools, the source of which cannot be proven by standard proctosigmoido-

scopic and radiographic techniques. Colonoscopy also will be helpful in obtaining biopsy material from polyps to establish or eliminate
possibility of carcinoma in situ in such lesions. In selected cases,
colonoscopy is indicated for the purpose of performing a wire snare
polypectomy.

The Barium Enema as a Cancer Detection Procedure: Its Use and Abuse

ROSCOE E. MILLER, M.D.

Department of Radiology, Indiana University School of Medicine, Indianapolis, Indiana

ACCORDING TO THE LATEST ESTIMATE of the American Cancer Society (1974), new cases of cancer of the colon and rectum will be found in 99,000 Americans this coming year. In 1 year, 48,000 Americans will die of that disease. Since cancer of the colon is highly curable if it is treated early, the picture need not be this grim. Selected studies report 71 per cent survival with surgical therapy for localized disease.

Franklin and McSwain (1970) studied more than 1,000 cases and reported an absolute 5-year survival rate of 71 per cent for early lesions as contrasted to 13 per cent survival for extensive lesions. Therefore, early diagnosis of and treatment for colonic and rectal cancer is definitely related to increased survival rates.

General surgeons have improved the 5-year survival rate remarkably by using the "no touch" technique (Turnbull, Kyle, Watson, and Spratt, 1968). Radiologists now have the opportunity to make an equally impressive contribution by diagnosing the lesion earlier and reducing the percentage of missed lesions to practically zero.

The barium enema is the principal method of detecting colonic cancer other than direct observation with the sigmoidoscope and colonoscope. Regrettably, the barium enema is probably the most neglected and poorly done examination in the field of radiology. All

277

too often what passes for a normal colon study is 2 or 3 views of fecal-filled large bowel that shows no grossly obstructing carcinoma.

The startling fact must now be faced that more than 18 per cent of carcinomas of the colon are completely missed on the initial barium enema examination. Saunders and MacEwen (1971) reported this fact and discussed the reasons for delay in diagnosing colonic carcinoma. One of the major reasons for delay in diagnosis was that the tumor was missed on the first barium enema examination. Eyler (1973) reported on a review of 15,000 studies where cancer was found at operation and a barium enema had been performed previously. The cases where the cancer had not been detected were segregated. In 75 percent of these missed carcinomas, the radiologist had mistaken the carcinoma for poor preparation or had described poor preparation but left the choice of repeat examination to the clinician. Sadly, we must assume that these patients had some sort of symptoms of colon disease which caused their physicians to request the examination in the first place.

We agree with Rogers (1971) that the radiologist too often tries to cover himself with a disclaimer concerning inadequate preparation and redundancy, but in doing so he has done a disservice to himself, his patient, and that patient's physician. A poor colon examination is immeasurably worse than no examination at all, since a report of a barium enema, any barium enema, is immediately translated by the clinician unfamiliar with radiologic problems as "normal colon." This phrase fits much more neatly on a discharge summary than the unwieldy and embarrassing statement that the colon was inadequately prepared and examined. The assumption of a normal colon can cause dangerous delay in the diagnosis of carcinoma. Persistent rectal bleeding or anemia is too easily consigned to hemorrhoids or simple iron deficiency. The poor examination is an abuse of the barium enema.

Early diagnosis of colonic carcinoma is of much more than academic interest. As noted earlier, the absolute 5-year survival for early carcinoma is 71 per cent as contrasted to 13 per cent survival for extensive lesions (Franklin and McSwain, 1970). With this differential, we radiologists must assume the major responsibility for finding early lesions. We have the proven tools at hand if we will only assume the responsibility for proper preparation and technique. We can no longer delegate this to some well meaning, but ill-informed referring physician. We do not do it in angiography, and we must not do it for gastrointestinal examinations. The payoff in cured or controlled cancer from gastrointestinal examinations is far greater than that from angiography because of the quantity of these lesions and the earlier, easier, and higher volume of barium enema examinations; 85 per cent of all fluoroscopy is gastrointestinal (Volume of X-Ray Visits, United States—April–September 1970, U. S. Public Health Service). We can no longer wait for the alteration of its vascular pattern on an angiogram to enable us to diagnose cancer of the colon. Most missed lesions in the colon are the result of poor preparation, faulty technique, and inadequate attention to detail rather than an inherent invisibility.

Choice of Method

The diagnostic yield in radiographic examinations of the colon depends primarily on a reliable technique. While human factors play an important role in all X-ray examinations, the efforts of a competent examiner can be wasted if he does not know and employ the best available techniques. Because a high percentage of malignant lesions found in the colon are operable, and resection of early lesions usually means cure, technique in finding the tumor becomes extremely important.

Some authors consider the air-contrast examination of the colon as an "entity of the past" (Pantone and Berlin, 1967). Their objections to the air-contrast method include failure to obtain a good barium coating of the bowel wall, a high incidence of false lesions caused by retained fecal material, obscuring the sigmoid by barium-filled ileal loops, discomfort to the patient, and extra time and effort for the examiner. Instead, they advocate the use of a full-column barium enema technique with high kilovoltage and multiple-pressure spot films.

Apart from other considerations, it first should be recognized that compression can be nullified by obesity. Often it will be ineffective because of overlying skeletal structures in 4 important areas: the splenic flexure, the hepatic flexure, the sigmoid, and the rectum. Unfortunately, these areas are frequently the site of both benign and malignant lesions.

Admittedly, air-contrast studies require a little additional effort, in time and equipment, on the part of the examiner. The patient's discomfort, however, will be very slight after the administration of 2 mg. of glucagon 10 minutes prior to the examination (Miller *et al.*, 1973).

We agree that a poor air-contrast study is worthless. However, so are other studies using poor techniques. Conversely, a first-rate air-contrast study is no doubt the most accurate technique available. Ample evidence of this will be presented later in this article.

Technique

To achieve adequate air-contrast studies, 5 requirements, all attainable, must be fulfilled: (1) a clean colon, (2) a suitable barium suspension that will coat well and not bubble or "flake out," (3) adequate insufflation of the bowel, (4) drainage of excess barium from the rectum, and (5) an adequate number of films with good radiological technique. We will examine these items briefly.

PREPARATION

The colon must be well prepared. This is a primary requirement for all colon examinations. Fecal matter simulating polyps will be seen in any type of examination if the colon is not clean. Retained fecal matter is more obvious in air-contrast studies, but so are the pathological lesions. A combination of diet, laxatives, and enemas must be used for successful cleansing of the colon.

A low residue or liquid diet is used as often as possible and, if possible, for several days preceding the study.

We routinely use 2 laxatives the day preceding the examination. Two ounces (60 ml.) of castor oil at noon or shortly thereafter plus 2½ oz. (75 ml.) of X-Prep liquid at 6:00 p.m. is reliable. We sometimes substitute 10 oz. of magnesium citrate or 20 gm. of magnesium sulfate for one or the other of these cathartics (*e.g.* in diabetics). A large volume of oral liquids also must be given to assist an effective purge. We urge a full 8 oz. glass of liquids each hour for 6 to 7 hours the day preceding the examination.

In addition to laxatives, a single 2,000 ml. water enema given in the X-ray department the morning of the study has proven to be as effective as any method we have tried for obtaining a clean colon for study. Very good evacuation usually follows the 2,000 ml. water enema, whereas a 500 or 1,000 ml. enema may be retained in the rectum and sigmoid. In a double blind study of 100 patients, Clysodrast (Barnes-Hind Diagnostics, Inc., Carolina, Puerto Rico) in the cleansing enema did not seem to make any difference except in the 60- to 70-year-old age group where it appeared quite effective (Skucas, Personal communication). We allow a full 30 minutes for evacuation before giving glucagon. Occasionally, there is some retained water in the colon which can be tolerated because of the high radiographic density of the barium.

The nature of the specific laxative is not nearly as important as the relentless application of the inflexible rule that the colon must be clean before the examination will be done. As an adjunct to enforcement, we routinely schedule the upper gastrointestinal tract first when both examinations are requested. Barium from the upper gastrointestinal tract is used as a "marker" to see if the colon is clean before we start the colon study. At times, this means we must bring the patient back the next day for a repeat study after having wasted 5 minutes on a preliminary film or 5 seconds on preliminary fluoroscopy. We agree with Eyler (1973) that the colon report should read, "positive, negative, or must be repeated."

The reports of Welin (1958, 1967), Carlile (1967), Rogers (1972), and Eyler (1973), in addition to our own, have shown that the colon can be cleaned in the department of radiology. It is the radiologist who should be responsible for this aspect of the examination. Probably one of the reasons this author is so adamant about a clean colon is that he, too, before routine cleansing enemas were done in the department, has misinterpreted tumor as fecal material. A tumor should not be missed because the radiologist does not take full responsibility for a clean colon, including a cleansing enema in his department. In fact, in cases of missed carcinoma this omission may soon be considered very poor medicine and probably malpractice because reports such as those above prove it can be done.

Figiel (1973), at a Colon Conference for the Detection of Colon Lesions, said that if a cancer turns up at surgery or autopsy and a barium enema which was called "normal" had been performed in the previous 2 years, then that is an error. However, he takes responsibility only for lesions above the sigmoid and does not include the rectum and rectosigmoid colon. Since that conference, this author has taken the attitude that if the patient has a carcinoma found at autopsy or surgery or by any other means, such as proctosigmoidoscopy or colonoscopy, and the patient had an air-contrast colon study within the previous 3 years, then that is an error. We believe this time span is reasonable because of the slow growth rate of tumors of the colon. Furthermore, we assume responsibility for the entire colon from the anus to the appendix.

We recently reviewed all of our cases of colonic cancer since 1966 and there has been 1 examination that was initially called "normal," which upon subsequent consultation with the gastroenterologist and review of the films, demonstrated 2 small tumors, 1 in the rectosigmoid and 1 in the cecum. This was done before operation, and with that exception, we have missed, to our knowledge, no tumors of the colon in an air-contrast examination using the criteria cited. In 1 additional case, the resident thought there was no tumor; however, the chief of the radiological gastrointestinal service thought there was a tumor. The barium coating was very thin, and the examination was repeated. A small villous adenoma was found in the rectosigmoid colon and reported before surgery. Repeat examination in case of doubt is a proper use of the barium enema.

It is possible that less drastic measures for cleansing of the colon may be discovered. At the present time, however, there has been no scientific double blind study of a large nature to evaluate cleansing of the colon on a truly scientific basis. We believe such studies will begin in the near future, but until then, we are dissatisfied with anything less than 2 cathartics and a 2,000 cc. cleansing enema given under the direction of the radiologist. Radiologists, heads of departments, and hospital administrators must realize that adequate facilities for cleansing of the colon in the department of radiology must be made available. Obviously, these facilities can also be used in preparation for other examinations such as gallbladder studies, IVP's, angiograms, and other studies of the abdomen and pelvis. Before we had special facilities, we gave the cleansing enema on the X-ray table.

Using our present colon cleansing technique, we have less than 5 per cent of individuals of all types who do not have satisfactorily clean colons. Studies of these are repeated the next day, generally with a change in the type of cathartic used, and a repeat cleansing enema given.

THE BARIUM SUSPENSION

To coat the bowel wall in air-contrast colon examinations, one must use a barium sulfate suspension that will adhere well but not bubble, flake, or flocculate. This factor will vary from place to place according to the calcium and other dissolved material in the water supply. Lack of good coatability is seen too often in the literature with illustrations that show flaking-out of the barium and absence of coating of the mucosa (Hartzell, 1964). It is the examiner's job to search and find the brands or mixture of barium sulfates that will function properly at his hospital (Miller, 1967, 1973). At Indiana University, about 2.5 parts of Intropaque (Lafayette Pharmacal, Lafayette, Indiana) are combined with one part of Barosperse (Mallinckrodt Chemical Works, St. Louis, Missouri) (by weight) and enough water is added to bring the mixture to 65 per cent weight/volume. In practice, 25 lbs. of Intropaque is weighed and thoroughly blended in 9 lbs. of Barosperse. This mixture can be divided into 1–lb. portions and kept in small plastic bags. To each 1–lb. portion, 500 cc.

of water is added. The 65 per cent weight/volume mixture can be stored in 1-gallon plastic jugs or, for your convenience, is available prepackaged (E-Z-Em Company, Inc., Westbury, New York). For quality control, each batch is checked with a Ba-Test hydrometer (Philips Medical Systems, Inc., Indianapolis, Indiana). A specific gravity of 65 is proper. The resultant suspension is about as thick as sour cream (the viscosity measure 60 to 90 seconds on a No. 4 Ford cup [Gardner Laboratory, Inc., Bethesda, Maryland]) and must be squeezed through large bore ⅜-inch internal diameter tubing with manual pressure on the plastic bag. The 2 brands of barium mixed together are eminently superior to either brand used alone. The reason for this is probably the ratio of barium to suspending agents in each preparation. A blend of the 2 brings this ratio to what is optimal for air-contrast colon studies. In a few instances where the local water supply was very soft, several drops of Mylicon (Stuart Pharmaceuticals, Wilmington, Delaware) added to the barium suspension has solved the problem of foaming or bubbles. We also urge that the water for the suspension be taken from the cold water tap because in many hospitals the hot water is softened.

An alternate contrast medium, almost as satisfactory, is to mix 1 gallon or container of Novopaque (Picker X-Ray Corporation, Cleveland, Ohio) with ½ gallon or container of Liquiapaque (General Electric Corporation, Milwaukee, Wisconsin). This can be done easily in a clean 2½ gallon plastic gasoline or water container.

AIR INSUFFLATION

Adequate insufflation adds greatly to the visibility of lesions but very little to patient discomfort after bowel relaxation with 2 mg, of glucagon given intramuscularly. In adults, 2,000 or more cubic centimeters of air is usually necessary. This equals 50 to 75 or more full compressions of a sphygmomanometer bulb (Fig. 1 *A*, *B*, *C*, and *D*).

DRAINAGE

Excellent demonstration of the rectum and distal sigmoid lesions is one of the superior aspects of good air-contrast studies. This requires only drainage of excess barium through the enema tip before air instillation and a short final check just before film exposure. It is a simple and rewarding maneuver. This is done by placing the enema bag below the table top and releasing the tubing clamp. Some air will also escape, but this is easily reinstilled, especially when using

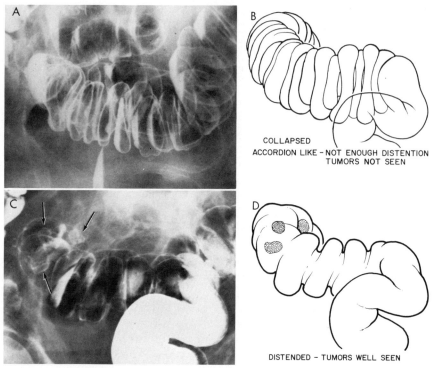

FIG. 1.—*A*, radiograph of the rectosigmoid colon in a 76-year-old male with bleeding from the rectum. Lack of sufficient distention by air causes an accordion-like condition that hides small lesions. *B*, schematic drawing of the radiograph illustrated in Figure 1*A*, *C*, radiograph of the same patient on the same day as in Figure 1*A*, but with more air and greater distention. Three small tumors are seen that were obscured in the previously partially distended rectosigmoid colon. With poor distention, this same phenomenon can occur in any segment of the colon. *D*, schematic drawing of the radiograph illustrated in Figure 1*C*.

the "Miller" air tip (E-Z-Em Company, Inc., Westbury, New York) (Miller, 1969). This tip allows complete control of barium, air, and rectal drainage at any point in the examination. Since the tube for instilling the air extends to the end of the enema tip, the instillation of air does not force residual barium in the enema tubing into the patient. Instead, the air can assist in draining the barium from the rectum (Fig. 2).

The importance of the rectosigmoid films cannot be overemphasized. Although it has been customary to consider the rectum and lower sigmoid the responsibility of the proctosigmoidoscopist, this is

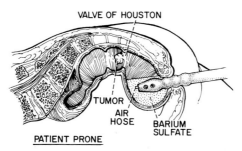

FIG. 2.—Schematic sectional drawing showing the rectum, with the patient in prone position for air-contrast study of the colon. Gravity causes the barium sulfate to drain toward the anus and enema tip. Note the small air tube at the end of the enema tip. Air entering at this site does not force residual barium in the barium enema tubing back into the patient. Instead, air instilled at this point assists in drainage of the barium from the rectum. Tumors in the rectum are easily hidden by rectal folds and frequently missed by sigmoidoscopy when they are situated near the valve of Houston.

no longer true. Andren (1956), Welin (1958, 1967), Carlile (1967), and Miller (1964) have demonstrated convincingly that the radiologist should take the responsibility for the total examination of the sigmoid and rectum. Because these areas cannot be compressed, lesions here are notoriously missed by full column techniques. However, multiple studies have shown that bleeding benign polyps, cancer, villous adenomas, and other lesions of the rectum, all within reach of the sigmoidoscope and finger, have been missed by competent people but diagnosed on adequate air-contrast colon examinations with drainage of the rectum. The reverse is sometimes true and each method is a check on the other, much to the benefit of the patient. The 2 methods of examination are not mutually exclusive. While we agree completely that radiologic examination of this area is not a substitute for the digital or sigmoidoscopic examination, it is certainly complementary. The radiologist must take responsibility for the entire colon from anus to appendix!

Technique

Adequate films in sufficient number are necessary to obtain reliable information on all segments of the colon. As opposed to the conventional barium enema techniques, the barium should be instilled with the patient in the prone position (Fig. 3 *A*, *B*, and Fig. 4). This prevents barium from entering the ileum for the first 5 critical films of the rectum and rectosigmoid area. After the colon is inflated,

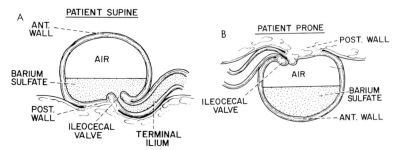

FIG. 3.—A, schematic cross-sectional drawing of the terminal ileum entering the colon with the patient supine. The terminal ileum usually enters the colon medially from the left side and terminates posteriorly. With the patient supine or on his left side, barium sulfate suspension will enter the terminal ileum easily. This is to be avoided in the early stages of an air-contrast colon examination because it can result in barium-filled loops of small bowel obscuring the rectum and rectosigmoid colon. B, schematic cross-sectional drawing of the terminal ileum entering the colon with the patient prone. Air distention of the cecum and ascending colon lifts the terminal ileum and ileocecal valve away from the barium sulfate suspension. Air can enter the terminal ileum (which does not matter), but not the barium sulfate suspension. Thus, barium sulfate does not enter the small bowel and overlie and obscure the rectum and rectosigmoid for the first 5 radiographs of this important part of the examination.

FIG. 4.—This is a radiograph of an autopsy specimen of cecum and terminal ileum. A hemostatic clip was placed on the most anterior aspect of the cecum (upper arrow) before removal from the cadaver. After removal of the cecum and terminal ileum, 2 clips (lower arrows) were placed inside the cecum on the lips of the ileocecal valve. The ascending colon was tied shut. A short angiographic catheter was placed through the terminal ileum into the cecum and the cecum was inflated with air. The specimen was then radiographed with a horizontal ray. The resultant radiograph is only 1 of several similar specimens taken in the same fashion. It shows that the ileum enters the colon from its medial (L) side and that the most distal part opens into the cecum posteriorly.

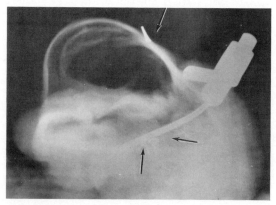

the patient can be rotated with little risk of barium reflux into the small bowel provided care is used to avoid excess barium in the cecum, and the supine position is avoided in the first stage of the examination.

The Examination Proper

The 65 per cent weight/volume barium-water mixture is squeezed into the colon (with the patient prone) until barium reaches the splenic flexure. At that point, the enema bag is quickly dropped to the floor and the barium drained from the rectum. As the air is insufflated, the table can be tilted, first head down, then foot down, while having the patient rotate so that the barium can flow to the dependent uncoated part of the colon. This is best done by watching the head of the barium column and following the course of the colon. One can easily manipulate the barium so that it runs its course by gravity to the cecum. Two thousand cc. or more of air is instilled (50 to 75 or more full squeezes of the sphygmomanometer bulb) and this often by itself forces the barium around to the cecum. Air in front of the barium causes us no concern because this lifts the ileocecal valve and prevents barium from entering the terminal ileum (Fig. 3 *A, B*). The patient is not sent to the toilet for evacuation either before the instillation of air or at completion of the study. Standing upright, then sitting and straining during defecation may force barium into the terminal ileum and ruin an otherwise competent study.

The following 14″ × 17″ films are exposed in the following order at 100 KV with single-phase equipment or at 90 KV with 3-phase equipment: First, prone angle view of the rectum and sigmoid with the tube tilted 30° toward the feet, PA with a vertical ray, prone 20° LAO, prone 20° RAO, and a 10″ × 12″ right lateral view, all of which include the rectum, are taken. Then the supine, 20° LPO, 20° RPO, all 3 to include both colonic flexures, are taken (45° oblique films cause too much superimposition and only 20° oblique views are taken). Finally, both lateral decubitus views, which again include the rectum, are taken with a stationary 6:1 crisscross grid.

The table is then raised upright and 9½″ × 9½″ or larger spot films are taken of each flexure, transverse colon, and cecum. Additional spot films will be taken of any suspicious lesions. This totals 14 radiographs in a 1-stage procedure. All our fluoroscopes are equipped with 6:1 crisscross or 12:1 linear 80– to 103–line aluminum interspaced grids in both table Bucky and spot film devices (Liebel-

Flarsheim Company, Cincinnati, Ohio). We also have a lateral decubitus apparatus that can be attached to any fluoroscopic table. It permits decubitus films to be made in a few seconds (Miller, 1970).

CRITICAL INITIAL FILM REVIEW

These films must be evaluated carefully by the radiologist before the patient leaves the department in case further overhead or spot films are required to evaluate suspicious or frankly abnormal areas. The pliability of this barium preparation allows a thorough film examination without haste. The barium will not clump for at least an hour. Air is cheap and the colon can easily be reinflated. In many cases, the film review is made before the patient evacuates and little or no additional air is needed.

FLUOROSCOPY

Fluoroscopy with spot films is still an important part of our technique of examining the colon. We simply reverse the usual order, reserving intensive fluoroscopy and spot films for suspicious areas seen in the initial 14 radiographs. Fluoroscopy with compression is just as valuable in the air-contrast technique as in the conventional filled-colon study. It has enabled us to confirm or reject a large number of suspicious lesions.

Comment

Obviously, it takes a little effort and some know-how on the part of the examiner to develop a reliable and consistent air-contrast technique. Are the results of high quality air-contrast studies worth these efforts?

The facts, not opinions, are these:

Probably by far the most conscientious practitioner of the high kilovoltage type of examination is Figiel. He reported at a Gastrointestinal Seminar at Indiana University in 1966 that, with his routine studies, he found polyps in 7.5 per cent of patients (Figiel, 1973).

Welin reported at a similar conference in Miami in 1965 and also in 1967 that in 13 years he has performed more than 36,000 consecutive air-contrast studies of the colon, and found polyps in 3,101 studies on 24,783 patients, or 12.5 per cent. This equaled the frequency of polyps found at routine autopsies at the same hospital (Welin, 1967). The only way he could find all these tumors, many of which were malignant, and determine their precise characteristics was by the use of good air-contrast techniques.

These 2 studies were performed by the acknowledged leaders in each technique. In the best hands and under the best circumstances, the high kilovoltage technique missed 40 per cent of polypoid lesions of the colon. We believe this is a significant percentage.

When compared to the multiple-compression spot film, full-column, high kilovoltage techniques, the use of adequate air-contrast colon examinations resulted in a 40 per cent greater diagnostic yield. To date, no other examination has been proved to give such precise information about the entire colon as does the good air-contrast technique. In addition, inflammatory lesions in the mucosa will also show up in great detail with air-contrast studies (Welin and Brahme, 1961).

At the very least, there is a high-risk group of patients that we consider should have an air-contrast colon examination as the primary examination. These are: (1) Any patient with rectal bleeding for any reason, or any patient with a history of bleeding. (2) Patients with polyps on proctoscopic examination. (3) Patients with a previous history of polyps or carcinoma. (4) Patients with a strong family history of polyps of carcinoma. (5) Patients in whom there is a high index of suspicion on the part of the clinician or radiologist, based on a change in bowel habits, weight loss, unexplained anemia, or other reason.

Noncompatible Techniques

Frequently, the question arises whether a regular barium enema and an air-contrast enema can be done on the same day. To do a good job and combine the 2 is certainly a rare exception, because these are 2 entirely separate types of examinations. The reasons are:

(1) The regular barium enema is given for emergency purposes and generally for bowel obstruction in either the large or small bowel. In these cases, no preparation is given. One is not looking for small tumors or even large tumors, but for obstruction.

(2) The regular barium enema should use a 15 to 20 per cent weight/volume concentration of barium sulfate which is indeed a low density type barium suspension. The X ray must penetrate this low density through a column sometimes 10 or more centimeters thick. Such a thin barium will not coat satisfactorily for an air-contrast examination because less than a millimeter-thick coat is deposited on the bowel wall when the colon is distended with air.

(3) In regular barium enemas, the radiologist ordinarily tries to

visualize the terminal ileum and see something of the small bowel. This is particularly true in Crohn's disease and cases of ulcerative colitis.

(4) With the full-column technique, the patient is examined supine so that barium easily goes into the terminal ileum through the ileocecal valve. Compression and palpation must be done to separate large and small bowel loops. There is no drainage of the rectum.

(5) The postevacuation film is important and valuable for early diagnosis of ulcerative colitis. In the case of a regular barium examination, no drug to relax the colon is given.

On the contrary, the air-contrast examination is entirely different. The reasons are:

(1) With air-contrast techniques, the radiologist is not looking for complete obstruction, but for small as well as large lesions, and the bowel is well prepared.

(2) The examination is started with the patient in the prone position to prevent and avoid reflux into the terminal ileum. This avoids covering up and obscuring the rectosigmoid and rectum.

(3) In the prone position, the rectum is easily drained and this is quickly accomplished by gravity.

(4) A heavy barium suspension of 65 per cent weight/volume or more is used so that a thin layer less than a millimeter thick can be deposited upon the bowel wall and still absorb enough X-rays to be easily seen on the radiographs.

(5) A drug is used to relax the bowel. With 2 mg. of glucagon given intramuscularly, the patient's discomfort is much less than in a full-column enema. In addition, the pressure inside the colon is less than in regular barium enemas without relaxant drugs. With relaxant drugs, one cannot depend upon postevacuation films.

The rare exception when the air-contrast enema can follow the regular barium enema is when no barium enters the terminal ileum and there is good evacuation. The regular barium enema is used as the cleansing enema. Only in these unusual circumstances can a satisfactory air-contrast enema with dense barium and a bowel relaxant follow a regular barium enema. This has been rare in my experience. Just 1 or 2 films after thin barium and a little air will not do and is an abuse of an excellent method.

Summary

The radiologist must assume complete responsibility for the preparation and examination of the entire colon including the rectum.

When one considers the increasing patient load and the relative scarcity of radiologists, one cannot expect that all radiologists will be willing or able to assume the additional effort to produce Welin's precise results routinely. However, even with these examiners, the air-contrast method can still fulfill the role of a precise and ultimate examination, especially in certain selected high-risk groups. We agree with Ochsner (1964) that it is indeed a poor examiner who has but one arrow in his diagnostic quiver.

Lastly, I want to emphasize strongly that what Dr. Leo Rigler said earlier at this symposium about lung cancer also applies to tumors of the colon. No matter how great or sophisticated the mental ability and our tools in differential diagnosis, it is all in vain if we do not find the lesion. We can and must find the 18 per cent of cancers currently missed on initial colon examinations. Not to find the lesion is the irrevocable error, and an abuse of the barium enema.

REFERENCES

American Cancer Society: *'74 Cancer Facts and Figures*. New York, New York, 1974, 31 pp.

Andren, L., and Frieberg, S.: Roentgen diagnosis of the rectum. *Gastroenterology*, 31:566–570, November 1956.

Brahme, F.: Granulomatous colitis. *The American Journal of Roentgenology, Radium Therapy and Nuclear Medicine*, 99:35–44, January 1967.

Carlile, T.: The roentgenologic diagnosis of carcinoma of the colon. In *Cancer of the Gastrointestinal Tract*. Chicago, Illinois, Year Book Medical Publishers, Inc., 1967, pp. 187–211.

Eyler, W.: *Detection of Colon Lesions, First Standardization Conference 1969*. Chicago, Illinois, American College of Radiology, 1973, p. 108.

Figiel, S. J.: Colon examination technique. In *Detection of Colon Lesions, First Standardization Conference 1969*. Chicago, Illinois, American College of Radiology, 1973, pp. 132–143.

Figiel, S. J., Figiel, L. S., and Rush, D. K.: Study of the colon by use of high-kilovoltage spot-compression technic. *The Journal of the American Medical Association*, 166:1269–1275, March 15, 1958.

————: High-kilovoltage spot-compression studies. A new approach to colonic polyp detection. *Medical Radiography and Photography*, 34:34–39, 1958.

Franklin, R., and McSwain, B.: Carcinoma of the colon, rectum, and anus. *Annals of Surgery*, 171:811–818, June 1970.

Hartzell, H. B.: To err with air. *The Journal of the American Medical Association*, 187:455–456, February 8, 1964.

Miller, R. E.: Barium enema examinations with large-bore tubing and drainage. *Radiology*, 82:905–911, May 1964.

————: Barium sulfate suspensions. *Radiology*, 84:241–251, February 1965.

————: Barium sulfate. *Postgraduate Medicine*, 41:A-91–96, January 1967.

———: A new enema tip. *Radiology*, 92:1492, June 1969.

———: Simple apparatus for decubitus films with horizontal beam. *Radiology*, 97:682–683, December 1970.

———: Barium sulfate as a contrast medium. In Margulis, A., and Burhenne, H., Eds.: *Alimentary Tract Roentgenology.* 2nd edition. St. Louis, Missouri, C. V. Mosby Company, 1973, Vol. I., pp. 114–126.

———: Examination of the rectum. In *Detection of Colon Lesions, First Standardization Conference 1969.* Chicago, Illinois, American College of Radiology, 1973, pp. 162–171.

Miller, R. E., Chernish, S. M., Skucas, J., Rosenak, B. D., and Rodda, B. E.: Hypotonic colon examination with glucagon. Exhibit and paper presented at the Radiological Society of North America Meeting, Chicago, Illinois, 1973. Radiology. (In press.)

Ochsner, S. F.: Barium or air for examination of the colon. *The American Journal of Roentgenology, Radium Therapy and Nuclear Medicine*, 92: 1200–1201, November 1964.

Pantone, A. M., and Berlin, L.: Air-contrast examination of the colon. An entity of the past. *American Journal of Digestive Diseases*, 12:110–112, January 1967.

Rogers, C. W.: Radiology's stepchild—The colon. *The Journal of the American Medical Association*, 216:1855–1856, June 14, 1971.

———: Early discovery of cancer of the colon. A radiographic method. *Southern Medical Journal*, 65:957–963, August 1972.

Saunders, C. G., and MacEwen, D. W.: Delay in diagnosis of colonic cancer —A continuing challenge. *Radiology*, 101:207–208, October 1971.

Skucas, J.: Personal communication.

Turnbull, R. B., Jr., Kyle, K., Watson, F. R., and Spratt, J.: Cancer of the colon. *Cancer*, 18:82–87, March–April 1968.

Volume of X-Ray Visits, United States—April-September 1970. Rockville, Maryland, National Center for Health Statistics, Office of Information, U. S. Public Health Service.

Welin, S.: Modern trends in diagnostic roentgenology of the colon. *British Journal of Radiology*, 31:453–464, September 1958.

———: Results of the Malmö technique of colon examination. *The Journal of the American Medical Association*, 199:369–371, February 6, 1967.

Welin, S., and Brahme, F.: The double contrast method in ulcerative colitis. *Acta Radiologica*, 55:257–271, April 1961.

Ultrasonic B-Scanning in the Evaluation of Abdominal Malignancy

GEORGE R. LEOPOLD, M.D.
Department of Radiology, Division of Ultrasound,
University of California San Diego, School of Medicine;
University Hospital, San Diego, California

ULTRASONIC B-SCANNING, which involves the production of 2-dimensional images of soft tissue structures by reflected sound waves, has recently achieved popularity in many areas of diagnosis (Holm, 1971). Although the technique is particularly well suited to the detection of fluid-filled lesions within the abdomen and pelvis, significant information also can be obtained in reference to tumor masses, both in and around the solid organs. Since the method is capable of outlining most of the soft tissue organs and assessing their internal composition in a noninvasive fashion, it has become a valuable adjunct to those who care for patients with a wide variety of malignant diseases of the abdomen.

Technique

The details of image production by this method have been well outlined (Lehman, 1966). Briefly, an ultrasonic pulse is created by the stimulation of a piezo-electric crystal, usually a synthetic polarized ceramic material. The sound frequency employed for most abdominal work is about 2 million cycles per second (2 megahertz). At this frequency, the sound beam can be focused into narrow beams and obeys many of the laws that ordinarily apply to light beams. As the beam passes through the body, small amounts of energy are re-

293

flected back to the transducer from areas of density change within the structure in question. By sweeping the transducer across a predetermined path and accumulating the information received, a 2-dimensional image along the scan path is constructed. In the average study of the abdomen, 8 or 10 transverse scan paths, usually 1 to 2 cm. apart, are performed and recorded. This ordinarily is followed by several longitudinal or sagittal scans to confirm the findings in a different spatial plane, just as with conventional X-ray studies and nuclear medicine techniques.

Ultrasonic analysis of abdominal structure possesses a significant advantage over routine X-ray examination since it is capable of distinguishing many subdensities within the radiographic category of "water" density. Cysts, for example, are quite different from solid masses since the former remain free of internal echoes even at very high levels of receiver sensitivity (Goldberg, 1971). Solid masses, by virtue of their complex internal structure, usually will demonstrate considerable echo formation when examined at the same sensitivity setting.

Ultrasonic analysis is limited by excessive gaseous distension, barium-filled bowel, or interposition of bone between transducer and target. All provide virtually complete reflection of the incident beam and render the structures behind them invisible. To eliminate air at the skin-transducer interface, a thin coating of mineral oil is ordinarily applied.

To date, expert scanning still requires considerable experience and a familiarity with both the equipment and the normal anatomy usually encountered in the area in question. It is hoped that the next generation of ultrasonic equipment will be much less operator dependent.

Malignant Diseases of the Liver

Using a routine series of 10 to 12 scans, the liver can be imaged satisfactorily in almost all patients. From these scans, the size and shape of the organ may be accurately predicted. A knowledge of the more frequently involved anatomic variants, such as Riedel's lobe, large or small caudate lobe, and large or small left lobe, is of great importance in the proper interpretation of such studies.

In addition to abnormal liver shape, patients with intrahepatic malignant disease often show alteration in the internal echo pattern of the organ. A transverse scan of a normal patient is shown in Figure 1, demonstrating a large amount of the central portion of the liver. It will be noted that the vast majority of the parenchyma is echo-free.

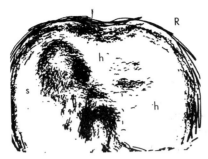

FIG. 1.—Transverse scan of the upper abdomen taken from a normal patient. Note that the liver (h) is free of internal echoes with the exception of the central, hilar area. R = patient's right side, V = vertebral body, s = spleen.

This is an indication of the homogeneity of the tissue being traversed. Current equipment, then, is incapable of resolving the smaller structures of the portal triads. The hilar echoes are prominent, normal structures that most likely arise from the larger portal venous radicles and biliary ducts.

The scan shown in Figure 2 demonstrates a circular collection of echoes near the center of the organ which arise from a lymphoma in that location. Here the difference in density produced at the margin of the lesion is sufficient to produce a detectable interface. Both primary and metastatic lesions are frequently capable of producing such a disruption of the normal pattern (McCarthy, 1967). Although metastases can be recognized by the presence of foci of discrete strong echoes in normally echo-free areas, in many cases they are not detected. These cases apparently represent situations where the density of the tumor too closely approximates the density of the liver. Much experimental work remains to be done on the specific density

FIG. 2.—Scan showing irregular, echo-producing mass (m) located centrally within the liver.

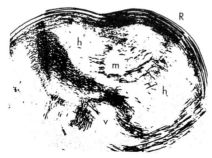

of various types of tumors to determine which ones are most likely to produce recognizable abnormalities.

Unfortunately, other entities such as cirrhosis, scar, benign tumors, and bile stasis may produce similar abnormal patterns. The role of ultrasound at present is probably in confirming the solid or cystic nature of lesions suggested on isotope scans and in elucidating those problems of interpretation which arise from unusual shape and position of the liver (Leyton, 1973).

An additional use of the technique is the spatial information obtained in reference to an abnormal focus of echoes. If percutaneous biopsy is performed using the localization obtained from ultrasonic scans, the yield is considerably increased over the customary blind technique (Holm, 1973).

Malignant Diseases of the Spleen

Like the liver, the spleen is composed of very homogeneous tissue that seldom produces internal echoes. The spleen can be demonstrated satisfactorily in either the supine or the prone position. Although the major emphasis in splenic diagnosis has been in the evaluation of trauma, abscess, or cyst, abnormal solid patterns have been reported with infarct as well as with the rare primary and metastatic tumors that involve that organ.

By far the greatest use of ultrasound in the evaluation of malignant disease has been in the depermination of splenic size or volume. Some authors have advocated the summation of multiple cross-sectional areas of the spleen to arrive at an estimated volume (Kardel, 1971). Such figures derive usefulness in the evaluation of therapy for certain hematologic disorders. Figure 3 is a scan of a patient with gross splenomegaly secondary to leukemia. Enlargement of the

FIG. 3.—Upper abdominal scan in a patient with myelogenous leukemia and massive splenomegaly (s). Other abbreviations: k = left kidney, a = aorta.

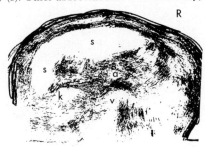

spleen is easily recognized since the organ tends to retain its characteristic crescentic shape.

Malignant Diseases of the Pancreas

The increase in frequency of carcinoma of the pancreas has emphasized the importance of applying new techniques for exploring that area. Ultrasound, in addition to having a major role in the diagnosis of pancreatitis and pseudocyst, is capable of demonstrating many pancreatic cancers (Englehart, 1970). Most workers agree that the normal pancreas usually cannot be visualized ultrasonically. Unlike the liver and spleen, pancreatic parenchyma is composed of considerable interlacing fibrous tissue which produces many internal echoes. Because the pancreas is normally covered with echo-producing small bowel, a distinction between the 2 is not possible. In the presence of edema or mass in the gland, however, the involved segment frequently becomes visible. Tumors present as lobular, relatively sonolucent spaces in the area where the pancreas is normally found. Figure 4 is a scan of a small carcinoma of the head of the pancreas. Tumors that occupy the head of the gland are easier to demonstrate than those of the body and tail, since the overlying liver serves as an excellent shield through which to examine. In general, such tumors must be 4 cm. or larger in diameter to be visible. The major diagnostic dilemma which arises is the separation of patients with chronically inflamed, edematous pancreatic heads from those with carcinoma.

FIG. 4 *(left)*. – Upper abdominal scan demonstrating a small mass in the area of the head of the pancreas (pf). Note that the pancreatic head lies relatively far anterior and to the right of the aorta (a).

FIG. 5 *(right)*. – Midabdominal scan showing the aorta (a) displaced forward from the spine (v) by a circumferential echo-free mass of lymph nodes (n).

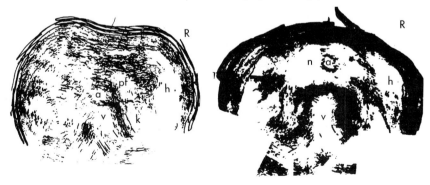

Detection of Retroperitoneal Nodes

Since the presence or absence of retroperitoneal lymph node metastases often determines the course of therapy, their detection is a critical matter. Although lymphangiography has been the method of choice, it is technically demanding and not suitable as a screening procedure. Furthermore, the accuracy of the technique in detecting malignant diseases other than lymphoma is debated by many. Ultrasonic scanning can frequently show periaortic and pericaval lymph nodes, provided they are 3 cm. or greater in size (Asher, 1969). Because of the homogeneity of lymphatic tissue, they usually appear as oval, echo-free masses clustered around the great vessels (Fig. 5). At times, it may be difficult to identify the elastic walls of the vessels because of their similarity in density to the nodal tissue.

Lymphangiography and ultrasonic lymph node scanning should be thought of as complementary techniques. While ultrasound is quicker and easier, enlarged nodes may be hyperplastic and not frankly malignant. More importantly, nodes may be involved with tumor and yet be normal in size. Nevertheless, the usefulness of the ultrasonic technique is clear in following the course of patients with known malignant disease invading the retroperitoneal nodes.

Radiation Therapy Planning

The ultrasonic technique is capable of outlining a wide variety of masses involving the mesentery. Figure 6 is a scan of a large lymphosarcoma of the mesentery which was being evaluated prior to radiation therapy. From the scans, the lateral margins of the port may be established easily. By performing sagittal scans, the top and bottom of the port also may be accurately placed. Calculation of depth dose

FIG. 6.—Low abdominal scan showing a large solid mass (m) of the mesentery which was localized for radiation therapy.

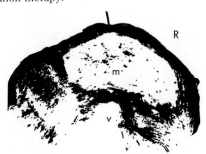

to both the tumor and the surrounding normal viscera is greatly facilitated by the spatial display of the scan. As treatment progresses and the tumor shrinks, scans may be employed to trim the port and further reduce dosage to normal structures (Brascho, 1972).

REFERENCES

Asher, W., and Freimanis, A.: Echographic diagnosis of retroperitoneal lymph node enlargement. *The American Journal of Roentgenology, Radium Therapy and Nuclear Medicine,* 105:438–445, February 1969.

Brascho, D.: Clinical applications of diagnostic ultrasound in abdominal malignancy. *Southern Medical Journal,* 65:1331–1339, November 1972.

Engelhart, G., and Blauenstein, U.: Ultrasound in the diagnosis of malignant pancreatic tumours. *The Journal of the British Society of Gastroenterology,* 11:443–449, May 1970.

Goldberg, B. B., and Pollack, H. M.: Differentiation of renal masses using A-mode ultrasound. *Journal of Urology,* 105:765–777, June 1971.

Holm, H. H.: Ultrasonically guided percutaneous puncture technique. *Journal of Clinical Ultrasound,* 1:27, March 1973.

Holm, H. H., Rasmussen, S. N., and Kristensen, J. K.: Ultrasonic scanning in the diagnosis of space-occupying lesions of the upper abdomen. *British Journal of Radiology,* 44:24–36, January 1971.

Kardel, T., Holm, H. H., Rasmussen, S. N., and Mortensen, T.: Ultrasonic determination of liver and spleen volumes. *Scandinavian Journal of Clinical and Laboratory Investigation,* 27:123–128, April 1971.

Lehman, J. S.: Ultrasound in the diagnosis of hepatobiliary disease. *Radiologic Clinics of North America,* 4:605–623, December 1966.

Leyton, B., Halpern, S., Leopold, G., and Hagen, S.: Correlation of ultrasound and colloid scintiscan studies of the normal and diseased liver. *Journal of Nuclear Medicine,* 14:27–33, June 1973.

McCarthy, C. E., Read, A. E., Ross, F. G., and Wells, P. N.: Ultrasonic scanning of the liver. *Quarterly Journal of Medicine,* 36:517–524, October 1967.

Endoscopic Visualization of Pancreatic and Bile Ducts in Malignant Disease

JACK A. VENNES, M.D.
*Department of Medicine, University of Minnesota,
Minneapolis, Minnesota*

THE BILIARY TREE AND PANCREAS are 2 areas which remain very inaccessible to precise nonsurgical evaluation. Improved techniques for the detection of early morphologic changes are needed to determine the existence, site, and etiology of disease. An endoscopic method has been developed by which one or both ductal systems can be outlined well with contrast material. Initial Japanese experience has now been augmented by experience in other countries, including the United States (Oi, 1970; Classen, 1971; Cotton, 1972; Vennes and Silvis, 1972; Ogoshi, Niwa, and Hara, 1973). Some of our preliminary observations with endoscopic ductal cannulation and visualization in patients proven to have malignant disease of these systems will be reviewed and discussed in this paper.

Briefly, the instrument used is a flexible side-viewing duodenoscope 10 mm. in diameter. We have used the Olympus JF instrument which permits passage of a 1.6 mm. Teflon cannula whose distal tip can be precisely maneuvered with biplane controls in a visual field of high resolution.

The procedure is performed in a radiology examining room equipped with padded table, spot film device, and high-resolution fluoroscopic monitor. After sedation and smooth muscle atony are

301

pharmacologically achieved, the duodenoscope is gently passed through the stomach and duodenal bulb into the descending duodenum. The papilla is expeditiously located and is searched closely for location of the ductal orifice. The cannula tip is positioned squarely opposite and close to the ductal orifice and the cannula is passed into one or both ducts. Under close fluoroscopic control, 60 per cent Renografin is cautiously injected. If only the pancreatic ductal system is being opacified, 2 to 5 ml. are injected slowly enough to avoid over-distension but completely enough to fill all patent ducts including lateral branches. If the common bile duct is entered, 5 to 40 ml. of contrast medium will be required for good structural detail; the larger amounts are required, preferably of lesser concentration, if a gallbladder or very dilated common duct is to be visualized. If the clinically desired ductal system is not entered initially, the cannula is repositioned and the contrast agent injected into the other system. The technical details of the necessary maneuvers have been largely mastered. Other details have been previously reported (Vennes and Silvis, 1972).

The procedure is well tolerated by patients, and usually requires less than 60 minutes. In our first 300 procedures, mild pancreatitis was induced in 10 patients; this is now largely avoided by slow, gentle ductal filling with careful monitoring. The cholangitis that occurred in 10 instances also has largely disappeared, as we have recommended surgical decompression of extrahepatic obstruction within 24 hours of instilling contrast agent in a semiclosed obstructed ductal system. Asymptomatic hyperamylasuria remains a transient sequel to 40 per cent of ductal cannulation procedures (Blackwood, Vennes, and Silvis, 1973).

Our first 300 procedures have been partially evaluated and reported (Silvis, Rohrmann, and Vennes, 1973; Vennes, Jacobson, and Silvis, 1974). Patients were studied because a clinical problem of extra-

Table
Proven Malignant Diseases Studied

Primary Tumor	
Pancreas	28
Bile Duct	8
Gallbladder	2
Hodgkin's Disease	2
Metastatic Disease	2
Total	42

hepatic obstruction or pancreatic disease remained after an otherwise completed evaluation. The clinically desired duct was visualized in 255 patients, or 85 per cent. This rose to 93 per cent when the last half of the examinations (150 studies) were considered separately.

Forty-two patients with malignant disease have been studied (Table); 39 had evident stricture and/or obstruction of one or both

FIG. 1 *(top left).*—Normal pancreaticocholangiogram. Note the fiberscope in place with tip in air-filled descending duodenum.

FIG. 2 *(top right).*—Common bile duct stricture located distally, within pancreatic tumor. Note the dilated common duct partially filled with contrast medium and the superimposed dilated cystic duct remnant.

FIG. 3 *(bottom left).*—Common bile duct stricture at level of cystic duct, resulting from gallbladder carcinoma. Note partially emptied normal pancreatic duct.

FIG. 4 *(bottom right).*—Common bile duct stricture at bifurcation of hepatic ducts, caused by bile duct carcinoma.

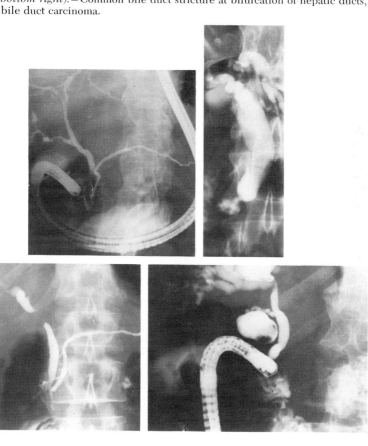

ductal systems. Although this experience is too preliminary for critical evaluation, the high incidence is noteworthy.

Figure 1 is a composite of normal pancreatic and bile duct systems filled simultaneously through a common channel. The pancreatic duct tapers normally with filled lateral branches, most evident in the head and uncinate process. The bile duct pursues a normal course along the duodenal wall. Intraphepatic branches are incompletely filled because of a lower pressure "run off" through the cystic duct which courses to the gallbladder outside the picture.

Strictures of the common duct may occur at the distal duct, near the cystic duct, or at the bifurcation. Figure 2 illustrates a short distal stricture as part of a pancreatic carcinoma. A smooth tapered stricture near the cystic duct, seen in Figure 3, is caused by a primary gallbladder carcinoma. In Figure 4, the stricture at the bifurcation of right and left hepatic ducts is the site of a primary bile duct carcinoma.

Total obstruction of the common duct (Fig. 5) is seen as an irregular cut-off. The primary pancreatic tumor has also strictured the pancreatic duct in the head before it terminates in a small pool of contrast medium.

Stricture and obstruction of the pancreatic duct are the most frequent characteristics of malignant disease in that system also. Figure 6 depicts a pancreatic duct which begins normally at the papilla, *i.e.* with smooth outline and normal lateral branches. It terminates in a tapering fashion devoid of lateral branches within the tumor mass. The partially emptied common duct is of normal caliber and is uninvolved by tumor. A similar tapering obstruction within pancreatic adenocarcinoma is seen in Figure 7. For comparison, a bluntly obstructed duct in Figure 8 is part of a benign inflammatory ductal occlusion, beyond which a noncommunicating pseudocyst was found surgically. Whether tapering or "rat-tail" deformity will prove to be a hallmark of malignant obstruction in these systems, is suggested but unproven by our experience to date.

Our first point of emphasis is that endoscopic contrast visualization of both biliary and pancreatic ductal systems is a promising method for providing excellent diagnostic details. The method will become more generally available. It has good patient tolerance and low morbidity. Second, ductal characteristics of a specific disease must be critically confirmed and developed. Stricture and obstruction, the 2 characteristics exemplified here in malignant disease, also occur as a result of benign causes such as previous surgical defect or inflammation. With more experience, it will be important to determine any

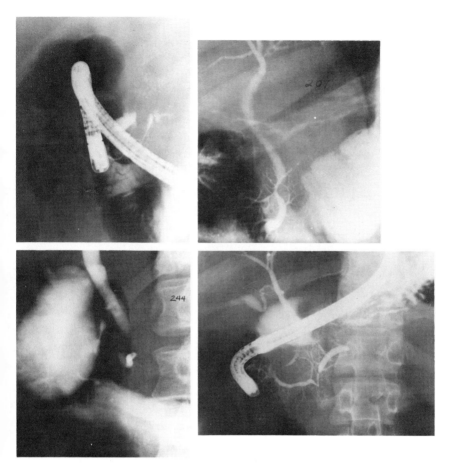

FIG. 5 *(top left).* — Complete obstruction of common bile duct caused by pancreatic carcinoma. Note jagged cut-off of common duct, stricture of pancreatic duct. Ampulla normal, not as large as contrast halo effect makes it appear.

FIG. 6 *(top right).* — Pancreatic duct obstructed by pancreatic tumor mass. Note narrowing, tapering, termination and disappearance of lateral branches.

FIG. 7 *(bottom left).* — Pancreatic duct obstructed by pancreatic tumor mass. Note lack of lateral branches, tapering obstruction. Normal common duct partially emptied, large gallbladder incidentally opacified.

FIG. 8 *(bottom right).* — Pancreatic duct obstructed by recurrent pancreatitis. Pseudocyst present at operation which, unusually, obstructed the duct but did not communicate with it.

identifiable characteristics of benign-versus-malignant stricture or obstruction. This is particularly true of pancreatic disease, since pancreatograms generally have not been available until now and other diagnostic methods lack precision.

REFERENCES

Blackwood, W. D., Vennes, J. A., and Silvis, S. E.: Post endoscopy pancreatitis and hyperamylasuria. *Gastrointestinal Endoscopy*, 20:56–58, November 1973.

Classen, M.: Fibroendoscopy of the intestines. *The Journal of the British Society of Gastroenterology*, 12:330–338, April 1971.

Cotton, P. B.: Cannulation of the papilla of Vater by endoscopy and retrograde cholangiopancreatography (ERCP). *The Journal of the British Society of Gastroenterology*, 13:1014–1025, December 1972.

Ogoshi, K., Niwa, M., Hara, Y., and Nebel, O. T.: Endoscopic pancreatocholangiography in the evaluation of pancreatic and biliary disease. *Gastroenterology*, 64:210–216, February 1973.

Oi, I.: Fiberduodenoscopy and endoscopic pancreatocholangiography. *Gastrointestinal Endoscopy*, 17:59–62, November 1970.

Silvis, S. E., Rohrmann, C. A., and Vennes, J. A.: Diagnostic criteria for the evaluation of the endoscopic pancreatogram. *Gastrointestinal Endoscopy*, 20:51–55, November 1973.

Vennes, J. A., Jacobson, J. R., and Silvis, S. E.: Endoscopic cholangiography for biliary system diagnosis. *Annals of Internal Medicine*, 80:61–64, January 1974.

Vennes, J. A., and Silvis, S. E.: Endoscopic visualization of bile and pancreatic ducts. *Gastrointestinal Endoscopy*, 18:149–152, May 1972.

Liver, Spleen, and Pancreas Scanning

THOMAS P. HAYNIE, M.D., SURAINDER K. AJMANI,
M.D., and MONROE F. JAHNS, Ph.D.
*Departments of Medicine and Physics, The University
of Texas System Cancer Center M. D. Anderson
Hospital and Tumor Institute, Houston, Texas*

NUCLEAR IMAGING TECHNIQUES find part of their usefulness in tumor diagnosis by permitting the visualization of organs not readily seen with conventional roentgenographic techniques. The liver, spleen, and pancreas qualify under this criterion. Because of their similar densities, these organs are difficult to differentiate from surrounding structures on plain X-ray films. For this reason, and because these organs are frequently involved in malignant processes, the staff members of the sections of Nuclear Medicine and Radioisotopes of M. D. Anderson Hospital have spent considerable effort in the study of these organs. This presentation will describe our current techniques, present some case reports to illustrate their usefulness, and discuss our opinion of the indications and limitations of these scans.

Material and Methods

Table 1 is a tabulation of the radionuclide imaging procedures most frequently performed in our Radioisotope Laboratory during the first half of the year 1973. Of a total of approximately 3,200 scans performed during this period, 54 per cent were of the liver and spleen and 3 per cent were of the pancreas, for an average of about 15 liver scans per working day and 15 pancreatic scans per month.

Table 1
Radionuclide Imaging Procedures Used at
MDAH in Detecting and Staging of Cancer

Table 1
Radionuclide Imaging Procedures Used at
MDAH in Detecting and Staging of Cancer

	% of Studies*
Liver-Spleen	54.3
Brain	22.0
Tumor (Gallium)	8.5
Bone	7.2
Thyroid	4.2
Pancreas	3.0
Kidney	0.5
Cardiac	0.3

*3,232 Scans January–July 1973

Table 2 is an outline of the liver-spleen scan technique that we currently employ. The radionuclide is technetium-99m in the chemical form of a sulfur colloid. This tracer localizes in the reticuloendothelial cells of the liver and spleen. The physical half-life of technetium-99m is 6 hours and physical decay is accompanied by emission of gamma rays of 140 keV. The imaging procedure is performed 20 minutes following an intravenous injection of 3 mCi. of this agent. The radiation dose to the patient is maximally 1 rad to the liver and spleen. No special preparation of the patient is required. We use a gamma camera and record the images on Polaroid film through a triple lens giving 3 similtaneous levels of exposure. Routinely, 5 views are obtained: anterior liver with and without costal margin markers, right lateral, and posterior views of the liver and spleen.

Table 3 outlines the pancreatic scan procedure. The radionuclide selenium-75 is utilized in the chemical form of selenomethionine, an amino acid analogue. The physical half-life of selenium-75 is 120

Table 2
Liver-Spleen Scan Technique

^{99m}Tc
Sulfur colloid
6-hour T$^{1/2}$ physical
140 keV
3 mCi IV
20 minute postdose
1 rad (liver-spleen)
No preparation
Polaroid camera
Anterior, posterior, and
 lateral views

Table 3
Pancreatic Scan Technique

^{75}Se
Selenomethionine
120-day $T^{1/2}$ physical
265 keV gamma
250 μCi IV
5 minutes postdose
1.5 rad (whole body)
High protein feeding
Polaroid camera
Anterior view

days and the gamma energy emitted is principally 265 keV. This gamma ray is sufficiently distinct from technetium-99m to permit simultaneous liver and pancreatic imaging. A dose of 250 μCi. is administered intravenously and imaging is begun 5 minutes after the injection. The radiation dose to the patient from the selenium-75 is maximally 1.5 rads to the whole body. Patient preparation consists of a high-protein feeding 30 minutes prior to the injection. The images are obtained with a gamma camera and Polaroid film. An anterior view is obtained with the detector angled to direct the collimator under the liver edge.

Case Reports

LIVER-SPLEEN SCANS.—A normal liver-spleen scan in a 53-year-old man with malignant melanoma is seen in Figure 1. The 5 views in Figure 1 are arranged with anterior views on the left, right lateral and posterior liver on the right, and posterior spleen at the bottom. Each view has 3 exposures, with an optimally exposed view on the left, underexposed on the right, and overexposed at the bottom. Note the costal margin markers in the anterior view (upper left image) which are strips of lead-impregnated rubber taped to the patient. In this scan, the liver and spleen appear normal in size and shape with homogeneous uptake. The patient expired several months after this study and no metastases were present in these organs.

Figure 2 is the liver-spleen scan of a 62-year-old woman who presented with gastric bleeding and hepatosplenomegaly. Hematologic study was suspicious for chronic myelogenous leukemia. The liver was enlarged on the scan, extending 14 cm. below the costal margin. There was also a large defect in the lateral right lobe, 8 cm. in diame-

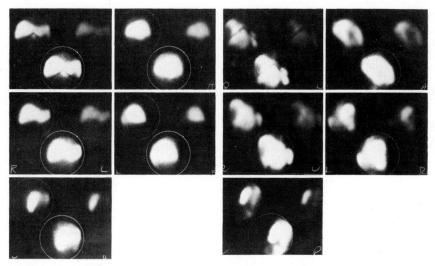

FIG. 1 *(left).* — Normal liver and spleen. See text for explanation.
FIG. 2 *(right).* — Pancreatic carcinoma metastatic to the liver.

ter. The spleen was not enlarged, but was displaced 5 cm. below the costal margin. The cause of this displacement was not apparent. The patient expired 2 days after the scan, and at autopsy there was a carcinoma of the head of the pancreas metastatic to the liver. This was a 7.5-cm. tumor mass on the superior surface of the right lobe.

Figure 3 is the scan of a 30-year-old man with widely disseminated

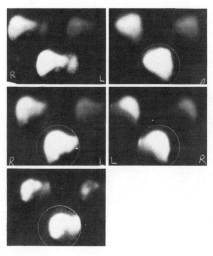

FIG. 3. — Malignant melanoma metastatic to liver and spleen.

malignant melanoma. The liver scan was interpreted as showing uneven uptake, and the spleen was enlarged with 2 focal defects. The patient expired several months later and there was metastatic melanoma in both organs.

Figure 4 is the scan of a patient with carcinoma of the esophagus who was also diabetic and hypertensive. The liver scan demonstrated a diffuse hepatomegaly without defects. At the time of surgical therapy, the liver was grossly enlarged and congested but no tumor was found involving the organ.

PANCREATIC SCANS. — A normal pancreatic scan obtained in a 34-year-old man with metastatic adenocarcinoma to the femur of unknown primary is seen in Figure 5A. A technetium-99m colloid image is recorded in the upper left panel and demonstrates the position of liver and spleen. The camera energy selection window is then changed to the selenium-75 peak and the selenomethionine injection is made. Four 15-minute exposures are made sequentially and, in this case, promptly visualized the liver and pancreas, which appear separated on the scans. Figure 5B shows a computer memory display of data obtained on this patient during the technetium scan (upper left) and selenium scan (lower left). The upper right panel shows a subtraction scan made by electronically removing the liver counts on the selenium scan, using the technetium scan for subtraction. The patient subsequently was found to have a primary tumor of the lung with no pancreatic involvement.

Figure 6A is a pancreatic scan of a 50-year-old man with epigastric

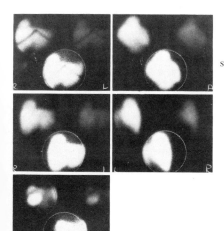

FIG. 4.—Congestive hepatomegaly secondary to cardiac decompensation.

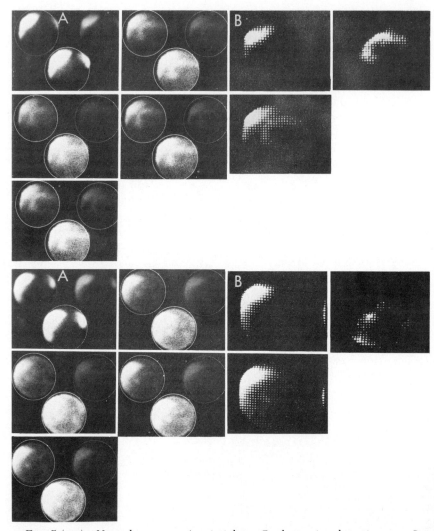

FIG. 5 *(top)*.—Normal pancreas. *A,* scintiphoto; *B,* electronic subtraction scan. See text for explanation.

FIG. 6 *(bottom)*.—Pancreatic adenocarcinoma. *A,* scintiphotos; *B,* subtraction scan.

pain and obstructive jaundice. The scan shows a marked irregularity in the concentration of selenomethionine in the pancreas. Figure 6B is the subtraction scan which shows that a portion of the head of the pancreas is visualized but the body and tail are not seen. At operation, the patient had adenocarcinoma of the pancreas.

Figure 7A is the pancreatic scan of a 61-year-old man with jaundice and a mass in the right upper abdomen. The pancreas is visualized normally on the scan. Figure 7B, the subtraction scan, confirmed normal uptake throughout. The area of decreased uptake between the head and body is a common variation in normal patients.

FIG. 7 *(top).*—Obstructive jaundice secondary to gallstones in common bile duct. A, scintiphotos; B, subtraction scan.

FIG. 8 *(bottom).*—Upper gastrointestinal tract disease and diabetes. A, scintiphoto; B, subtraction scan.

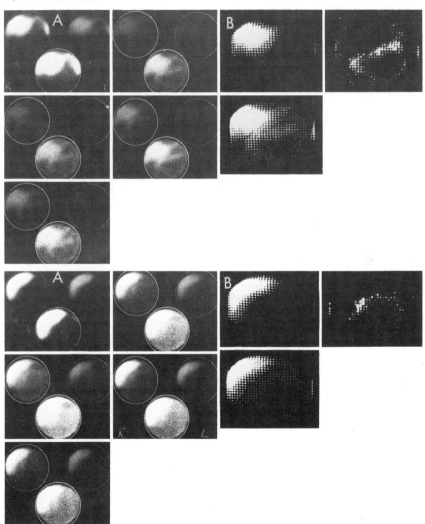

An IV cholangiogram revealed multiple stones in the common bile duct which were removed surgically with good results.

Figure 8A is a scan which was obtained from a 62-year-old man with diabetes, weight loss, and pain in the right side. The scan showed poor visualization of the pancreas. In Figure 8B, the subtraction procedure displayed the organ suboptimally. The patient underwent exploratory laparotomy and pyloroplasty with good result. No pancreatic abnormality was identified at the time of surgery.

Discussion

Table 4 lists some indications for liver-spleen scanning in cancer patients. These scans may provide the answers to questions regarding the size, position, and configuration of the liver and spleen. They may detect accessory splenic tissue, help in the differential diagnosis of abdominal masses, or detect metastatic or primary cancer or other liver diseases. They may be helpful as a guide to biopsy or in follow-up after surgery or chemotherapy. Table 5 indicates some limitations inherent in the liver-spleen scan technique. Depending on the type and location, tumors smaller than 3 cm. probably will not be seen. It is difficult to differentiate benign masses from cancer. Normal anatomic variations may simulate or hide pathologic abnormalities, and activity in the liver may mimic and be confused with splenic tissue and vice versa.

Table 6 shows the indications for pancreatic scanning—patients suspected of having pancreatic cancer or pancreatitis. Table 7 indicates the limitations of pancreatic scanning. A number of anatomic variations and concentration of radionuclide in liver and intestinal tract may mimic or hide pathologic abnormalities. Extrapancreatic

Table 4
Indications for Liver-Spleen Scanning

Size
Position
Configuration
Accessory spleen
Abdominal mass
Metastatic cancer
Primary tumor
Cirrhosis or other parenchymal disease
Infarct
Abscess
Before biopsy
After surgery or chemotherapy

Table 5
Limitations of Liver-Spleen Scanning

Resolution ~ 3 cm.
Benign mass mimics cancer
Anatomic variation
Liver-spleen confusion

disease, for example upper gastrointestinal tract lesions, may result in an abnormal pancreatic scan without direct involvement of the pancreas. The limit on lesion size that can be detected is hard to establish for this small organ, as some lesions that arise peripherally may be quite large and go undetected, while other small lesions may produce significant abnormality by obstruction of pancreatic ducts. In general, the inherent resolution is about the same as for liver scanning.

The following points should be emphasized: (1) The resolution of liver-spleen and pancreatic scanning is limited and the procedures cannot detect cancer in its earliest stages. They are of most use in the symptomatic or high-risk patient. (2) The procedures are nonspecific and cannot be relied upon alone in establishing an etiologic diagnosis. Their best use is as an adjunct to other diagnostic procedures. Because of their safety, they often are of use as early outpatient procedures and for follow-up.

I have not attempted to review the percentage over-all accuracy and specificity of these procedures. These are available in the literature for liver (Jhingran, Jordan, Jahns, and Haynie, 1971; Lipton, DeNardo, Silverman, and Glatstein, 1972; Ludbrook, Slavotinek, and Ronai, 1972; Drum and Christacopoulos, 1972; Leyton, Halpern, Leopold, and Hagen, 1973; Milder *et al.*, 1973; Rosenthal and Kaufman, 1973; and Mangum and Powell, 1973), spleen (Petasnick and Gottschalk, 1966; Larson, Tuell, Moores, and Nelp, 1971; Westin, Lanner, Larson, and Weinfeld, 1972; and Silverman, DeNardo, Glatstein, and Lipton, 1972), and pancreas (Blanquet *et al.*, 1969; Staab, Babb, Klatte, and Brill, 1971; Heslip and Overton, 1971; Landman, Polcyn, and Gottschalk, 1971; Hatchette, Shuler, and Murison, 1972;

Table 6
Indication for Pancreatic Scanning

Suspected pancreatic cancer
Suspected pancreatitis

Table 7
Limitations of Pancreatic Scanning

Anatomic-functional variation
Intestinal and liver obscuration
  and confusion
Upper gastrointestional tract
  (nonpancreatic) lesion confusion

---

and Maile, Rodriguez-Antunez, and Gill, 1972). Results vary with the techniques employed, the patient population under study, and the threshold for abnormality according to the scan-interpreter; however, in spite of their limitations, the procedures can be valuable aids in oncologic practice.

REFERENCES

Blanquet, P. P., Dubarry, J. J., Beck, C., Pegneaux, J., Lebras, M., and Hecquet, M. F.: Scintigraphie pancreatique par soustraction electronique a propos de 200 examens. *La Presse Medicale*, 30:1237–1240, September 6, 1969.

Drum, D. E., and Christacopoulos, J. S.: Hepatic scintigraphy in clinical decision making. *Journal of Nuclear Medicine*, 13:908–915, December 1972.

Hatchette, J. B., Shuler, S. E., and Murison, P. J.: Scintiphotos of the pancreas: Analysis of 134 studies. *Journal of Nuclear Medicine*, 13:51–57, January 1972.

Heslip, P. G., and Overton, T. R.: The value of radioisotope scanning in the investigation of suspected carcinoma of the pancreas. *The American Journal of Roentgenology, Radium Therapy and Nuclear Medicine*, 112:667–677, August 1971.

Jhingran, S. G., Jordan, L., Jahns, M. F., and Haynie, T. P.: Liver scintigrams compared with alkaline phosphatase and BSP determinations in the detection of metastatic carcinoma. *Journal of Nuclear Medicine*, 12:227–230, May 1971.

Landman, S., Polcyn, R. E., and Gottschalk, A.: Pancreas imaging—is it worth it? *Radiology*, 100:631–636, September 1971.

Larson, S. M. Tuell, S. H., Moores, K. D., and Nelp, W. B.: Dimensions of the normal adult spleen scan and prediction of spleen weight. *Journal of Nuclear Medicine*, 12:123–126, March 1971.

Leyton, B., Halpern, S., Leopold, G., and Hagen, S.: Correlation of ultrasound and colloid scintiscan studies of the normal and diseased liver. *Journal of Nuclear Medicine*, 14:27–33, January 1973.

Lipton, M. J., DeNardo, G. L., Silverman, S., and Glatstein, E.: Evaluation of the liver and spleen in Hodgkin's disease. I. The value of hepatic scintigraphy. *American Journal of Medicine*, 52:356–361, March 1972.

Ludbrook, J., Slavotinek, A. H., and Ronai, P. M.: Observer error in reporting on liver scans for space-occupying lesions. *Gastroenterology*, 62: 1013–1019, May 1972.

Maile, A., Jr., Rodriguez-Antunez, A., and Gill, W. M., Jr.: Pancreas scanning after ten years. *Seminars in Nuclear Medicine*, 2:201–219, July 1972.

Mangum, J. F., and Powell, M. R.: Liver scintiphotography as an index of liver abnormality. *Journal of Nuclear Medicine*, 14:484–489, July 1973.

Milder, M. S., Larson, S. M., Bagley, C. M., Jr., DeVita, V. T., Jr., Johnson, R. E., and Johnston, G. S.: Liver-spleen scan in Hodgkin's disease. *Cancer*, 31:826–834, April 1973.

Petasnick, J. P., and Gottschalk, A.: Spleen scintiphotography with technetium-99m sulfur colloid and the gamma ray scintillation camera. *Journal of Nuclear Medicine*, 7:733–739, October 1966.

Rosenthal, S., and Kaufman, S.: The liver scan in metastatic disease. *Archives of Surgery*, 106:656–659, May 1973.

Silverman, S., DeNardo, G. L., Glatstein, E., and Lipton, M. J.: Evaluation of the liver and spleen in Hodgkin's disease. II. The value of splenic scintigraphy. *American Journal of Medicine*, 52:362–366, March 1972.

Staab, E. V., Babb, A. O., Klatte, E. C., and Brill, A. B.: Pancreatic radionuclide imaging using electronic subtraction technique. *Radiology*, 99:633–640, June 1971.

Westin, J., Lanner, L. O., Larsson, A., and Weinfeld, A.: Spleen size in polycythemia. *Acta Medica Scandinavica*, 191:263–271, March 1972.

Arteriography in the Diagnosis of Tumors of the Liver, Spleen, and Pancreas

JOSEF RÖSCH, M.D.
Department of Diagnostic Radiology, University of
Oregon Medical School, Portland, Oregon

ARTERIOGRAPHY HAS A CENTRAL ROLE in the diagnosis of tumors of the liver, spleen, and pancreas. Detailed visualization of the vasculature of these organs enables detection of tumors in the early stage of growth and their differentiation from nontumorous lesions. By yielding information about the nature, size, and multiplicity of tumors and the secondary involvement of other organs, arteriography

Table 1
Accuracy of Arteriography in Diagnosis of Hepatic, Splenic, and Pancreatic Tumors—
150 Consecutive Proven Cases

Tumor Location	Number of Patients	Correct Number	Diagnosis Per Cent	False-Negative Diagnosis
Liver	75	73	97%	2 metastatic tumors with simultaneous obstructive jaundice
Spleen	7	7	100%	—
Pancreas	68	65	95%	2 avascular islet cell tumors, 1 carcinoma with simultaneous pancreatitis and pancreatolithiasis

Table 2
Accuracy of Arteriography in Excluding Hepatic and Pancreatic Tumors —
50 Consecutive Proven Cases

Organ	Number of Patients	Correct Number	Diagnosis Per cent	False-Positive Diagnosis of Tumor
Liver	38	37	97%	1 hepatitis with microabscessi
Pancreas	12	10	83%	1 aberrant pancreas 1 enlarged lymph node

also contributes substantially to therapeutic decisions, particularly in the planning of surgical treatment.

The accuracy of arteriography in the diagnosis of hepatic, splenic, and pancreatic tumors depends on their vascularity and size. Arteriography has a high rate of accuracy in the diagnosis of hypervascular tumors and may identify a tumor 5 to 10 mm. in diameter. Avascular tumors are usually found later, while growing to 2 cm. or more in diameter. In our series of 150 consecutive patients with proven hepatic, splenic, or pancreatic tumors, arteriographic accuracy reached 97 per cent (Table 1). It was highest in splenic diagnosis, where none of 7 splenic tumors was missed. In diagnosis of the liver, we failed to find metastatic tumors in 2 patients where simultaneous biliary involvement with intrahepatic bile duct enlargement masked the tumor changes. Underlying changes of advanced pancreatitis and pancreatolithiasis were the cause of a false-negative diagnosis in 1 patient with a small carcinoma of the pancreas. Also, 2 nondiagnosed islet cell tumors were predominantly fibrotic and hypovascular, and their size ($\frac{1}{2}$ cm. and 1 cm., respectively) was below the arteriographic diagnostic limits.

Arteriography also has a high rate of accuracy in the exclusion of tumors. In our series of 50 consecutive cases examined for suspected hepatic or pancreatic tumors, with final diagnosis proven by surgery and/or autopsy, diagnosis was correct in 97 per cent of cases with suspected hepatic tumors and 83 per cent of cases with suspected pancreatic tumors (Table 2). One false-positive diagnosis of hepatic metastases was made in a patient with hepatitis and microabscessi. In 2 patients with clinically suspected islet cell tumor, an aberrant pancreas and an enlarged lymph node, respectively, were misdiagnosed as tumor.

Hepatic Tumors

Angioma of the liver occasionally may be of the capillary type and form a small, well-demarcated focus consisting of minute and tortuous vessels. The cavernous type of angioma occurs more often, however, and may present as a solitary lesion or multiple foci, or may involve a large portion of the liver (Fig. 1). It is supplied by normal or only slightly enlarged arteries, and its filling appears in the late arterial phase. Variously dilated vascular spaces (lakes), which are irregularly crowded together, form its typical angiographic appearance. Cavernous hemangioma often has an irregular shape and sometimes may have an irregular demarcation from normal tissue. Defects occasionally appear, particularly in large hemangiomas, and these are caused by bleeding into the tumor. Large angiomas often displace adjacent hepatic vessels. Filling of cavernous hemangiomas typically persists into the late capillary or even the venous phase. No filling of draining veins appears in hemangiomas, except in children with giant tumors.

Adenomas or hamartomas of the liver, consisting of well-formed hepatic and bile duct cells, are moderately vascular (Fig. 2). They form rounded foci with variously large, tortuous vessels, and sometimes even small lakes. They are well demarcated from the hepatic tissue, and often a capsule is seen around them as a translucent ring. In the capillary phase, they become opacified and show higher density at the surrounding parenchyma.

Cyst of the liver, regardless of its etiology, presents as an avascular focus with displaced and deformed adjacent intrahepatic vessels. A giant cyst may even deform extrahepatic arteries (Fig. 3). A sharply marginated, usually round defect is seen in the capillary phase and may have a denser rim, particularly in hydatoid cyst. Polycystic liver disease is demonstrated by multiple avascular areas surrounded by deformed branches and a typical finding of numerous regular defects in the capillary phase.

Hepatoma (hepatocell carcinoma) may present as a massive solitary tumor, multiple noduli, or diffuse infiltrative tumor. Enlargement of the feeding hepatic arteries, deformity of the hepatic branches, rich tumor neovascularity, tumor stain, and infiltration of portal radicles are characteristic angiographic features of hepatoma which are variously prominent, depending on the form of its growth.

Enlargement of the feeding arteries occurs mainly in a large solitary hepatoma. The branches adjacent to the tumor may be less filled

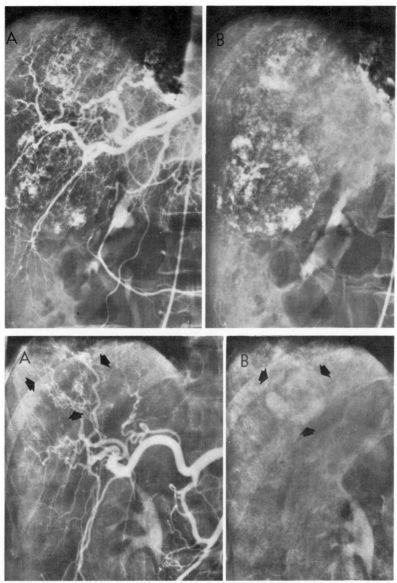

FIG. 1 *(top)*.—Large multifocal hepatic hemangioma involving most of the right lobe and part of the left lobe. *A*, arterial phase; *B*, capillary phase.

FIG. 2 *(bottom)*.—Hepatoadenoma in the upper part of the right lobe (arrows). *A*, arterial phase; *B*, capillary phase.

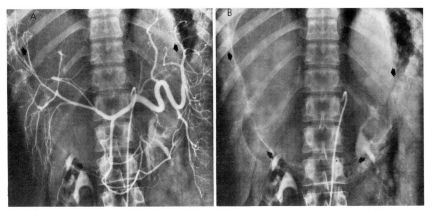

FIG. 3.—Giant echinococcal cyst of the liver (arrows). *A*, arterial phase; *B*, capillary phase.

because of shunting of flow into the hepatoma and are variously deformed. A major solitary tumor usually displaces adjacent branches. Distortion, straightening, irregular narrowing, direct invasion, or even obstruction of intrahepatic arteries are more often prominent in the multinodular or diffuse form of hepatoma.

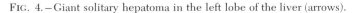

FIG. 4.—Giant solitary hepatoma in the left lobe of the liver (arrows).

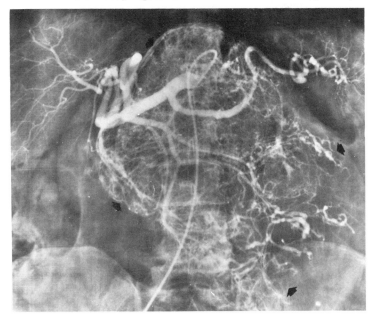

Rich neovascularity is the most characteristic feature of hepatoma. Tumor vessels in a solitary hepatoma are usually large, tortuous, and irregular, and form bizarre vascular networks (Fig. 4). Vascular lakes and arteriovenous shunts with early filling of veins are often present also. An infiltrating hepatoma usually consists of smaller, irregular, tortuous tumor vessels which are intermingled with distorted hepatic branches, giving a completely anarchic appearance on the hepatogram (Fig. 5). Hypovascular or avascular areas also are often found in hepatomas and result from secondary necrosis or hemorrhage.

The capillary phase usually shows dense and irregular tumor stain and often also visualizes early venous filling. In the venous phase, there is sometimes retrograde visualization of intrahepatic portal radicles and even of the portal vein. They may show luminal defects secondary to tumor thrombosis.

Cholangiocarcinoma presents in a solitary or infiltrative form. The solitary form has a predominantly expansive growth and displaces

FIG. 5.—Diffuse hepatoma involving the whole right lobe of the liver. A, arterial phase; B, early capillary phase.

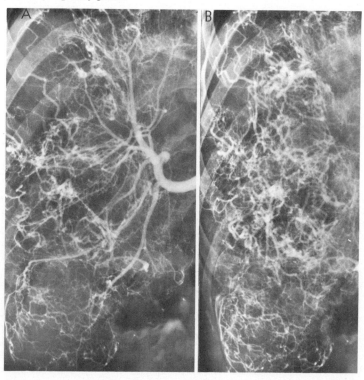

surrounding hepatic vessels. It is slightly hypervascular and its neovascularity consists of fine tortuous vessels. They are sometimes poorly seen individually, but the tumor becomes evident in the capillary phase as a dense focus standing out against the normal hepatic parenchyma. The infiltrative form of cholangiocarcinoma of the liver is poorly vascularized and presents by infiltration, distortion, irregular narrowing, or even complete obstruction of intrahepatic arteries.

Metastatic tumors have a variable angiographic appearance, depending on their vascularity. Metastases of hemangiosarcoma, hypernephroma, or choriocarcinoma are highly vascular and their vascularity consists of irregular, large, tortuous vessels or lakes (Fig. 6). They often are irregular in shape and have indistinct margins. Their visualization begins in the early arterial phase and persists into the late capillary phase, during which a distinct tumor stain and sometimes venous filling also are seen. Metastases of an islet cell or carcinoid tumor also are hypervascular, but their tumor vessels usually are fine and merge together forming dense, rounded, and sharply delineated

FIG. 6. – Multiple metastases of hypernephroma into the liver and pancreas. A, arterial phase; B, capillary phase.

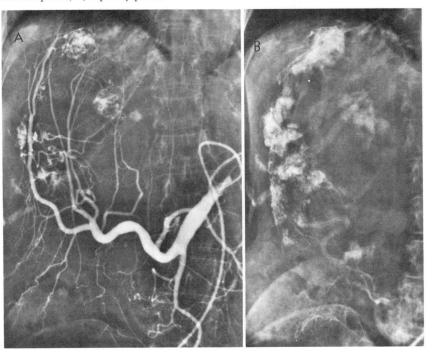

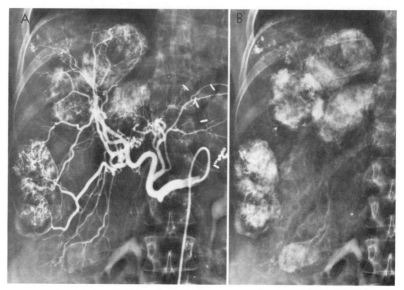

FIG. 7.—Multiple liver metastases of islet cell carcinoma. *A*, arterial phase; *B*, capillary phase.

FIG. 8.—Multiple liver metastases of colonic carcinoma. *A*, arterial phase; *B*, capillary phase.

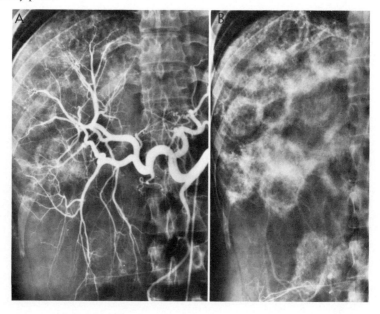

foci (Fig. 7). They appear in the late arterial phase and often persist into the venous phase. Metastases of colonic, breast, or adrenal carcinoma usually show moderate vascularity, with minor tumor vessels, and become moderately dense in the capillary phase (Fig. 8). All hypervascular metastases may show central defects, particularly the fast-growing ones which are caused by tumor necrosis or bleeding. The hepatogram shows variable deformities of the intrahepatic arteries also, depending on the size, number, and character of the metastases. They may be displaced, stretched, narrowed, infiltrated, or completely obstructed.

Hypovascular metastases, as from lung, gastric, esophageal, or pancreatic carcinoma, usually are diagnosed by deformity of intrahepatic branches and defects in liver opacity. Depending on the size of the metastases, small or middle-sized hepatic branches are displaced, arched, stretched, narrowed, invaded, or completely obstructed. With multiple metastases, the smaller arteries are not visualized at all; the hepatogram is poor and formed by stretched and narrowed major and middle-sized branches. The capillary phase shows translucent defects and may have a "Swiss cheese" appearance, with multiple metastases.

Splenic Tumors

Cyst of the spleen presents the typical appearance of an avascular area, displaced splenic branches, and a regularly shaped, well-delineated defect in the splenic opacity. These changes are variously prominent, depending on the location, size, and number of cysts. A cyst in a subcapsular location displaces superficial branches only and causes minor marginal defect. An intrasplenic cyst usually distorts major splenic branches and causes an evident defect in the splenic opacity. In a giant cyst, the adjacent arteries are displaced, narrowed, and reduced in number because of atrophy of the adjacent splenic parenchyma. This appearance distinctly contrasts against the unaffected parenchyma, which remains well vascularized. Multiple cysts distort the whole splenic arterial architecture, and the individual branches are displaced, narrowed, and arched as they encircle avascular areas. The capillary phase then shows distinct regular defects.

Adenoma or hamartoma of the spleen which is formed by unorganized splenic tissue usually presents as a round, well-localized, vascular tumor, displacing adjacent splenic branches. Its vascularity consists of small, tortuous vessels forming an irregular network. In the capillary phase, it reveals diffuse density similar to the surrounding parenchyma, and it may be delineated by a translucent ring.

Primary sarcomas of the spleen are usually vascular and reveal both expansive and infiltrative growth. Tumor vessels may be fine or large, but are often irregular and tortuous; even vascular lakes with arteriovenous shunts and early filling of the splenic vein sometimes may be seen (Fig. 9). The adjacent splenic branches are displaced and often irregularly narrowed, infiltrated, and sometimes completely obstructed. The capillary phase shows irregular tumor stain. Filling of collateral circulation may appear in the venous phase in cases of tumorous obstruction of the splenic vein.

Metastases in the spleen retain the character of the primary tumor. Metastases of a lymphoma or bronchogenic carcinoma are hypovascular and present by displacement, deformity, infiltration, or amputation of splenic branches and multiple defects in splenic opacity. Metastases of a sarcoma or melanoma have a similar appearance, but small tumor vessels are seen in individual foci (Fig. 10). Metastases of hypervascular tumors, such as hemangioendothelioma or hypernephroma, form irregular dense foci, which may persist or drain early in enlarged veins. Tumor invading the spleen from adjacent organs appears as an irregular avascular zone with displaced, infiltrated, or obstructed splenic branches and an irregular defect in splenic opacity.

FIG. 9.—Reticulum cell sarcoma of the spleen (arrows). *A*, arterial phase; *B*, capillary phase.

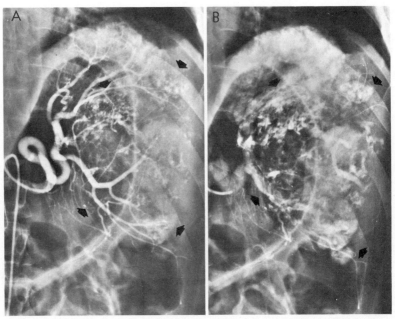

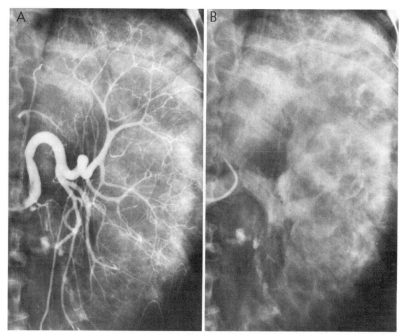

Fig. 10.—Multiple metastases of melanoma in the spleen. *A*, arterial phase; *B*, capillary phase.

Pancreatic Tumors

Pseudocyst of the pancreas presents as an avascular zone with displaced adjacent vessels (Fig. 11). A small cyst inside the pancreas distorts only pancreatic branches. A large cyst affects major arterial trunks around the pancreas as well. The gastroduodenal, common hepatic, and superior mesenteric arteries become distorted by a pseudocyst in the head of the pancreas. The splenic artery and the superior mesenteric artery with its jejunal branches are affected by a cyst in the body and tail of the pancreas. The displaced arteries are stretched, arched, and sometimes diffusely narrowed, but remain smooth in outline. Around a fresh pseudocyst, a hypervascular rim may be seen.

The portion of the pancreatic parenchyma not involved by pseudocyst often shows signs of pancreatitis with vessel deformity and hypervascularity. The venous phase often reveals deformity or even occlusion of adjacent major venous trunks with filling of collateral circulation. The splenic vein is affected by pseudocyst in the tail of the pancreas, while a cyst in the head of the pancreas usually distorts the superior mesenteric vein.

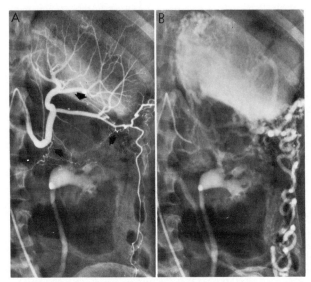

FIG. 11.—Pseudocyst of the tail of the pancreas (arrows) with obstruction of the splenic vein. A, arterial phase; B, venous phase.

Cystadenoma and cystadenocarcinoma of the pancreas are tumors with expansive growth and high vascularity (Fig. 12). They displace adjacent vessels as pseudocysts, but contain numerous small or large, irregular, tortuous vessels, forming a rich network. In the capillary

FIG. 12.—Cystadenoma in the tail of the pancreas (arrows). A, arterial phase; B, capillary phase.

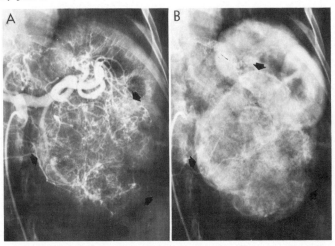

phase, the tumor shows dense blush; however, its opacity is not homogenous and usually contains ill-defined defects caused by cysts inside the tumor.

Islet cell adenoma has various appearances, depending on its vascularity and size. A small hypervascular tumor presents as a dense, well-circumscribed focus which appears in the late arterial phase and persists through the capillary phase. It is most often localized in the tail or body of the pancreas, but also may be found in the adjacent organs growing in an aberrant pancreas (Fig. 13). A large hyper-

Fig. 13 *(top).*—Small hypervascular islet cell adenoma in the descending duodenum (arrow). *A*, arterial phase; *B*, capillary phase.

Fig. 14 *(bottom).*—Three avascular islet cell tumors in the tail and body and one in the head of the pancreas (arrows).

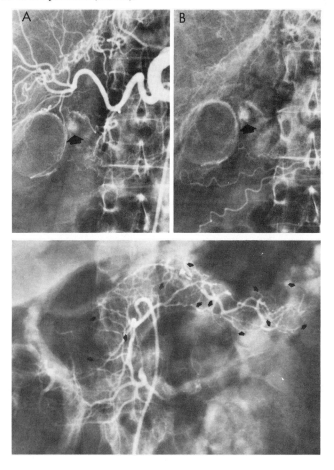

vascular tumor usually is supplied by an enlarged artery and, in the early arterial phase, already shows neovascularity consisting of irregular, tortuous vessels. It is often round and well delineated.

An avascular islet cell tumor presents by a mass effect on surrounding vessels, and small intrapancreatic arteries are most often affected. They are displaced and arched around a round, avascular area (Fig. 14). A well-circumscribed defect also may be seen in the parenchymatous blush.

Islet cell carcinoma may have a similar appearance as adenoma of a dense, well-circumscribed focus and differs from it only by metastases which usually are found in the liver. More often, however, an islet cell carcinoma presents as a large tumor with an irregular shape, extensive vascularity, and involvement of surrounding structures, particularly major portal trunks (Fig. 15). Its metastases usually form dense, well-circumscribed foci.

Adenocarcinoma of the pancreas is an infiltrative, poorly vascularized tumor and invasion of arteries is its primary angiographic feature. Small intrapancreatic arteries are affected first. Their irregularity in outlines and diameter with abrupt angulations are often described as a serrated or serpinginous encasement. A cutoff of pancreatic branches also may be seen and is typical for carcinoma. These changes are localized to a small area, and a differentiation from pancreatitis usually can be made. A major tumor also involves major arteries around the pancreas, and the gastroduodenal, common hepat-

FIG. 15.—Giant islet cell carcinoma in the tail and body of the pancreas (arrows).

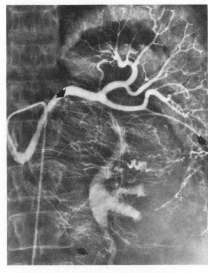

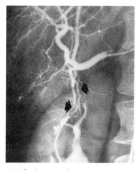 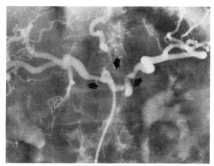

FIG. 16 *(left).* — Adenocarcinoma of the head of the pancreas with infiltration of the gastroduodenal artery and its pancreatic branches (arrows).

FIG. 17 *(right).* — Adenocarcinoma of the body of the pancreas with infiltration of the hepatic, splenic, and left gastric arteries (arrows).

ic, and superior mesenteric arteries are involved by a tumor in the head of the pancreas (Fig. 16). A tumor in the body and tail of the pancreas primarily invades the splenic artery (Fig. 17).

Tumor vessels may be demonstrated in pancreatic carcinoma with superselective arteriography and are usually small and tortuous. The capillary phase may then show a slight tumor blush. The venous phase shows another typical feature of pancreatic carcinoma, venous invasion, and obstruction. The splenic vein or the superior mesenteric vein, and occasionally the portal vein, are affected, depending upon the location and extension of the tumor.

Metastases into the pancreas from a distant tumor retain its character and present as hypervascular foci or by mass effects. Malignant tumors from adjacent organs growing into the pancreas, particularly carcinoma of the stomach or colon, present by invasion and obstruction of the pancreatic and peripancreatic arteries and major portal trunks.

Acknowledgments

Aided in part by United States Public Health Service Grants HL03275 and HL05828.

REFERENCES

Boijsen, E.: Selective hepatic angiography in primary and secondary tumors of liver. *Review Internationale Hepatologie,* 15:385–395, 1965.

Lunderquist, A.: Angiography in carcinoma of the pancreas. *Acta Radiologica Supplement,* 235:1–132, 1965.

Madsen, B.: Demonstration of pancreatic insulinomas by angiography. *British Journal of Radiology*, 39:488–493, July 1966.

Nebesar, R. A., Pollard, J. J., and Stone, D. L.: Angiographic diagnosis of malignant disease of the liver. *Radiology*. 86:284–292, February 1966.

Odman, P.: Percutaneous selective angiography of the coeliac artery. *Acta Radiologica Supplement*, 159:1–168, 1958.

Reuter, S. T., and Redman, H. C.: *Gastrointestinal Angiography*. Philadelphia, Pennsylvania, W. B. Saunders Co., 1972, 292 pp.

Rösch, J.: *Roentgenology of the Spleen and Pancreas*. Springfield, Illinois, Charles C Thomas, 1967, 365 pp.

Rösch, J., and Steckel, R. J.: Selective angiography of the abdominal viscera. W. H. Hanafee, Ed.: In *Golden's Diagnostic Radiology, Section 18*. Baltimore, Maryland, The Williams and Wilkins Co., 1972, pp. 17–87.

Radiation Changes in the Liver Demonstrated by Angiography

SIDNEY WALLACE, M.D.
*Department of Diagnostic Radiology, The University of
Texas System Cancer Center M. D. Anderson Hospital
and Tumor Institute, Houston, Texas*

THE EFFECTS OF IONIZING RADIATION on the liver depend upon the volume of the liver irradiated, the dosage, and the time during which the radiation takes place, as well as on the condition of the hepatic cells at the time of the irradiation (Dettmer, Kramer, Driscoll, and Aponte, 1968; Witcofski, Pizzarello, and Everhart, 1972). Clinically, these effects may be obscured because of the functional reserve and regenerative capacity of the liver (Dettmer, Kramer, Driscoll, and Aponte, 1968; Tefft *et al.*, 1970; Tefft, Traggis, and Filler, 1969).

Irradiation of a portion of the liver with a time-dose relationship of 1,000 rads per week for 4 to 5 weeks usually occurs as a side effect of radiation therapy to adjacent structures. The patient is usually asymptomatic referrable to the liver as long as the unirradiated portion of the liver is healthy (Filler *et al.*, 1969; Nebesar, Tefft, Vawter, and Filler, 1969; Tefft *et al.*, 1970; Tefft, Traggis, and Filler, 1969). As with surgical hepatectomy, a minimum of 15 per cent of normal unirradiated liver is probably necessary to maintain normal liver function and allow for compensatory hypertrophy (Filler *et al.*, 1969; Tefft *et al.*, 1970). Awareness of liver damage may be manifested only by radioisotopic hepatic scanning revealing a segmental area of diminished uptake coinciding with the portal of irradiation (Spencer and Kligerman, 1970; Wordsworth and Dykes, 1969).

Total liver irradiation is extremely dangerous and is encountered most often with total abdominal radiation therapy. A group of 65 patients with ovarian carcinoma was treated at M. D. Anderson Hospital between January 1965 and August 1967 by the moving strip technique with cobalt 60 with doses ranging from 2,450 to 2,920 rads in 12 days; 14 patients apparently cured of cancer were noted to have the clinical findings of radiation hepatitis. Of these 14 patients, 11 died either directly or indirectly of radiation injury (Wharton, Delclos, Gallager, and Smith, 1973).

This communication presents the angiographic findings correlated with histologic changes during the acute and chronic phases of partial and total liver irradiation.

Illustrative Cases

Partial Hepatic Irradiation

Acute. — Acute radiation changes are illustrated by the findings in a 39-year-old male patient with carcinoma of the left kidney and pulmonary metastases. In an attempt to decrease the size of the primary neoplasm and palliate the patient's disease, radiation therapy was given to the left kidney to a dose of 5,500 rads in 6½ weeks. Repeat renal, celiac, and superior mesenteric arteriography was performed at the end of treatment to assess the effect. The right hepatic artery originated from the superior mesenteric artery supplying the right lobe of the liver and demonstrated normal arterial and venous phases. The left hepatic artery, a branch of the common hepatic artery, arose from the celiac axis. The left lateral segmental branches were elongated and widely separated as the result of enlargement of the left lobe. Portal venous branches were opacified within the first 2 seconds, while the left hepatic arterial branches were still visualized, indicating that arteriovenous shunting was present. The portal venous radicles filled in a retrograde fashion from the periphery toward the hilum. There was slow and prolonged opacification of these vessels. A vascular blush was seen in the enlarged left lateral segment of the liver in the distribution of the radiation portal with the margins of the irradiated area sharply defined (Fig. 1).

Chronic. — Chronic changes seen in partial hepatic irradiation were demonstrated by angiography performed 1 year after irradiation therapy to a portion of the right lobe of the liver which was included in the treatment portal. The patient was a 13-year-old female with carcinoma of the left adrenal gland. Three months after removal of

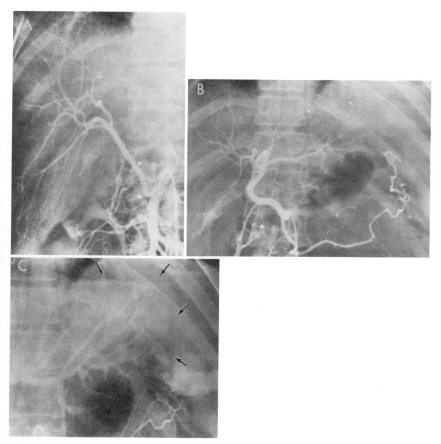

Fig. 1.—Partial liver irradiation. Acute changes. A, nonirradiated right lobe of the liver. The right hepatic artery originated from the superior mesenteric artery. No significant abnormalities are noted in the vasculature of the right lobe. B, irradiated lateral segment of the left lobe of the liver. The left lateral branches are enlarged and separated. C, irradiated left lateral segment. There was opacification and retrograde flow in the portal venous radicles of the left lobe of the liver. The radiation portal is delineated by the vascularity.

the left adrenal carcinoma, a paracaval mass was noted possibly originating from the right adrenal. This mass, as well as a segment of the right lobe of the liver, was treated by radiotherapy to a dose of 5,000 rads in 5 weeks; 3½ months later a hepatic scan utilizing ^{99m}Tc colloid revealed a zone of decreased uptake in the area treated (Fig. 2A, B). The scan remained unchanged on a repeat examination performed 7 months later. At that time, 1 year after radiation therapy to the liver, a celiac arteriogram demonstrated marked tortuosity or

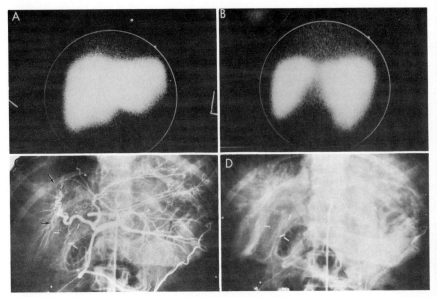

FIG. 2.—Partial liver irradiation. Chronic changes. *A*, hepatic scan prior to irradiation. *B*, hepatic scan 7 months later after a portion of the right lobe had been irradiated. Note the defect in the right lobe and enlargement of the left lobe. *C*, arteriogram 1 year after irradiation. The treated portion of the right lobe is contracted as demonstrated by tortuous right hepatic arteries. The left hepatic arteries are elongated in association with the compensatory hypertrophy. *D*, the hepatogram and venous phase again reveal the small right lobe and enlarged left lobe.

"configuration of the corkscrew vessels" in a contracted area of the right lobe of the liver within the treated zone. The arterial branches of the left hepatic artery supplied a notably enlarged left lobe, and the vessels were separated and elongated (Fig. 2*C*, *D*). The hepatogram revealed a contracted portion of the right lobe in the treated area, and the direction of venous flow was normal. The liver function studies remained normal throughout this period of time.

In contrast to these patients, treated by partial hepatic irradiation and remaining asymptomatic referrable to the liver with normal liver function studies, the patients whose entire liver was treated manifested clinical findings of radiation hepatitis. In a series of 65 patients treated for carcinoma of the ovary at M. D. Anderson Hospital and Tumor Institute between 1965 and 1967, 14 who were apparently cured of their neoplasm were noted to have clinical findings attributable to the irradiation of their liver. The treatment by ^{60}Co teletherapy with the moving strip technique delivered an estimated dose of 2,450 to 2,920 rads in 12 days and resulted in 11 fatalities. Based upon the onset of clinical symptoms, length of survival, and histologic changes, these 11 cases of radiation hepatitis can be divided into 3 groups—Group I, Group II, and Group III.

With total liver irradiation of this magnitude, the onset of symptoms was seen in 4 to 24 weeks, with death following in 3 to 10 months in Group I, those who died in the acute stage. In Group II, symptoms became obvious in 8 to 24 weeks, with a survival of 18 to 37 months. Group III, those who died with chronic changes, manifested symptoms at 24 to 44 months. The clinical findings of radiation hepatitis during the acute stage consist of hepatomegaly, ascites, and pleural effusion. In the chronic phase, the liver was contracted and the patients presented with ascites and pleural effusion. Liver function studies were abnormal in all parameters and the clinical picture was that of venous occlusive disease and cirrhosis. Liver failure and/or hematemesis was the usual cause of death.

The angiographic changes are illustrated in a 43-year-old female receiving abdominal irradiation for the treatment of ovarian carci-

FIG. 3.—Total liver irradiation. Chronic changes. *A*, arterial phase. *B*, venous phase. The arteries are tortuous, probably as the result of hepatic fibrosis. The direction of venous flow is normal. The liver is small and is separated from the abdominal wall. This is probably caused by the liver size and ascites. *C*, the same finding of tortuous vessels is seen in another patient receiving total hepatic irradiation. *D*, the liver and spleen are small. The direction of venous flow is normal.

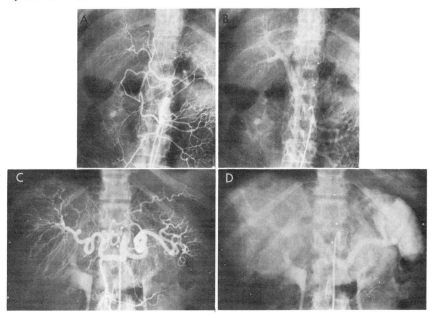

noma. The patient was treated to 2,800 rads in 12 days and did well until 3½ years later when she was admitted because of ascites. Paracentesis revealed yellowish fluid with no evidence of tumor cells. The BSP was 60 per cent, alkaline phosphatase 170, and SGOT 165. Arteriography revealed a small liver, exhibiting tortuous arteries. The venous phase was well opacified and the direction of flow was normal (Fig. 3*A*, *B*). At exploratory laparotomy, the liver was fibrotic, perhaps 50 to 60 per cent of normal size. Although there was no evidence of recurrent or metastatic tumor, the patient's condition worsened with the addition of bilateral pleural effusion, progressive ascites, and icterus. She died 3 months later of liver failure with hepatic fibrosis and esophageal varices. Another patient with a similar sequence of events is illustrated in Figure 3*C* and *D*. The liver and spleen were small and fibrotic as the result of radiation therapy. The separation between the contracted liver and the abdominal wall was caused by ascites.

Discussion

In appraising radiation injury to the liver, an appreciation of the histologic findings is necessary to fully understand the angiographic picture (Wharton, Delclos, Gallager, and Smith, 1973; Nebesar, Tefft, Vawter, and Filler, 1969). The histologic changes consist of a progression of events which is partially reversible, dependent upon the extent of damage and the condition of the liver prior to therapy (Dettmer, Kramer, Driscoll, and Aponte, 1968; Witcofski, Pizzarello, and Everhart, 1972). The hallmark of radiation hepatitis is the fibrinous occlusion of the central hepatic vein with sinusoidal congestion and parenchymal atrophy. These may progress to dense fibrous occlusion of the central vein and hepatic fibrosis (Ackerman, 1972; Dettmer, Kramer, Driscoll, and Aponte, 1968; Nebesar, Tefft, Vawter, and Filler, 1969; Wharton, Delclos, Gallager, and Smith, 1973).

Congestion of the sinusoids is most intense near the center of the hepatic lobule. The etiology is the result of a combination of the direct effect on the hepatic cells as well as of vascular injury primarily affecting the smaller hepatic venous branches (Ariyama, Fausto, Tamvakopoulos, and Van Lancker, 1970; Cammarano, Pons, Chinale, and Gaetani, 1969; Dettmer, Kramer, Driscoll, and Aponte, 1968; Fabrikant, 1969; Looney and Chang, 1969a and b; Witcofski, Pizzarello, and Everhart, 1972). The hepatic veins demonstrate subintimal fibrous thickening, endothelial denudation, and intraluminal fibrin deposition leading to obliteration by proliferation of collagen. When congestion is severe, necrosis of liver cells and local atrophy frequently follow. Congestion may also extend to involve the portal bed with secondary splenomegaly and, occasionally, hypersplenism.

Hepatic venous thromboses may organize, resulting in the formation of circumscribed fibrous nodules in the lobular centers. The hepatic veins may recover by recanalization or there is development of collateral circulation. Congestion then subsides and in mild cases, complete cellular repair may occur. With severe injury, the irradiated portion becomes contracted and firm and the surface of the liver is granular. Histologically, there is central lobular fibrosis, sublobular venous fibrosis, and venous occlusion. Fibrosis also extends to the portal triads with involvement of the portal vein radicles, hepatic arteries, and bile ducts (Ackermann, 1972; Dettmer, Kramer, Driscoll, and Aponte, 1968; Filler *et al.*, 1969; Nebesar, Tefft, Vawter, and Filler, 1969; Tefft *et al.*, 1970; Tefft, Traggis, and Filler, 1969; Wharton, Delclos, Gallager, and Smith, 1973).

The histologic findings seen in radiation hepatitis are reflected in the arteriographic changes. In the acute phase, the enlargement of that portion of the liver receiving radiation is represented by elongation and increased separation of the branches of the hepatic arteries. The sinusoidal congestion in the distribution of the radiation portal is manifested during angiography by a sharply defined zone of hypervascularity. Occlusion of the intralobular hepatic veins results in an obstruction to outflow which is reflected in rapid shunting from the hepatic artery to the portal vein with its retrograde filling toward the nonirradiated areas. Under normal circumstances, there are communications between the hepatic artery and portal vein, but these are seldom opacified unless there is obstruction to hepatic vein outflow as is seen in venous occlusive diseases like hepatic vein thrombosis and cirrhosis or in hepatomas (Nebesar and Pollard, 1969). Arteriovenous fistulas between the hepatic artery and portal vein also have been seen in trauma, but opacification of the portal veins proceeds in a hepatofugal direction, opposite to that seen in radiation changes. The decrease of normal functioning hepatic parenchymal and reticuloendothelial cells is reflected in the isotopic scans which reveal a decrease in uptake in the treated area (Nebesar, Tefft, Vawter, and Filler, 1969; Spencer and Kligerman, 1970). The acute phase lasts approximately 3 to 6 months.

Repair and regeneration is initiated almost immediately, depending upon the extent and severity of the injury. However, with progressive damage, chronic changes become obvious in approximately 6 months. Fibrosis and contraction of the irradiated portion of the liver are associated with tortuosity of the branches of the hepatic artery. Shunting to the portal vein is no longer seen, probably because of recanalization of hepatic veins. The branches of the portal vein in the treated area are tortuous, in contrast to their elongation and separation in the remainder of the liver. In the nonirradiated liver, compensatory hypertrophy is evidenced by stretching and separation of the normal hepatic arteries. The portal venous flow is normal in direction but diverted to the veins in the nonirradiated areas (Nebesar, Tefft, Vawter, and Filler, 1969).

Total hepatic irradiation results in the same sequence of histologic changes (Wharton, Delclos, Gallager, and Smith, 1973). With dosages ranging from 2,500 to 3,000 rads in 2½ weeks, the effects are slowly progressive, ultimately terminating in extensive hepatic fibrosis. The hepatic arteries are tortuous, reflecting the increase in peripheral vascular resistance. The direction of flow in the portal circulation is normal, although hepatic fibrosis was considered the etiology of the tortuosity of the intrahepatic branches of the portal vein.

Summary

Irradiation of the liver is manifested by sinusoidal congestion, parenchymal atrophy, subintimal fibrous thickening of the central veins, and, eventually, dense fibrous occlusion of the hepatic veins. The angiographic findings reflect these histologic changes.

REFERENCES

Ackerman, L. V.: The pathology of radiation effect of normal and neoplastic tissue. *The American Journal of Roentgenology, Radium Therapy and Nuclear Medicine,* 114:447–458, March 1972.

Ariyama, K., Fausto, N., Tamvakopoulos, E., and Van Lancker, J. L.: Effects of x-radiation on amino acid incorporation into regenerating liver proteins. *Radiation Research,* 42:528–538, June 1970.

Cammarano, P., Pons, S., Chinale, G., and Gaetani, S.: Effect of x-irradiation on polyribosome organization and RNA labeling in the liver of normal and adrenalectomized rats. *Radiation Research,* 39:289–304, August 1969.

Dettmer, C. M., Kramer, S., Driscoll, D. H., and Aponte, G. E.: A comparison of the chronic effects of irradiation upon the normal, damaged and regenerating rat liver. *Radiology,* 91:993–997, November 1968.

Fabrikant, J. I.: Radiation response in relation to the cell cycle in vivo. *The American Journal of Roentgenology, Radium Therapy and Nuclear Medicine,* 105:734–745, April 1969.

Filler, R. M., Tefft, M., Vawter, G. F., Maddock, C., and Mitus, A.: Hepatic lobectomy in childhood: Effects of x-ray and chemotherapy. *Journal of Pediatric Surgery,* 4:31–41, February 1969.

Looney, W. B., and Chang, L. O.: The effects of x-radiation on thymidine-labeled DNA of regenerating rat liver. *Radiation Research*, 37:525–530, March 1969a.

———: The recovery in vivo of DNA synthesis following radiation. *Cancer Research*, 29:1156–1158, May 1969b.

Nebesar, R. A., and Pollard, J. J.: A critical evaluation of selective celiac and superior mesenteric angiography in the diagnosis of pancreatic diseases, particularly malignant tumor: facts and artefacts. *Radiology*, 89:1017–1027, December 1967.

Nebesar, R. A., Tefft, M., Vawter, G. F., and Filler, R. M.: Angiography in radiation hepatitis. Presented at the fifty-fifth annual meeting of the Radiological Society of North America, Dec. 1969.

Spencer, R. P., and Kligerman, M. M.: Scan evidence of hepatic "refunction" after tumor irradiation. *Journal of Nuclear Medicine*, 11:140–141, March 1970.

Tefft, M., Mitus, A., Das, L., Vawter, G. F., and Filler, R. M.: Irradiation of the liver in children: Review of experience in the acute and chronic phases, and in the intact normal and partially resected. *The American Journal of Roentgenology, Radium Therapy and Nuclear Medicine*, 108:365–385, February 1970.

Tefft, M., Traggis, D., and Filler, R. M.: Liver irradiation in children: acute changes with transient leukopenia and thrombocytopenia. *The American Journal of Roentgenology, Radium Therapy and Nuclear Medicine*, 106:750–765, August 1969.

Wharton, J. T., Delclos, L., Gallager, S., and Smith, J. P.: Radiation hepatitis induced by abdominal irradiation with the cobalt 60 moving strip technique. *The American Journal of Roentgenology, Radium Therapy and Nuclear Medicine*, 117:73–80, January, 1973.

Witcofski, R. L., Pizzarello, D. J., and Everhart, H.: Repair and latent injury in rat liver after x-irradiation. *Radiology*, 105:195–198, October 1972.

Wordsworth, O. J., and Dykes, P. W.: A functional and morphological study of liver radiation injury following intravenous injection with colloidal gold 198 Au. *International Journal of Radiation, Biology, and Related Studies*, 14(6):497–515, 1969.

Roentgen Diagnosis of Radiation Injury of the Gastrointestinal Tract

LEE F. ROGERS, M.D.*, and
HARVEY M. GOLDSTEIN, M.D.†
*Departments of Diagnostic Radiology, *The University
of Texas Medical School at Houston, and †The
University of Texas System Cancer Center M. D.
Anderson Hospital and Tumor Institute, Houston,
Texas*

THE PHYSICIAN IS CONSTANTLY made aware of the delicate therapeutic balance between cure and complication – the risk of treatment
against the gain of control of disease. In the treatment for life-threatening disease, the physician and the patient must be willing to accept a certain percentage of complications. An unwillingness to do
so may consign the patient to an earlier or even needless demise and
will deprive the physician of an opportunity to cure his patient. In
order to achieve the optimum therapeutic balance, one must strive to
maximize the rate of cure while simultaneously maintaining the rate
of complications at an acceptable minimum. Still, even under the
best of circumstances, some injury to normal surrounding tissues is
inevitable. Radiation injuries of the alimentary tract have proven particularly vexing to all physicians involved in their diagnosis and
management, including the diagnostic radiologist. Despite the presence of severe clinical symptoms, the radiological changes may be
subtle and easily overlooked. Moreover, extensive changes may be
easily confused with those created by recurrent malignant disease

or postoperative adhesions (Localio, Stone, and Friedman, 1969; Perkins and Spjut, 1962; Todd, 1938).

The purpose of this report is to provide some understanding of the factors involved in radiation injury of the alimentary tract, present the spectrum of radiological findings, call attention to significant features in the differential diagnosis, and correlate the resultant pathology with the radiologic findings.

Pathogenesis

The factors involved in the production of radiation injury of the intestinal tract may be divided into 2 categories (Rubin and Casarett, 1968; Strockbine, Hancock, and Fletcher, 1970). The first is related to the treatment modality. In general, the greater the dose, the shorter the time, and the larger the treatment volume, the greater the likelihood of injury. Radiation injuries of the alimentary tract are seldom encountered with tumor doses below 4,200 to 4,500 rads delivered to whole pelvic fields of approximately 15 × 15 cm. (Localio, Stone, and Friedman, 1969; Strockbine, Hancock, and Fletcher, 1970). The rate of injury increases gradually between 4,500 and 6,000 rads and sharply thereafter (Roswit, Malsky, and Reid, 1972; Strockbine, Hancock, and Fletcher, 1970). In general, the tolerance of the normal tissues increases distally from the duodenum to the small bowel and, thence, to the colon and rectum.

The second category consists of factors inherent to the patient: a previous history of abdominal surgery or pelvic inflammatory disease (Joelsson, Raf, and Soderberg, 1971; Kaplan, Hudgins, and Wall, 1965) and concomitant arteriosclerosis, diabetes, and/or hypertension. The former is important, since adhesions limit motion of the small bowel and may fix loops within the pelvis. Normally, the small bowel is free to move and therefore in the absence of adhesions, it is quite unlikely that the same segment of bowel will be within the field of treatment each day. The latter facts are important since they adversely affect the vasculature of the bowel. It is also possible that previous surgery may have compromised the vascularity of the bowel. Radiation affects the small vessels so that tissues affected by pre-existing vascular disease are therefore more susceptible to injury (DeCosse *et al.*, 1969; Rubin and Casarett, 1968). Even then, there remains the important factor of the individual sensitivity. For reasons not presently apparent, some individuals undergo treatment without ill effects, while others similarly treated may develop radiation injury with its attendant morbidity and mortality.

While the radiation effect on the mucosa is potentially reversible, the effect on the vascular tissue is prolonged and gradually progressive. The ultimate outcome therefore is dependant upon the degree of injury of the vascular tissue. The extent of the obliterative endarteritis and the resultant tissue hypoxia are the critical factors in the pathogenesis of bowel injury.

Occurrence

Radiation injury of the intestinal tract has been reported in 0.6 to 17 per cent of all individuals receiving irradiation therapy for abdominal and pelvic malignant diseases (Joelsson, Raf, and Soderberg, 1971; Kottmeier, 1964; Smith *et al.*, 1968). The mean reported occurrence is approximately 6 per cent.

Previous treatment for carcinoma of the cervix accounts for approximately 75 per cent of radiation-induced gastrointestinal disease in most series (DeCosse *et al.*, 1969; Mason, Dietrich, Friedland, and Hanks, 1970; Rubin and Casarett, 1968). Carcinoma of the cervix requires a high central dose of approximately 7,000 rads to eradicate the disease. This requires the use of intracavitary X-ray sources which may result in high doses to the rectum and sigmoid, depending upon the adequacy of the pelvic anatomy. In far-advanced disease, the anatomy is significantly distorted and space is limited, increasing the likelihood of injury. Treatment for carcinomas of the ovary, bladder, and endometrium accounts for most of the remainder of the injuries while a small percentage results from treatment for carcinoma of the prostate, testicular tumor, renal and adrenal carcinoma, and lymphoma. It is obvious from the above that radiation enteritis and colitis occur predominantly in females. The ratio of females to males is approximately 9:1.

Clinical Features

Transient symptoms of nausea, vomiting, and diarrhea indicating acute injury are common during treatment and usually respond to conservative measures. The symptoms of a chronic injury usually occur within 2 years following the completion of treatment (DeCosse *et al.*, 1969; Strockbine, Hancock, and Fletcher, 1970); however, the onset may occur as early as a few months or, rarely, as late as many years after cessation of treatments. The symptoms of chronic small bowel injury are those of obstruction with crampy abdominal pain, nausea, and vomiting. Injuries of the colon and rectum may be accompanied by blood and mucus in the stool, painful defecation, te-nesmus, painless rectal bleeding, and/or reduction in the caliber of the stool. When the delay between irradiation and clinically appar-ent injury is prolonged, it may indicate the presence of a superven-ing vascular disease, *i.e.*, arteriosclerosis, upon the previously inap-parent effect of radiation on the vascular bed.

Since it is the the pelvic organs that are most commonly irradiated, it is logical to find that the rectum, sigmoid, and ileum are structures most commonly affected. Treatment is less commonly given to the upper abdomen and when it is, the total dose and treatment volumes are generally much lower than those utilized in malignant diseases of the pelvis. Radiation injury of the stomach, duodenum, jejunum, and transverse colon are therefore infrequent.

Pathology

Dense, peritoneal adhesions are present in the abdomen. The af-fected bowel is shortened and the mesentery is thickened and con-tracted. The surface of the bowel is gray and opaque, and telangiec-tases are evident (DeCosse *et al.*, 1969). The bowel wall is thickened and the lumen stenotic (Joelsson, Raf, and Soderberg, 1971). On cut-ting the bowel, the thickening is found to be predominantly in the submucosal layer, chiefly fibrous in nature, and with or without nod-ule formation. The mucosa is edematous, atrophic, and frequently ulcerated. Microscopically, the submucosal thickening consists of hyalinized fibroplastic proliferation. Examination of the small vessels demonstrates an obliterative endarteritis consisting of endothelial proliferation, hyaline rings, and subendothelial foam cells (Kaplan, Hudgins, and Wall, 1965; Perkins and Spjut, 1962; Rubin and Casarett, 1968).

Radiologic Features

The radiographic findings (Chau, Fletcher, Rutledge, and Dodd, 1962; Mason, Dietrich, Friedland, and Hanks, 1970; Perkins and Spjut, 1962; Roswit, Malsky, and Reid, 1972) of radiation injury to the gastrointestinal tract are largely the manifestations of an ischemic process. Distinct, sequential acute and chronic stages are not often seen; some overlap and combinations of inflammatory stages are more typical. In the majority of cases, small intestine and colon are both affected (DeCosse *et al.*, 1969), so that complete radiologic evaluation should include both a small bowel series and a barium enema.

ESOPHAGUS

The most common radiologic manifestation of esophagitis secondary to mediastinal irradiation is a diffuse motility abnormality. Failure to complete the primary peristaltic wave with initiation of both abnormal contractions is frequently noted, as is failure to relax the inferior esophageal sphincteric mechanism. In our experience, it is unusual to demonstrate morphologic findings of radiation esophagitis. Only a few cases of radiation-induced ulceration or stricture have been documented. Few follow-up esophagrams are performed, since a remission of the dysphagia usually occurs soon after the completion of therapy.

STOMACH

The lack of frequent gastric irradiation injury is explained only partly by the fact that the stomach area is not often included in the usual high dose therapy field. In addition, the stomach tolerates radiation relatively well compared to much of the small bowel and colon; however, when approaching a dosage of 5,000 rads, gastric ulcers begin to appear with increasing frequency (Lane, 1970; Roswit, Malsky, and Reid, 1972; Sylven, Vikterof, and Schnurer, 1969). The

FIG. 1 *(left).*—Benign pyloric channel ulcer (arrow) with associated inflammatory deformity of the distal stomach following abdominal radiation therapy. No healing occurred during a 3-month period.

FIG. 2 *(right).*—Radiation duodenitis. Postbulbar stricture in a young patient treated for a right adrenal neoplasm. Thickening of duodenal folds is present.

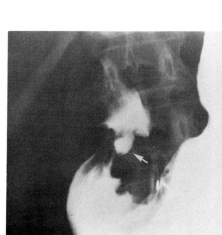
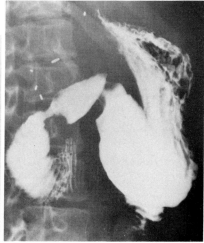

ulcers are usually in the distal portion of the stomach, which is included in the usual spinal and paraspinal radiation portals. These ulcers cannot be differentiated from the usual gastric ulcer in this location, except that healing is delayed (Fig. 1). When healing does occur, considerable scarring with antral narrowing and deformity may result. Unless associated with ulceration, radiation gastritis usually is not identified radiologically.

DUODENUM

As with radiation gastritis, radiation duodenitis is a relatively infrequent occurrence. When encountered, it may present with ulceration indistinguishable from peptic ulcer disease. More commonly, submucosal thickening of duodenal folds is present which may eventually result in stricture formation (Fig. 2).

SMALL INTESTINE

INTESTINAL MANIFESTATIONS. — In general, it is the distal small bowel loops that are involved since they lie within the pelvis. The jejunum may be primarily affected if the upper abdomen is irradiated. The typical appearance of radiation enteritis when first detected is straightening and thickening of the valvulae conniventes, which is produced primarily by submucosal edema and/or fibrosis. On occasion, actual nodular filling defects resulting from submucosal inflam-

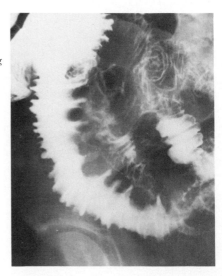

FIG. 3.—Notable radiation ileitis demonstrating mucosal fold thickening and actual nodular filling defects secondary to focal submucosal inflammation.

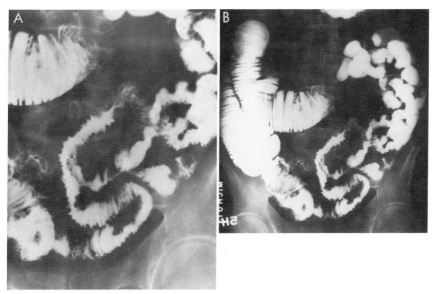

FIG. 4.—Radiation enteritis with proximal small bowel obstruction. *A*, close-up view demonstrates notable thickening and straightening of the mucosal folds with compression of the intervening barium-filled troughs. The affected loops were rigid, with little peristaltic activity. *B*, no focal point of narrowing was identified, but rather several long segments of rigid loops were present.

mation and fibrous nodule formation may be present (Fig. 3). In cases of notable submucosal thickening, the barium-filled troughs between mucosal folds are compressed and take on a spike-like appearance (Fig. 4*A*). Bowel wall thickening is characterized by separation of adjacent loops. At fluoroscopy, the affected bowel is narrowed and rigid with negligible peristaltic activity or change in luminal caliber. Frequently, there is evidence of proximal small bowel intestinal obstruction (Fig. 4*B*). Large ulcerations usually are not noted in the small intestine, but multiple, diffuse, "rose-thorn" ulcers similar to Crohn's disease may occur.

EXTRAINTESTINAL MANIFESTATIONS.—Extraintestinal features are a reflection of localized adhesions and mesenteric involvement. With fluoroscopic palpation, intestinal loops are seen to be matted together and may be displaced only *en masse*. Though not specific, sharp angulation of bowel loops, secondary to adhesions fixing the affected loops, rather than the usual gradual undulations may be present. Another potentially confusing radiographic manifestation of adhesions is spiculation of mucosal folds along one side of the bowel.

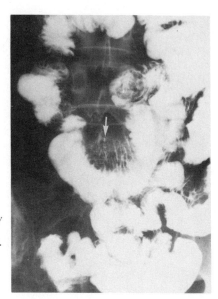

FIG. 5.—Thickening of the mesentery with traction changes on one side of a stretched loop of small intestine (arrow). This appearance mimics neoplasm.

This "tacked down" appearance is secondary to traction or pulling effect from adherent structures and is particularly prominent with any peristaltic activity of the involved loop. Foreshortening and thickening of portions of the mesentery tend to stretch intestinal loops, simulating a recurrent neoplastic mass. This is especially true when mucosal "tacking" accompanies this phenomenon (Fig. 5).

COLON

A smooth stricture of the sigmoid colon and/or rectum is the most common presenting finding in the large intestine (Fig. 6A, B). The affected bowel in this area is often straightened and elevated from the pelvis, presumably because of thickening of the pelvic soft tissues and associated adhesions. Ulceration of colonic mucosa is occasionally identified and usually associated with a narrowed area. The ulcerations may be multiple and relatively superficial, or they can be single and deep to the point of perforation (Fig. 7A, B). Submucosal edema and thickening may produce a "thumbprinting" effect making a differentiation from recurrent neoplastic deposits difficult. This is the pseudocarcinoma pattern as initially described by Todd (1938) of Manchester. On evacuation radiographs, the mucosal pattern may appear prominent from the inflammatory process but is seen to be intact.

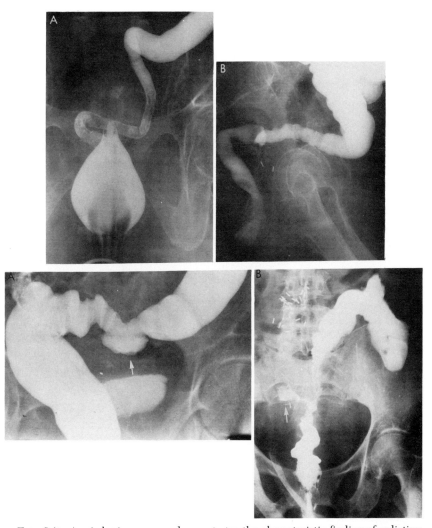

FIG. 6 *(top).*—A, barium enema demonstrates the characteristic finding of radiation colitis; a smooth stricture of the rectosigmoid and distal sigmoid colon. *B*, lateral view of a barium enema in another patient with radiation colitis, demonstrating a smooth, elongated stricture of the distal colon and rectum.

FIG. 7 *(bottom).*—Radiation colitis. *A*, barium enema demonstrates a large solitary distal sigmoid ulceration (arrow). *B*, barium enema in a different patient shows a blind ending perforation of the rectosigmoid colon (arrow) with limited distensibility of the colon in this area.

SEQUELAE

OBSTRUCTION. — The most commonly occurring gastrointestinal sequela of radiation is obstruction. This usually occurs in the distal small bowel or sigmoid colon. Obstruction may result from significant narrowing caused by intrinsic stenosis or adhesions at one or more focal points, but an obstructive picture of equal severity also occurs from longer segments of more modestly narrowed but rigid bowel loops (Fig. 4*A*, *B*).

ULCERATION. — Single or multiple ulcerations of varying sizes occur in both the small and large intestines (Fig. 7*A*). Bleeding, usually chronic in nature, may result, although bleeding may be present even without radiologic demonstration of ulceration. Perforation with abscess formation is another sequel to ulceration (Fig. 7*B*).

FISTULAE. — Fistula formation is another frequent consequence of radiation enteritis and colitis, which may occur between any nearby hollow viscus. Besides adjacent bowel, fistulae may occur between the rectum, bladder, vagina, and skin in any combination, *i.e.*, enterovaginal (Fig. 8*A*), enterovesical (Fig. 8*B*), coloenteric, rectovaginal, *etc.* Careful examination of the small bowel at short intervals during barium transit is critical to the accurate assessment of fistulae. In our experience, both upright and lateral views of the pelvis have been most helpful in delineation of fistulae involving the bladder, small bowel, vagina, and rectum.

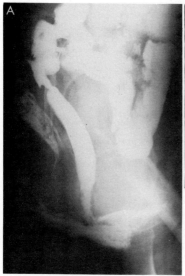
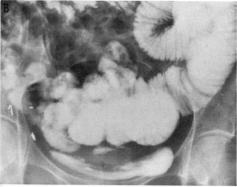

FIG. 8. — Radiation enteritis with fistula formation. *A*, lateral upright view of a small bowel series demonstrates a long fistulous tract communicating from the distal ileum to the vagina. *B*, enterovesical fistula arising from the distal ileum.

CARCINOMA OF THE RECTUM AND COLON. — Carcinoma of the rectum or sigmoid has been reported to arise within areas of chronic irradiation injury (Black and Acker, 1965; DeCosse *et al.*, 1969; McMahon and Rowe, 1971). Whether this is a sequela of irradiation injury or a *de novo* carcinoma is a subject of dispute. We have had no experience with this entity at M. D. Anderson Hospital. The frequency of carcinoma of the colon or rectum has not increased in our patients treated for carcinoma of the cervix. In those cases reported in the literature, the tumors are said to arise within an area of stenosis and frequently demonstrate irregular, abrupt margination with mucosal destruction.

DIFFERENTIAL DIAGNOSIS

Differential diagnosis varies considerably depending upon the location and degree of the radiation injury. Particular diagnostic difficulties may be encountered in the acute-subacute phase of radiation enteritis where a thickened, nodular, fixed, and possibly ulcerated bowel may be easily confused with infiltrative enteropathies, regional enteritis, lymphoma, and especially recurrent metastatic neoplasm. When extraintestinal mesenteric involvement is prominent, differentiation from recurrent neoplasm is particularly difficult. Acute colonic changes also must be differentiated from recurrent pelvic neoplasm and inflammatory colitis, while more chronic, smooth strictures are similar to other causes of colonic strictures including large vessels ischemia and chronic inflammatory colitis. Somewhat abrupt, irregular colonic strictures may even closely resemble primary annular carcinomas.

ANGIOGRAPHY

Angiographic investigation of radiation-induced gastrointestinal disease has been limited. Both animal and human studies have demonstrated vascular spasm and hyperemia during the course of radiation (Bosniak, Hardy, Quint, and Ghossein, 1969; Dencker *et al.*, 1972; Sprayregen and Glotzer, 1971). This is uniformly followed by both arterial and venous stenoses and occlusions at the site of the affected bowel segments.

Summary

The salient clinical and pathological features of radiation enteritis and colitis have been reviewed and correlated with the resultant radiographic findings. When radiation injury is suspected, both the large and small bowel should be examined to determine the full extent of injury. The differential diagnosis between recurrent and/or metastatic disease and radiation injury may be quite difficult. Some distinguishing radiographic features are presented.

Acknowledgments

The authors are indebted to Gilbert M. Fletcher, M.D., and Gerald D. Dodd, Jr., M. D., for their encouragement, support, and assistance in the preparation of this manuscript.

REFERENCES

Black, W. C., and Acker, L. V.: Carcinoma of the large intestine as a late complication of pelvic radiotherapy. *Clinical Radiology*, 16:278–281, July 1965.

Bosniak, M. A., Hardy, M. A., Quint, J., and Ghossein, N. A.: Demonstration of the effect of irradiation on canine bowel using in vivo photographic magnification angiography. *Radiology*, 93:1361–1368, December 1969.

Chau, P. M., Fletcher, G. H., Rutledge, F. N., and Dodd, G. D., Jr.: Complications in high dose whole pelvis irradiation in female pelvic cancer. *The American Journal of Roentgenology, Radium Therapy and Nuclear Medicine*, 87:22–40, January 1962.

DeCosse, J. J., Rhodes, R. S., Wentz, W. B., Reagan, J. W., Dworken, H. J., and Holden, W. D.: The natural history and management of radiation induced injury of the gastrointestinal tract. *Annals of Surgery*, 170:369–384, September 1969.

Dencker, H., Holmdahl, K. H., Lunderquist, A., Olivecrona, H., and Tylen, U.: Mesenteric angiography in patients with radiation injury of the bowel after pelvis irradiation. *The American Journal of Roentgenology, Radium Therapy and Nuclear Medicine.* 114:476–481, March 1972.

Joelsson, I., Raf, L., and Soderberg, G.: Stenosis of the small bowel as a complication in radiation therapy of carcinoma of the uterine cervix. *Acta Radiologica Therapy*, 10:593–604, December 1971.

Kaplan, A. L., Hudgins, P. T., and Wall, J. A.: Injury of the small intestine following irradiation for gynecologic cancer. *Southern Medical Journal*, 58:1109–1114, September, 1965.

Kottmeier, H. L.: Complications following radiation therapy in carcinoma of the cervix and their treatment. *American Journal of Obstetrics and Gynecology*, 88:854–866, April 1964.

Lane, D.: Irradiation gastritis simulating carcinoma. *Medical Journal of Australia*, 2:576–577, September 1970.

Localio, S. A., Stone, A., and Friedman, M.: Surgical aspects of radiation enteritis. *Surgery, Gynecology and Obstetrics*, 129:1163–1172, December 1969.

Mason, G. R., Dietrich, P., Friedland, G. W., and Hanks, G.E.: The radiological findings in radiation-induced enteritis and colitis, a review of 30 cases. *Clinical Radiology,* 21:232–247, June 1970.

McMahon, C. E., and Rowe, J. W.: Rectal reaction following radiation therapy of cervical carcinoma: Particular reference to subsequent occurrence of rectal carcinoma. *Annals of Surgery,* 173:264–269, February 1971.

Perkins, D. E., and Spjut, H. J.: Intestinal stenosis following radiation therapy, a roentgenologic-pathologic study. *The American Journal of Roentgenology, Radium Therapy and Nuclear Medicine,* 88:953–966, November 1962

Roswit, B., Malsky, S. J., and Reid, C. B.: Severe radiation injuries of the stomach, small intestine, colon and rectum. *The American Journal of Roentgenology, Radium Therapy and Nuclear Medicine,* 114:460–475 March 1972.

Rubin, P., and Casarett, G.: Alimentary tract: Small and large intestines and rectum. In *Clinical Radiation Pathology.* Philadelphia, Pennsylvania, London, England, and Toronto, Ontario, Canada, W. B. Saunders Company, 1968, pp. 193–240.

Smith, A. N., Douglas, M., McLean, N., Ruckley, C. V., and Bruce, J.: Intestinal complications of pelvic irradiation for gynecologic cancer. *Surgery, Gynecology and Obstetrics,* 127:721–728, October 1968.

Sprayregen, S., and Glotzer, P.: Angiographic demonstration of radiation colitis. *The American Journal of Roentgenology, Radium Therapy and Nuclear Medicine,* 113:335–337, October 1971.

Strockbine, M. F., Hancock, J. E., and Fletcher, G. H.: Complications in 831 patients with squamous cell carcinoma of the intact uterine cervix treated with 3,000 rads or more whole pelvis irradiation. *The American Journal of Roentgenology, Radium Therapy and Nuclear Medicine,* 108:293–304, February 1970.

Sylven, B., Vikterlof, K. J., and Schnurer, L. B.: Gastric ulceration following cobalt teletherapy, estimation of the tolerance dose, *Acta Radiologica,* 8: 183–188, June 1969.

Todd, T. F.: Rectal ulceration following irradiation treatment of carcinoma of the cervix uteri, pseudo-carcinoma of the rectum. *Surgery, Gynecology, and Obstetrics,* 67:617–631, November 1938.

Thermography and Parathyroid Venous Sampling in the Diagnosis and Localization of Parathyroid Tumor

NAGUIB A. SAMAAN, M.D., Ph.D., ROBERT C. HICKEY, M.D., C. STRATTON HILL, Jr., M.D., and SIDNEY WALLACE, M.D.
Departments of Medicine, Surgery, and Radiology, The University of Texas System Cancer Center M. D. Anderson Hospital and Tumor Insitute, Houston Texas

HYPERCALCEMIA PRODUCES bizarre clincial syndromes because calcium is involved in many cellular mechanisms. However, since the SMA was introduced, physicians are able to discover the presence of hypercalcemia in nonsymptomatic patients as well. The early symptoms of hypercalcemia are nonspecific, such as polyuria, polydipsia, vague muscular aches, easy fatigability, muscle weakness, muscle hypotonia, abdominal pain, nausea, vomiting, constipation, and lethargy or insomnia. Eventually, overt dehydration occurs as do central nervous system changes in the form of disorientation, confusion, and lethargy, often leading to coma. Renal damage with azotemia or bone changes are more common features of long-term hypercalcemia.

Differential Diagnosis

The most common causes of hypercalcemia in a general hospital are malignant diseases with metastases and multiple myeloma. Next in frequency are primary hyperparathyroidism and pseudohyperparathyroidism, which is hypercalcemia resulting from production of a parathyroid-like hormone by a tumor. Other less common causes of hypercalcemia include vitamin D intoxication, sarcoidosis, Addisonian crisis, milk-alkali syndrome, and idiopathic hypercalcemia of infancy (Lafferty, 1966; Myers, 1973).

DIAGNOSIS OF HYPERPARATHYROIDISM

ALTERATION IN SERUM COMPOSITION. — In hyperparathyroidism, the serum calcium level is usually high while the serum phosphorous level is usually low. The alkaline phosphatase activity is high in patients with overt bone disease. Repeated determinations of fasting serum blood samples are required. Blood should be withdrawn after release of the tourniquet because venous stasis may give a false high value for serum calcium. The normal serum calcium level is 9.5 to 10.5 mg./100 ml. Small but persistent elevation above this level is significant. Each laboratory must establish its own range with its own method. In primary hyperparathyroidism, the ionizable or filterable calcium is high; plasma magnesium is normal or low. The plasma chloride is usually above 102 mEq./liter in patients with hyperparathyroidism and less than that in other forms of hypercalcemia.

ALTERATION IN URINE COMPOSITION. — As a result of high circulating parathyroid hormone, hypercalciuria and hyperphosphaturia occur. Hypercalciuria is defined as urinary output of calcium of more than 180 mg. per day on a normal diet, unless the glomerular filtration rate is substantially reduced. High daily urinary output of phosphorous appears to be of no value in the diagnosis since the overlap between normal and hyperparathyroidism is great. The presence of renal insufficiency interferes with the indices of phosphate excretion to a great extent and negates the diagnostic value of phosphorous clearance which is the ratio of phosphorous clearance/creatinine clearance (P/C ratio).

RADIOLOGICAL CHANGES. — In hyperparathyroidism, subperiosteal bone resorption, bone cyst formation, pepperlike appearance of the skull, and pathological fractures may occur, but not all of these changes need to be present in all patients for a diagnosis of hyperparathyroidism to be established.

PREOPERATIVE LOCALIZATION OF THE HYPERFUNCTIONING PARA-
THYROID TISSUE. — The usual assessments by clinical, biochemical,
and radiographic measures are aided appreciably by the radioimmunoassy (RIA) to detect high parathyroid hormone (PTH) level. In our
laboratory, we established a radioimmunoassy of PTH which is sensitive to as low as 0.04 ng./ml. serum (Samaan *et al.*, in press). The
assay procedure is similar to that described by Samaan, Hill, Beceiro,
and Schultz (1973) for the measurement of human calcitonin.

High concentration of PTH in the peripheral blood is usually
found in patients with hyperparathyroidism, but normal levels of
parathyroid hormone have been found in patients with surgically
confirmed hyperparathyroidism. Massage of both sides of the neck
and measurement of PTH in the peripheral blood has been suggested by Reiss and Canterbury (1969) to be of value in the diagnosis of
the site of the parathyroid tumor. However, we found that this
method is unsatisfactory. In our institution, selective catheterization
and venous blood sampling of the parathyroid gland, introduced by
Reitz *et al.* (1969) facilitated not only the diagnosis of hyperparathyroidism but also the localization of hyperfunctioning parathyroid
tissue.

VENOUS SAMPLING TECHNIQUE. — Under local anesthesia and sterile conditions, a femoral vein was percutaneously punctured and
catheterized utilizing the Seldinger technique. Under fluoroscopic
control, a red preshaped Kifa catheter with a single end hole was
advanced into the inferior and superior vena cava, then into both
innominate veins and both internal jugular veins as well as the superior thryoid veins. In all patients, cannulation of the inferior thyroid
veins was attempted. Blood samples were taken, if possible, from 2
sites in the internal jugular veins, the innominate veins, the superior
vena cava, and the inferior vena cava. Samples were also obtained
from the inferior thyroid veins whenever possible. Contrast medium
was injected into the thyroid veins and serial films were taken to outline the venous system of the thyroid gland and to detect any anomaly in the thyroid venous system.

In all our patients who were studied and whose diagnoses of hyperparathyroidism were confirmed at surgery, the fasting serum level
of PTH in the peripheral blood was either higher than seen in normal subjects or at the upper limits of normal in the presence of hypercalcemia. The PTH level in 27 normal subjects (14 males and 13
females) was $1.01 \pm$ S.D. 0.52 ng./MRC bovine PTH/ml. In 40 of the
43 patients suspected of having hyperparathyroidism, the elevated
levels of PTH and the unilateral and bilateral PTH gradient of the

venous samples permitted correct localization of the hyperfunction-ing parathyroid tissue. In 1 patient who had been treated for breast carcinoma and who had no evidence of recurrence or metastasis, a high gradient of PTH was found in the left innominate vein, but at operation, a parathyroid tumor could not be found. A complete surgi-cal exploration was not done. Blood samples taken at the time of sur-gery from the venous system in the neck also showed the highest level of PTH in the left innominate vein. The 2 other patients showed a high level of PTH in the left innominate vein, and at sur-gery a right inferior parathyroid adenoma was found. However, in these 2 patients, the right inferior thyroid vein joined the left thyroid vein to form a common trunk which opened in the left innominate vein.

Of the 43 patients studied, 16 had tumor in other sites, while 5 pa-tients are members of a family with multiple endocrine adenoma-tosis.

The association of hyperfunctioning parathyroid tissue with tumors in other parts of the body is well explained in the following 2 cases:

CASE 1. – A 47-year-old white female had bilateral breast cancer treated recently by a right simple and left radical mastectomy fol-lowed by irradiation therapy. The axillary nodes contained metastat-ic deposits of cancer on both sides.

Biochemically, the patient displayed a hypercalcemic and hypo-phosphatemic state (11.3 to 12.7 mg. per cent and 2.4 to 3.2 mg. per cent respectively); there existed no overt clinical or radiographic evidence of metastatic disease. Peripheral serum showed a high lev-el of PTH. Selective sampling of the venous effluents in the neck showed the diagnostic high PTH in the left innominate vein. At sur-gery, a left inferior parathyroid adenoma was removed (Fig. 1).

CASE 2. – A 33-year-old football coach was referred to M. D. An-derson Hospital and Tumor Institute for investigation of pulmonary

FIG. 1. – The parathyroid hormone levels in blood obtained by venous catheter from different venous sites in the neck.

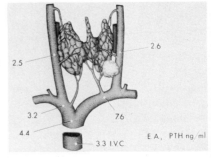

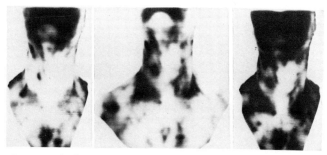

FIG. 2.—Sequential photographs of a thermogram showing a hot spot on the lower part of the neck on the right side.

metastatic deposits. He had a background of familial multiple endocrine adenomatosis. This patient was found to have nephrocalcinosis with a serum creatinine level of 3 mg. per cent, calcium of 11.2 to 12.8 mg. per cent, and phosphorus of 3 to 3.4 mg. per cent. On peripheral and selective venous catheterization, there was elevated PTH in the cervical venous effluents on both sides. Life-threatening azotemia secondary to renal stones demanded attention first; at surgery, total resection of 2 and partial resection of 2 other hyperplastic parathyroids were done, followed immediately by mediastinotomy which disclosed a metastatic, pancreatic nonbeta islet cell cancer. Two weeks after parathyroid extirpation, the patient became normocalcemic and the PTH level dropped to within normal range.

PARATHYROID THERMOGRAPHY.—Thermography is the visual representation of the differential disposition of infrared energy (heat) emitted from a body. Differences in skin temperature are scanned by a radiation detector and the detector signal is amplified and displayed on a cathode ray oscilloscope. A permanent record can then be made with a Polaroid camera. Sixteen of the patients suspected of having hyperparathyroidism were tested by thermography of the neck but only 6 showed the correct localization. A thermogram indicating a hot spot on the lower part of the right side of the neck is shown in Figure 2.

Conclusion

It is apparent from these studies that the radioimmunoassay of plasma PTH from selectively catheterized veins and large neck veins gave the correct preoperative localization in the majority of patients (40 of 43) with hyperfunctioning parathyroid tissue. Parathyroid thermography is not a reliable test for detection of hyperfunctioning parathyroid tissue. Primary hyperparathyroidism should be considered as one of the causes of hypercalcemia in malignant disease. Family history and examination of other family members of an affected patient may reveal the familial form of hyperparathyroidism, multiple endocrine adenomatosis.

Acknowledgments

This study was supported by the U.S.P.H.S., N.I.H. Grant No. CA 05831-12 and the American Cancer Society Grant No. CI-78B.

REFERENCES

Lafferty, F. W.: Pseudohyperparathyroidism. *Medicine,* 45:247–260, May 1966.

Myers, W. P. L.: Hypercalcemia associated with malignant disease. In *Endocrine and Nonendocrine Hormone-Producing Tumors* (A Collection of Papers Presented at the Sixteenth Annual Clinical Conference on Cancer, 1971, at The University of Texas at Houston M. D. Anderson Hospital and Tumor Institute, Houston, Texas). Chicago, Illinois, Year Book Medical Publishers, Inc., 1973, pp. 147–171.

Reiss, E., and Canterbury, J. M.: Primary hyperparathyroidism: Application of radioimmunoassay to differentiation of adenoma and hyperplasia and to preoperative localization of hyperfunctioning parathyroid glands. *New England Journal of Medicine,* 280:1381–1385, June 19, 1969.

Reitz, R. E., Pollard, J. J., Wang, C. A., Fleischli, D. J., Cope, O., Murry, T. M., Deftos, L. J., and Potts, J. T., Jr.: Localization of parathyroid adenomas by selective venous catheterization and radioimmunoassay. *New England Journal of Medicine,* 281:348–351, August 14, 1969.

Samaan, N. A., Hickey, R. C., Hill, C. S., Jr., Medellin, H., and Gates, R. C.: Parathyroid tumors: Preoperative localization and their association with other tumors. *Cancer.* (In press.)

Samaan, N. A., Hill, C. S., Jr., Beceiro, J. R., and Schultz, P. N.: Immunoreactive calcitonin in medullary carcinoma of the thyroid and in maternal and cord serum. *Journal of Laboratory and Clinical Medicine,* 81:671–681, May 1973.

The Diagnosis of Orbital Tumors by Ultrasonic Scanning

GILBERT BAUM, M.D.
*Ultrasound Laboratory, Albert Einstein College of
Medicine, Bronx, New York*

THE ORBIT is the forte of ophthalmic ultrasound. The difficulty of visualizing diseases of the soft tissue of the orbit on X-ray films is well known. This first case illustrates the point: The patient had had exophthalmus for approximately 4 years. He had been seen at numerous hospitals and had accumulated an X-ray studies folder of about 2 inches thick. In addition, he had had previous exploratory surgery at the time he was referred for ultrasonographic examination.

Ultrasonographic examination immediately displayed distortions characteristic of an orbital tumor (Fig. 1). From serial reconstructions of ultrasonograms through the tumor, we were able to reconstruct the gross anatomy of this tumor as shown on the artist's drawing and recommended that this tumor be removed by a transcranial route rather than by a Krönlien's procedure (Baum and Greenwood, 1961). The surgical findings substantiated the ultrasonographic findings. By means of serial ultrasonograms, one is able to produce a 3-dimensional reconstruction of the eye and orbit. Such a reconstruction enables one to precisely localize and measure the size and distribution of orbital tumors. The reconstruction showed that the mass lay outside of the muscle cone. A clue to this location is the clear space on the ultrasonogram between the mass and the echoes from the tissues of the orbital cone proper.

Orbital tumors may also occupy other areas outside of the muscle

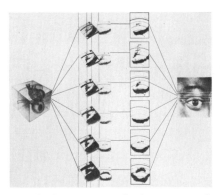

FIG. 1.—A 3-dimensional ultrasonogram displaying an oribtal tumor located between the periosteum and the roof of the orbit. On a 3-dimensional ultrasonogram, it is possible to outline the size, shape, and location of a tumor in any part of the orbit even though a tumor may escape detection by X-ray examination or even by surgical exploration. This composite photograph illustrates the changes in the appearance of the ultrasonograms taken through the levels of the exophthalmic eye. By constructing a 3-dimensional ultrasonogram, an artist is able to construct a phantom of the lesion to serve as a guide for the surgeon.

cone. Figure 2 demonstrates the ultrasonographic appearance of a benign mixed cell tumor of the lacrimal gland. The X-ray findings were negative in this case despite the obvious deformation which this tumor caused and the palpability of the tumor.

Figure 3 is an isophotodensitometric printout of a mixed cell tumor of the lacrimal gland shown in Figure 2, demonstrating the amplitude complexity of this type of tumor. We are trying, by this technique, to determine if it is possible to correlate the ultrasonographic pattern with a specific disease.

Figure 4 demonstrates a meningioma of a lid which again lies

FIG. 2.—A black and white ultrasonogram of a benign mixed cell tumor of the lacrimal gland.

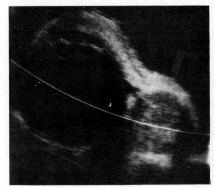

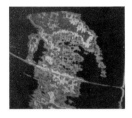

FIG. 3.—A color-coded isophotodensitometric printout of the tumor area of Figure 2. This figure demonstrates the amplitude complexity of this type of tumor.

above and outside of the muscle cone so that the retro-orbital space is free of echoes. In this case, note that the meningioma is virtually free of echoes and produces a break in the wall of the tumor. At surgery, an arm of this meningioma was found extending deep into the orbital cavity through this break.

The next section deals with tumors affecting the structures within the muscle cone of the orbit. Fundamental to interpretation and diagnosis of tumors in this region is an understanding of the ultrasonographic anatomy of the orbit (Baum and Greenwood, 1963; Baum, 1965). This is illustrated in Figure 5. The fat and musculature of the orbit lie within the bony walls of the orbit. Above and below the optic nerve they assume a crescentric "V" or "U" shape. At the level of the optic nerve, there is a tunnel through the orbital fat through which the optic nerve passes. If there is no disease of the orbit, the orbital fat patterns of the 2 eyes are symmetrical and virtually superimposable at corresponding positions of gaze. This is the foundation upon which ultrasonographic interpretation is based.

FIG. 4.—*Left,* an ultrasonogram of a meningioma of the lid. This tumor (arrow) lies above and outside the muscle cone so that the retro-orbital space is free of echoes. The meningioma demonstrates a high degree of absorption and weak internal echoes so that there is an apparent break in the wall of the tumor. At surgery, an arm of this meningioma projected deep into the orbital cavity through this break. The normal lid (*right*) is shown for comparison.

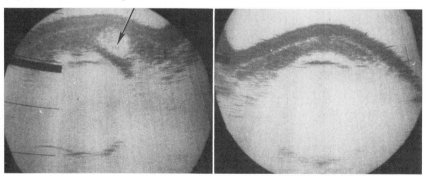

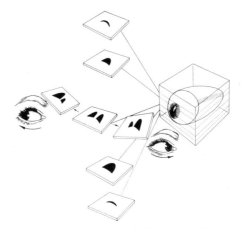

FIG. 5.—The ultrasonographic anatomy of the orbit. Above and below the optic nerve, the orbital fat assumes a "U" or "V" shape depending upon the bony configuration of the orbit. At the level of the optic nerve, an echo-free tunnel appears for the passage of the optic nerve. At corresponding levels of scan, the orbital fat patterns of the 2 eyes are symmetrical. The medial and lateral fat lobes of the orbit may be observed to expand and contract as the eye is rotated.

A horizontal plane of scan is used for examining the eye. Serial vertical scanning in 0.5 mm. steps is carried out, starting at the inferior border of the eyebrow. A scan through the center of the eye produces the tomogram shown in Figure 6. Note how this compound scan accurately reproduces the cross-sectional anatomy of the eye

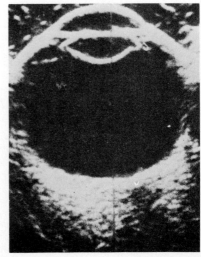

FIG. 6.—A compound scan of a human eye at the level of the optic nerve.

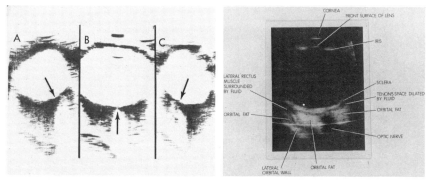

FIG. 7 *(left)*.—An ultrasonogram which demonstrates the passage of the central retinal vessel into the eyeball. The motion that the vessels of the eye undergo as the eye is rotated laterally *(A)* and medially *(B)* is demonstrated. The lateral orbital wall and the oblique musculature adjacent to the optic nerve also are demonstrated.

FIG. 8 *(right)*.—An ultrasonogram demonstrating fluid in Tenon's space and the muscle sheaths surrounding the lateral rectus muscle in a case of pseudotumor of the orbit.

and also demonstrates the orbital fat behind the eye as well as the optic nerve space. A single scan produces a tomogram measuring approximately 0.2 mm. in thickness.

Recent improvements in our ultrasonographic instrumentation have made it possible for us to routinely visualize the passage of the

FIG. 9.—*A*, an ultrasonogram demonstrating the compression and rotation of the optic nerve (arrow 1) by a recurrent neurilemmoma (arrow 2). *B*, the path of the optic nerve of the normal fellow eye is shown at arrow 1. *C*, a similar distortion of the optic nerve produced by hemangioma of the orbit.

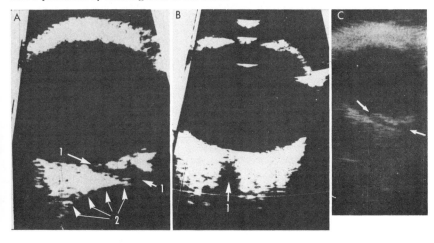

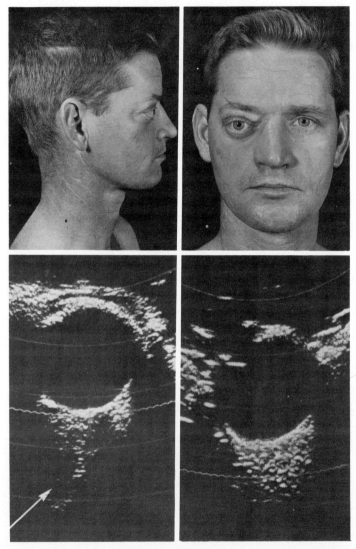

FIG. 10.—A patient with a myxoma of the orbit (arrow). A 3-dimensional reconstruction demonstrated that this tumor was positioned in a saddle fashion over the optic nerve as illustrated in the drawing. Ultrasonogram of normal eye is shown at OS.

central retinal arteries into the globe, the motion of the optic nerve, the lateral wall of the orbit, and the oblique musculature adjacent to the optic nerve (Fig. 7). This figure demonstrates that the optic nerve is a very dynamic structure; its position and orientation change as the eye is rotated from side to side. These improvements in instrumentation have also enabled us to visualize changes in the orbit which, to the best of our knowledge, have never before been visualized. Thus, in 3 consecutive cases of pseudotumor of the orbit in young males, we have been able to demonstrate fluid in Tenon's space behind the eye as well as fluid surrounding the lateral rectus muscle (Fig. 8).

The knowledge that the optic nerve should enter at right angles to the globe when the eye looks straight ahead also enables us to explain visual loss in cases of orbital tumors. In this case of a recurrent neurilemmoma of the orbit, ultrasonography demonstrates the compression and rotation of the optic nerve by the tumor (Fig. 9A and B). A similar finding is demonstrated in Figure 9C which shows the same phenomenon in a case of hemangioma of the orbit. Interestingly, in both of these cases, disc changes were absent. In the last case, the patient's visual acuity was 20/20 despite the compression of the optic nerve against the back surface of the globe. This interpretation of optic nerve compression was confirmed at surgery. We have observed this in other cases and have also observed a return of vision after the pressure on the optic nerve had been relieved.

Surgical sparing of the optic nerve is demonstrated in the following case: Again, this is a patient who had exophthalmus for a period of approximately 4 years, had been seen in numerous hospitals, and had also accumulated a voluminous folder of X-ray films (Krueger,

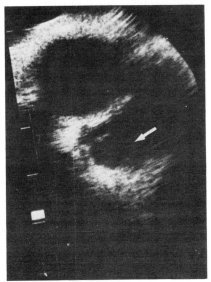

Fig. 11.—The loss of orbital echoes (arrow). Extension of the orbital mass to the medial side of the orbit is demonstrated.

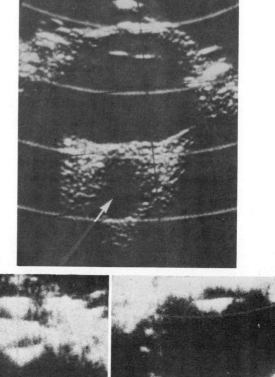

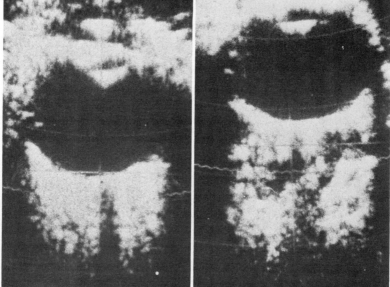

FIG. 12 *(top)*.—An ultrasonogram of an orbital cyst (arrow).
FIG. 13 *(bottom)*.—There is virtual total replacement of the orbital fat pattern in a case of a congenital neurofibroma, OD *(right)*. Normal is shown at OS *(left)*.

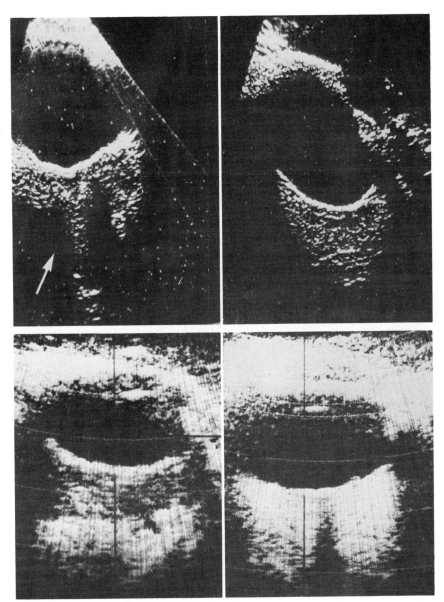

FIG. 14 *(top).—Left,* an ultrasonogram of a meningioma of the orbit (arrow). *Right,* normal eye.

FIG. 15 *(bottom).—Left,* lymphosarcoma invades and distorts the orbital fat pattern at all levels of scan. *Right,* normal eye.

Polifrone, and Baum, 1967). A 3-dimensional ultrasonographic examination indicated that this tumor had to be removed by a transcranial route rather than by a Krönlien's procedure (Fig. 10).

Orbital disease produces 4 types of change in the orbital fat pattern: an excess of echoes, echoes at an aberrant site, a loss of echoes, and/or a change of the internal texture of the fat pattern.

Figure 11 demonstrates a loss of orbital echo pattern (arrow). This ultrasonogram illustrates this loss of echoes in the center of the orbital fat pattern and the extension of an orbital mass to the medial side of the orbit.

Figure 12 illustrates an orbital cyst in a case of spontaneous hemorrhage of the orbit.

The distortion produced by a huge neurofibroma of the orbit which has virtually totally replaced the orbital fat pattern is shown in Figure 13.

Echoes in an aberrant site are shown by the distortion produced by meningioma of the orbit (Fig. 14). It has displaced the orbital fat pattern.

Lymphosarcoma produces a pattern in which all portions of the orbital fat appear to be invaded by the tumor (Fig. 15).

At its present stage of evolution, ultrasonography is unquestionably able to localize and determine the size of a soft-tissue mass within the orbit (Coleman, 1972). There is some indication that it may be possible to correlate the ultrasonographic appearance to a precise histopathological diagnosis, but more extensive experience must be gained before such a firm conclusion may be reached.

Ultrasonography is the single most important diagnostic examination in cases of exophthalmus, and its use is essential for adequate management of this condition.

Acknowledgment

This work was made possible by Grant GM-12460 from the National Institutes of Health, U. S. Public Health Service.

REFERENCES

Baum, G.: A reappraisal of orbital ultrasonography. Series II. *Transactions of the American Academy of Opthalmology and Otolaryngology*, 69:943–958, September–October 1965.

Baum, G., and Greenwood, I.: Orbital lesion localization by three dimensional ultrasonography. *New York State Journal of Medicine*, 61:4149–4157, Dec. 15, 1961.

Baum, G., and Greenwood, I.: Present status of orbital ultrasonography. *American Journal of Ophthalmology*, 56:98–104, July 1963.

Coleman, D. J.: Reliability of ocular and orbital diagnosis with B-scan ultrasound. *American Journal of Ophthalmology*, 74:704–718, October 1972.

Krueger, E. G., Polifrone, J. C., and Baum, G.: Retrobulbar orbital myxoma and its detection by ultrasonography. Case report. *Journal of Neurosurgery*, 26:87–91, January (part 1) 1967.

Nuclear Techniques in the Diagnosis of Thyroid Tumors

PHILIP C. JOHNSON, M.D.
Department of Medicine, Baylor College of Medicine,
Houston, Texas

To be surgically removed, thyroid nodules should be symptomatic, cosmetically displeasing, or carcinomas. Because localized carcinomas are not obvious and cause only a small percentage of palpable thyroid nodules, preoperative diagnostic criteria are necessary to decrease the number of thyroid surgical procedures performed for noncancerous, asymptomatic, or cosmetically acceptable nodules (Mustacchi and Cutler, 1956).

Pathology of Nodules

There are 4 pathological situations which produce palpable nodules in the thyroid gland.

COLLOID NODULES.—Adenomatous goiters are the most common cause of single and multiple thyroid nodules. The incidence of nodular goiters increases with the age of the patient. Formerly endemic in parts of the U.S., these goiters are still seen even though iodine deficiency has been eliminated. Increased dietary iodide has made these goiters smaller and their multinodularity less obvious to palpation; they are the only cause of autonomous nodules.

THYROIDITIS.—Chronic and subacute thyroiditis generally involve most of the thyroid gland, producing a diffuse enlargment. However, some thyroid glands will contain discrete areas of thyroiditis which give the examiner the impression that he is palpating a true nodule. When subacute thyroiditis has subsided, the gland may become irregular and nodules may be felt.

ADENOMAS. — The pathological subclassification of adenomas is of little clinical importance. Prior irradiation may be a cause of adenoma formation. Adenomas are not precancerous, and autonomous nodules are not adenomas.

CANCER. — Thyroid neoplasia appears in 5 general forms. (1) The well-differentiated types, papillary and/or follicular adenocarcinomas, are the least malignant. A major rationale for surgical therapy for thyroid nodules is to remove papillary follicular carcinoma before it becomes highly malignant undifferentiated carcinoma. More than 90 per cent of patients with early differentiated carcinoma can be cured. (2) Medullary carcinoma arises in the thyroid gland but not from thyroxine-producing cells. This cancer secretes thyrocalcitonin and histaminase. The presence of such tumors is proven and even predicted by finding detectable serum levels of thyrocalcitonin. They produce amyloid and are usually asymptomatic (Baylin, Beaven, Engelman, and Sjoerdsma, 1970; Catalona, Engelman, Ketcham, and Hammond, 1971). Medullary carcinomas are slow growing yet many times more malignant than papillary follicular carcinomas. Cure is not common. These cancers are often familial, being part of the multiple endocrine syndromes, with bilateral pheochromocytomas the most common. (3) Metastatic cancer in the thyroid gland is rarely noted (< 5 per cent of cancer cases). (4) Lymphosarcoma can develop primarily in the thyroid gland. Cure is possible by combining surgical removal of the thyroid gland and radiation therapy. Lymphosarcoma of the thyroid is associated with similar disease in the stomach (Woolner, McConahey, Beahrs, and Black, 1966). (5) Undifferentiated thyroid carcinomas, both small and large cell types, probably arise from and are a retrogressive change in papillary follicular carcinomas (Ibanez *et al.*, 1966). When undifferentiated cancer appears, there is no effective therapy.

Clinical Findings Suggestive of Cancer

Several preoperative clinical criteria can be used to help select patients for surgical biopsy while attempting to avoid excessive surgery for benign nodules.

AGE OF PATIENT. — Except in obvious colloid nodular thyroids, nodules appearing in females before the age of 25 should be considered as cancer. Nodules in males up to the age of 40 have a strong possibility of being cancer (Jhingran and Johnson, in preparation).

SOLITARY NODULES. — The presence of multiple palpable nodules is evidence against cancer. There is a clinical problem here, since we have found that 42 per cent of thyroid glands noted to have solitary nodules preoperatively are found to contain multiple nodules when examined at surgery or in pathology (Jhingran and Johnson, in preparation). This probably occurs because of the nodule's small size or because the nodule's consistency is similar to normal thyroid tissue.

PRESSURE SYMPTOMS. — Tracheal obstruction and difficulty in swallowing are common only in undifferentiated carcinomas. Occasional colloid nodular thyroids produce tracheal obstruction. In our experience, these are easily distinguished from cancer.

CERVICAL LYMPH NODE ADENOPATHY. — Except in children, palpable cancerous cervical lymph nodes are more likely to be nonthyroidal cancers. Metastatic thyroid carcinoma extensive enough to produce palpable lymph nodes may have come from an occult primary tumor.

VOCAL CORD PARALYSIS. — In the presence of thyroid carcinoma, paralysis indicates direct invasion of the recurrent laryngeal nerve. Therefore it is unusual in early differentiated carcinomas. Thyroid cancer is an uncommon cause of vocal cord paralysis unless a palpable mass is present in the neck.

PRIOR X-RAY OR RADIATION THERAPY. — Face, neck, or upper chest radiation therapy is followed by a high incidence of thyroid cancer 10 or so years later. However, we and others have found that nearly the same percentage of patients who have adenomas removed have had prior irradiation Jhingran and Johnson, in preparation; Clark, 1955; Rose, Hartfield, Kelsey, and Macdonald, 1963). Irradiation may initiate a thyroid neoplasm but it does not seem to act as a growth factor (Sampson *et al.*, 1970).

PRIOR PATHOLOGICAL ABNORMALITY. — Thyroid regrowth years after surgical removal of a nodule is a common cause of nodularlike swelling in the neck. In these cases, obtaining the original pathology report or slides is most important. It is characteristic of colloid nodular thyroids to produce new nodules years after a nodule has been removed by hemithyroidectomy.

THYROGLOSSAL DUCT CYST. — These are almost never cancer. Less than 40 cases have been described in the world literature (Shepard and Rosenfeld, 1968).

CONSISTENCY OF NODULE. — Three of 4 cancerous nodules feel hard to palpation, but only 38 per cent of hard nodules are cancers (Jhingran and Johnson, in preparation).

Less helpful in clinical diagnosis are a family history of thyroid disease, growth rate, and known duration of the nodule. Rapid growth does not occur in cancer unless the tumor has converted to an undifferentiated type. In our experience, hemorrhage into a colloid nodule is the most common cause of a rapidly growing thyroid nodule.

Radionuclear Techniques

Using clinical criteria, there is 10 per cent accuracy in predicting whether a surgically removed nodule will be carcinoma. Nuclear medicine techniques can be used to improve this percentage preoperatively to 20 per cent.

IMAGING AND SCANNING WITH ^{131}I. — Thyroid scanning or imaging is used to distinguish functional from nonfunctional nodules preoperatively. We have found no real difference of clinical importance between a thyroid scan performed with a rectilinear scanner and thyroid imaging using the Pho/Gamma camera; however, others are of the opposite opinion (Robinson, Collica, and Chang, 1968).

SCANNING AND IMAGING WITH OTHER RADIONUCLIDES. — Radioactive ^{131}I has disadvantages since it is beta emitter and produces a relatively high radiation dose per μCi. Several investigators have tried other iodine radionuclides or iodine-like ions as a substitute. The most commonly used is ^{99m}Tc pertechnetate (Black, 1972; Atkins and Richards, 1968). This anion is trapped by thyroid cells, but not organified. Thus, a high trapping rate in a nodule, even when no hormone is produced, would produce a hot nodule in a technetium scan. If no hormone were stored, the nodule would release the radioactivity, producing a cold nodule in a 24-hour ^{131}I scan. Instances where nodules were hot using technetium and cold using iodine have been reported (Steinberg, Cavalieri, and Choy, 1970; Usher and Arzoumanian, 1971). However, the high trapping rate has been used as a diagnostic aid in chronic thyroiditis (Hauser, Atkins, Eckelman, and Richards, 1971). Short half-life iodine ^{123}I has beeen used for thyroid scanning. It is nearly ideal because of its gamma ray energy and low radiation exposure per μCi; however, it is too expensive for general use.

FLUORESCENT SCANNING. — Fluorescent scanning has been used in thyroid diagnosis (Hoffer, Bernstein, and Gottschalk, 1971). In this procedure, a gamma ray point source with energies just above the binding energy of an iodine K electron is used to irradiate the thyroid gland. This irradiation causes iodine atoms to give off characteristic X rays. The source and detector are moved back and forth across the thyroid at a uniform speed as in routine radionuclide scanning. The quantity of X rays is proportional to iodine content. These scans can be used to classify nodules according to iodine content. As would be expected from pathological appearances, the colloid-rich nodules of a colloid nodular thyroid gland give higher count rates than do thyroid carcinomas. Low-iodine-containing nodules often are not cancers (LeBlanc and Johnson, 1973). The technique is particularly useful for thyroid glands where ^{131}I uptake is blocked by exogenous iodide. When ^{131}I uptake is blocked, it is difficult to obtain adequate conventional scans. Iodine blockade does not affect the quality of a fluorescent scan.

In the conventional ^{131}I scan and images, thyroid nodules usually are seen as areas of increased or decreased concentration. Some palpable nodules will not be seen because their radioactive concentration is similar to that of the surrounding thyroid gland. Cold nodules are areas within the thyroid which concentrate no radioactivity, or less than other thyroidal areas. Cold nodules have a 1 in 4 chance of being carcinomas. Hot nodules which concentrate nearly all of the iodide and suppress the surrounding gland are called autonomous nodules and have no chance of being cancer. While autonomous nodules are not cancers, cancer may be located nearby. The scan is of limited help with nodules showing concentrations between these 2 extremes. An important use of ^{131}I scanning is to locate thyroid metastases; metastases are located which are not seen or palpated by the surgeon at the time of thyroidectomy. We frequently find lymph node metastases in the scan even when no positive node was obtained at surgery.

RESULTS FROM THYROID SCANNING. — Shown in Table are the various clinical factors, combined with the radionuclide studies in a series of 224 patients. Preoperatively, these patients had nodules which on physical examination were not obviously cancer. A 22 per cent cancer incidence was found in the over-all series. The various factors produce percentages from 11 to 69 per cent. Hard nodules found to be cold on the thyroid scan show a 41 per cent incidence of cancer, with only a slight increase to 43 per cent for hard, cold, and single nodules, indicating that multinodularity is not evidence against cancer when a cold, hard nodule is palpated. The percentage incidence of adenoma varied from 11 per cent in the over-all series

Table
Association of Cancer and Adenoma with Preoperative Findings — 224 Patients

| | | Per cent at Surgery | |
	No.	Cancer	Adenoma
Single nodule	181	25	18
Cold nodule on scan	133	27	18
Hard nodule	91	38	11
Single, cold	79	32	19
Prior irradiation	22	32	27
Hard, cold	64	41	12
Hard, single	77	42	13
Hard, cold, single	51	43	16
Male < 40 years	16	69	25

to 25 per cent in males less than 40 years of age; except for patient age, there is little spread of these percentages.

Thyroid Radioimmunoassays

Radionuclides are used to perform radioimmunoassays which are important in the diagnosis of thyroid cancer.

THYROID STIMULATING HORMONE (TSH). — This pituitary hormone elevates when thyroxine levels are lower than needed to maintain a euthyroid state. TSH levels can be helpful in the diagnosis of some nodular thyroids. High levels are seen frequently in patients with chronic thyroiditis even though serum T–4 is normal. High TSH levels are not found with colloid nodular thyroids. We try not to scan for thyroid metastases except in the presence of elevated TSH levels, and ^{131}I therapy is not given for cancer except when TSH levels are elevated. Adequate TSH levels are produced with only minimal patient discomfort by having the patient substitute liothyronine, 50 μg. daily, for his usual thyroid replacement therapy. This is given for 4 weeks, which is enough time for the plasma-bound thyroxine to decrease to hypothyroid levels. The liothyronine is stopped abruptly and no replacement is given for 2 weeks. After the tenth day, most patients begin to develop symptomatic hypothyroidism. Scanning and therapy can be performed any time thereafter since TSH levels will be elevated.

THYROCALCITONIN. — Generally, thyrocalcitonin levels are nearly undetectable in normal individuals. Patients who will develop or who have developed medullary carcinoma will have easily measured levels. The continued elevation of thyrocalcitonin after removal of a medullary carcinoma indicates metastases.

Diagnostic and Therapeutic Program

DIAGNOSIS. — Most clinicians believe that a trial of thyroid therapy is indicated to test whether the nodule will decrease in size or disappear. The patient should realize that this is a slow process. When a nodule is associated with a high serum TSH, thyroiditis is likely and thyroid feeding should cause shrinkage of the gland and its nodule. Thyroid therapy does not shrink cancers and adenomas. Thyroid therapy ordinarily does not completely shrink colloid nodular thyroids and these thyroids will grow even while thyroid therapy is being taken, since growth does not require elevated TSH levels. A thyroid scan or imaging procedure while the patient is taking full doses of thyroid will show areas not suppressed in colloid nodular thyroid. Complete suppression occurs in thyroiditis. Thyroid therapy serves an important function after the diagnosis of thyroid carcinoma is made. It is generally believed that TSH is a growth factor of differentiated thyroid carcinomas. Therefore, full therapeutic doses of thyroid are administered continuously except for short periods when thyroid is stopped for radionuclide scanning and therapy. Plasma TSH levels are useful. Enough thyroid therapy must be administered to keep TSH levels low, except before scanning and therapy when TSH levels must be elevated to obtain adequate results. The recent introduction of the radioimmunoassay technique for measuring serum TSH has been a significant advance in the therapy for and diagnosis of thyroid cancer. This makes it possible to treat and scan for metastases when they are stimulated by endogenous TSH. Later, the TSH levels prove that thyroid replacement therapy is adequate to suppress endogenous TSH.

THERAPY. — When a thyroid neoplasm is found surgically, therapy is divided into 4 stages. First, all thyroid carcinomas should be surgically removed as completely as possible. Radical neck dissections are no longer justified as a primary procedure for differentiated thyroid carcinomas even in the presence of lymph node involvement. A near-total thyroidectomy is the treatment of choice for all malignant diseases of the thyroid. The surgeon should plan to leave any part of the gland necessary to prevent hypoparathyroidism and vocal cord paralysis. These thyroid remnants are removed later with radioactive iodine. The surgeon should remove all palpable lymph nodes.

Second, radioactive iodine therapy is an integral part of the treatment for differentiated carcinomas, *e.g.* papillary, follicular, or papillary-follicular carcinomas (Johnson and Beierwaltes, 1956; Haynie, Nofal, and Beierwaltes, 1963; Varma *et al.*, 1970; Krishnamurthy and

Blahd, 1972). Treatment should continue until areas of iodide concentration are no longer found in the posttreatment thyroid scan. However, unlike other cancers, a rapid therapeutic program is not necessary. Radioactive iodine treatments can be separated by months and even years with good results. Radioactive iodine is the treatment of choice for all thyroidal pulmonary metastases and bone metastases unless the metastases do not concentrate iodine. Radioactive iodine is not needed and should not be used for undifferentiated thyroid carcinoma, medullary carcinoma, and lymphosarcoma.

Third, external beam radiation is used for papillary follicular carcinomas which seem to be getting out of control in spite of adequate ^{131}I therapy, and for tumor deposits which do not concentrate ^{131}I, e.g. medullary and lymphosarcoma (Sheline, Galante, and Lindsay, 1966; Smedal, Salzman, and Meissner, 1967).

Fourth, chemotherapy can be used as a last effort in medullary and undifferentiated thyroid carcinomas (Gottlieb, Hill, Ibanez, and Clark, 1972); however, there have been no reported cures from chemotherapy in malignant disease of the thyroid.

Conclusion

Following a diagnostic program, as outlined briefly here, and a therapeutic program consisting of a modified total thyroidectomy and ^{131}I therapy, it should be possible to avoid excessive removal of noncancerous nodules, hypoparathyroidism, and postsurgical vocal card paralysis and still obtain a cure or at least a prolonged remission in over 90 per cent of the cases of differentiated thyroid carcinoma. When the carcinoma appears to be increasing in size in spite of surgical treatment and radioactive iodine, external irradiation is the only course open.

REFERENCES

Atkins, H. L., and Richards, P.: Assessment of thyroid function and anatomy with technetium-99 as pertechnetate. *Journal of Nuclear Medicine*, 9:7–15, January 1968.
Baylin, S. B., Beaven, M. A., Engelman, K., and Sjoerdsma, A.: Elevated histaminase activity in medullary carcinoma of the thyroid gland. *New England Journal of Medicine*, 283:1239–1244, December 3, 1970.
Black, M. B.: ^{99m}Tc pertechnetate flow study for evaluation of "cold" thyroid nodules. *Radiology*, 102:705–706, March 1972.
Catalona, W. J., Engelman, K., Ketcham, A. S., and Hammon, W. G.: Familial medullary thyroid carcinoma, pheochromocytoma and parathyroid adenoma (Sipple's syndrome). Study of a kindred. *Cancer*, 28:1245–1254, November 1971.

Clark, D. E.: Association of irradiation with cancer of the thyroid in children and adolescents. *The Journal of the American Medical Association*, 159: 1007–1009, November 5, 1955.

Gibbs, J. C., Jr., Halligan, E. J., Grieco, R. V., and McKeown, J. E.: Scintiscanning the thyroid nodule: An aid in its surgical management. *Archives of Surgery*, 90:323–328, March 1965.

Gottlieb, J. A., and Hill, C. S., Jr.: Chemotherapy of thyroid cancer with adriamycin. Experience with 30 patients. *New England Journal of Medicine*, 290:193–197, January 1974.

Hauser, W., Atkins, H. L., Eckelman, W. C., and Richards, P.: Thyroidal pertechnetate uptake in Hashimoto's disease. *The American Journal of Roentgenology, Radium Therapy and Nuclear Medicine*, 112:720–725, August 1971.

Haynie, T. P., Nofal, M. M., and Beierwaltes, W. H.: Treatment of thyroid carcinoma with I¹³¹. Results at fourteen years. *The Journal of the American Medical Association*, 183:303–306, February 1963.

Hoffer, P. B., Bernstein, J., and Gottschalk, A.: Fluorescent techniques in thyroid imaging. *Seminars in Nuclear Medicine*, 1:379–389, July 1971.

Horn, R. C., Jr., Welty, R. F., Brooks, F. P., Rhoads, J. E., and Pendergrass, E. P.: Carcinoma of the thyroid. *Annals of Surgery*, 126:140–155, August 1947.

Ibanez, M. L., Russell, W. O., Albores-Saavedra, J., Lampertico, P., White, E. C., and Clark, R. L.: Thyroid carcinoma—biologic behavior and mortality. Postmortem findings in 42 cases, including 27 in which the disease was fatal. *Cancer*, 19:1039–1052, August 1966.

Jhingran, S. G., and Johnson, P. C.: Thyroid nodules not obviously cancer. (In preparation.)

Johnson, P. C., and Beierwaltes, W. H.: Thyroid carcinoma treated with radioactive iodine, an eight year experience. *Journal of the Michigan Medical Society*, 55:410, 1956.

Krishnamurthy, G. T., and Blahd, W. H.: Diagnostic and therapeutic implications of long-term radioisotope scanning in the management of thyroid cancer. *Journal of Nuclear Medicine*, 13:924–927, December 1972.

LeBlanc, A. D., Bell, R. L., and Johnson, P. C.: Measurement of ¹²⁷I concentration in thyroid tissue by x-ray fluorescence. *Journal of Nuclear Medicine*, 14:816–819, November 1973.

Meadows, P. M.: Scintillation scanning in the management of clinically single thyroid nodule. *The Journal of the American Medical Association*, 177: 229–234, July 29, 1961.

Melvin, K. E., Miller, H. H., and Tashjian, A. H., Jr.: Early diagnosis of medullary carcinoma of the thyroid gland by means of calcitonin assay. *New England Journal of Medicine*, 285:1115–1120, November 11, 1971.

Mustacchi, P., and Cutler, S. J.: Some observations on the incidence of thyroid cancer in the United States. *New England Journal of Medicine*, 225: 889–893, November 8, 1956.

Robinson, T., Collica, C. J., and Chang, S.: Clinical comparison of scans and scintiphotos of the thyroid gland. *The American Journal of Roentgenology, Radium Therapy and Nuclear Medicine*, 103:738–745, August 1968.

Rose, R. G., Hartfield, J. E., Kelsey, M. P., and Macdonald, E. J.: The association of thyroid cancer and prior irradiation in infancy and childhood. *Journal of Nuclear Medicine*, 4:249–258, July 1963.

Sampson, R. J., Key, C. R., Buncher, C. R., Oka, H., and Iijima, S.: Papillary carcinoma of the thyroid gland. Sizes of 525 tumors found at autopsy in Hiroshima and Nagasaki. *Cancer*, 25:1391–1393, June 1970.

Sheline, G. E., Galante, M., and Lindsay, S.: Radiation therapy in the control of persistent thyroid cancer. *The American Journal of Roentgenology, Radium Therapy and Nuclear Medicine*, 97:923–930, August 1966.

Shepard, G. H., and Rosenfeld, L.: Carcinoma of thyroglossal duct remnants. Review of the literature and addition of two cases. *American Journal of Surgery*, 116:125–129, July 1968.

Shimaoka, K., and Sokal, J. E.: Differentiation of benign and malignant thyroid nodules by scintiscan. *Archives of Internal Medicine*, 114:36–39, July 1964.

Smedal, M. I., Salzman, F. A., and Meissner, W. A.: The value of 3 mv roentgen-ray therapy in differentiated thyroid carcinoma. *The American Journal of Roentgenology, Radium Therapy and Nuclear Medicine*, 99:352–364, February 1967.

Steinberg, M., Cavalieri, R. R., and Choy, S. H.: Uptake of technetium 99-pertechnetate in a primary thyroid carcinoma: Need for caution in evaluating nodules. *Journal of Clinical Endocrinology and Metabolism*, 30:800–803, June 1970.

Usher, M. S., and Arzoumanian, A. Y.: Thyroid nodule scans made with pertechnetate and iodine may give inconsistent results. *Journal of Nuclear Medicine*, 12:136–137, March 1971.

Varma, V. M., Beierwaltes, W. H., Nofal, M. M., Nishiyama, R. H., and Copp, J. E.: Treatment of thyroid cancer. Death rates after surgery and after surgery followed by sodium iodide I[131]. *The Journal of the American Medical Association*, 214:1437–1442, November 23, 1970.

Woolner, L. B., McConahey, W. M., Beahrs, O. H., and Black, B. M.: Primary malignant lymphoma of the thyroid. Review of forty-six cases. *American Journal of Surgery*, 111:502–523, April 1966.

Xerography and Film Mammography: A Comparative Evaluation

JOHN E. MARTIN, M.D., F.A.C.R.
*Departments of Radiology, St. Joseph Hospital; The
Univeristy of Texas System Cancer Center M. D.
Anderson Hospital and Tumor Insitute, Houston, Texas*

A NEW DIMENSION in the diagnosis of breast disease is now available in xeroradiography. There is considerably more information on
a xeroradiograph of the breast than on a comparable film mammogram, the difference in information could be equated to the difference that was noted between dark adaption fluoroscopy and image
amplification. The difference is like walking from a closet into a
lighted room.

The superiority of xeroradiography is based on the high resolution
of the process and the so-called "edge effect." Xeroradiography lacks
the broad-area contrast present in film, but the increased resolution
of imaging more than compensates for the lack of broad-area contrast.

Film mammography has been somewhat limited in its use because
of many factors. In conventional tungsten tube mammography, the
type "M" industrial film was the best type of film to use, but because
of the difficulty of hand processing in this period of automation, and
also because of increased stress on X-ray tubes, many physicians attempting to do mammography refused to use the industrial film. All
other films represented some type of compromise and none of them
contained the same amount of diagnostic information as the type
"M" film.

Radiographic diagnosis by film mammography was reputed to be
easy. This was true in fatty breasts where obvious infiltrative masses

were seen, but not true in dense breasts and for minimal or noninvasive carcinomas. As radiologists attempted to work with film, many became frustrated because of the difficulty of performing the examination and their lack of accuracy in diagnosis. This was particularly frustrating when large, clinically obvious lesions were not recognized in breasts with dense tissue. The film studies also required meticulous attention to the details of processing and exposure which many radiologists, because of their busy schedules, did not provide. As a result of these drawbacks, many radiologists did mammography only in a casual way or refused to do mammography at all. There were a limited number of radiologists throughout the country who were doing good mammography as it was understood at that time.

The senograph with the molybdenum target tube which was developed in France was then introduced into this country. Because of the high-contrast images with increased detail, "moly" imaging became popular with many radiologists as their diagnostic accuracy improved and the examination became easier to perform. There were some limitations to this type of equipment, such as a significant increase in radiation dosage and the fact that, almost without exception, the posterior portion of the breast was not imaged. A new cassette holder and pressure device is now available which is reputed to image the entire breast; however, even with the improvement in the molybdenum target equipment, there are still large areas of high-contrast uniform opacities in breasts in which no detail can be discerned, so that diagnostic evaluation of these areas is limited. Aside from lowering radiation dosages, "low dose" film has the same limitations as other film.

In xeroradiography, because of the high resolution of the process, these large dense areas of tissue are satisfactorily penetrated and there is enough differential tissue density so that satisfactory detail is seen (Fig. 1). In evaluating xeroradiographic images, a certain retraining process is necessary, because the radiologist is frequently somewhat confused by the tremendous amount of information present on the xeromammogram which is not present on film. There is a significant improvement in identification of calcifications within the breast with many more calcifications being seen (Figs. 2 and 3). Numerous small cysts or adenomas measuring 1 to 2 mm. are frequently seen. Seeing so many tiny masses leads to some initial apprehension on the part of the examiner until he realizes that this is a common finding and these tiny masses are, for the most part, of no significance. Subareolar duct detail is also clearly differentiated for the first time in xeroradiography. Probably the most important factor

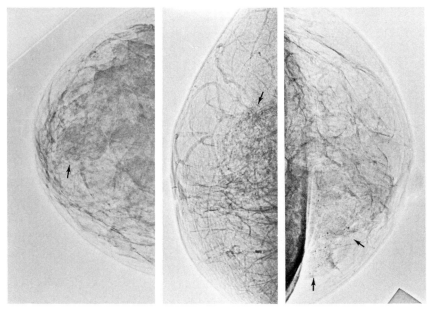

FIG. 1 *(left).* — Dense fibrocystic disease with prominent cyst (arrow).
FIG. 2 *(center).* — Small stellate carcinoma with intraductal calcification (arrow).
FIG. 3 *(right).* — Intraductal carcinoma identified only by intraductal calcification (arrows).

is the resolving power in large areas of dense opacity of fibrosis or other forms of fibrocystic disease so that definitive detail is present.

Xeroradiography lacks the broad-area contrast that film has but more than makes up for this in the resolution of detail. Although broad-area contrast is important in film, it also causes some of our major problems in the large areas of dense opacification.

Xeroradiography may presently be at the place that film was 40 years ago, in that it is a new science. Although selenium plates have been present for many years, the high resolution required in radiology was not built into selenium drums or plates before the mammography studies began. As a result, research experience in xeroradiography is limited and still in its infancy. The entire process is more sensitive than film, but as yet, nothing comparable to the intensifying screen has been developed for xeroradiography. The system has a potential resolution of 200 line pairs per mm. At the present, the selenium plates have 4–8 line pairs of resolution per mm. with high contrast X-ray techniques (350 Ma. S.), the resolution on the xero image is approximately 16 line pairs of resolution per mm. Another factor in xeroradiography which has caused some adverse criticism is the wide latitude of the xeroradiographic process as well as the high resolution. This wide latitute allows the possibility of imaging over a large range of exposure factors. The images all have an esthetic quality, but a pretty image is not necessarily a good image.

For a satisfactory xeromammogram, a very narrow corridor of exposure is necessary. Once this corridor is established, there should be no difficulty in having consistent repeatable images. It is best to use the smallest focal spot possible and to have controls of ½ kv. steps; 1 kv. step is absolutely mandatory. The tungsten tube is preferable with inherent filtration only. Technicians can usually tell by feeling the breast what the proper technique is. After making the initial image, because of the short processing time, the technician quickly knows whether the image needs to be repeated or the technique changed for the following images.

The criterion for a good image is good detail; detail is mandatory in xeroradiography. There has been a tendency on the part of some radiologists to underpenetrate the images, and when the images are underpenetrated they are too blue and the skin is not imaged. By the same token, if an image is overexposed, all of the skin is imaged as is all of the breast tissue, but there is a lack of detail. Again, to re-emphasize, detail is mandatory in xeroradiography and if detail is not present there is something wrong with the technical or mechanical factors in imaging.

Once satisfactory techniques are arrived at and good detail images are obtained, these images can be read rapidly with confidence and high diagnostic accuracy. Most of the radiologists doing good xeromammography are obtaining an accurate rate of diagnosis of carcinoma of 95 per cent or better. There are few examinations, if any, in radiology where such accuracy can be obtained. The xeromammograms have particular appeal to surgeons because for the first time the surgeon can see the carcinomas or benign processes that the radiologist identifies. As a result, those radiologists doing good xeromammography have noticed a significant increase in the number of patient examinations.

Initially, a comparative evaluation of film and xeroradiographic studies was begun. The comparative evaluation was stopped after 100 cases, as there was so much more information on the xeroradiograms than on the comparable film mammograms, particularly in view of finding 2 carcinomas by xeroradiography which were not identified on the film mammograms. Before the study was completed, the examiner was looking with reluctance and skepticism at the film studies.

In our experience, many small carcinomas measuring anywhere from 2 mm. to 5 mm. are being found consistently in xeroradiography. The wide latitude and extremely high resolution of the process should continue to help us find small carcinomas in the breast and in this way improve the cure rate in carcinoma of the breast.

The Present Status of Thermography in Detection of Cancer of the Breast

GERALD D. DODD, Jr., M.D.
*Department of Diagnostic Radiology, The University of
Texas System Cancer Center M. D. Anderson Hospital
and Tumor Institute, Houston, Texas*

THE USE OF THERMOGRAPHY as a breast cancer detection procedure is based upon the observation of Lawson (1956) and others (Lloyd Williams, Lloyd Williams, and Handley, 1961) that the majority of cancers of the breast emit more heat than the surrounding normal tissues. Although the first clinical thermographic study was performed in 1956, it is only within the last 5 to 10 years that significant numbers of patients have been examined. Much of the equipment used during the earlier clinical trials was crude, and only limited information was developed relative to thermogenesis and interpretive criteria. In recent years, improvements in the scanning devices have subsequently increased our knowledge in these areas as well as making apparent certain deficiencies in the technique which substantially affect its use as a case-finding procedure. These developments largely relate to the circadian rhythms of tumors, the mechanisms of heat transfer involved in the production of surface temperatures, and the specificity of the examination. All of these must be understood if the present status of thermography is to be placed in its proper perspective.

The Physiologic Basis for Thermography

The interpretation of a thermogram is based upon a comparison of surface temperatures of corresponding parts of the body. The prescan cooling of the patient produces a relatively stable thermal background against which temperature symmetry may be judged. Abnormally warm areas are relatively unaffected by the cooling process and may be identified against the diminished background temperature.

The human skin plays an all-important role in the heat regulatory process. Under stable conditions, heat flows at uniform rates from sites of production to cooler tissue or blood which in turn carry the heat to the body surface. From the surface, it is dissipated to the external environment by the processes of radiation (45 per cent), convection (25 per cent), and evaporation (30 per cent) (Samuel, 1970). Since heat loss by sweating does not occur below 30°C., the major avenues of heat dissipation at lower temperatures are radiation and convection. Control of heat loss at temperatures below 30°C. is effected by constriction of the superficial blood vessels, a factor which is utilized in the prescan cooling of patients.

The role of the cutaneous blood vessels is of fundamental importance in the production of thermographic patterns. The skin may be considered as an insulated cover surrounded by a halo of water vapor (Lloyd Williams, 1964). Blood vessels passing through the insulating layer provide, in their finer ramifications, an efficient heat exchange system. Cooper, Randall, and Hertzman (1959) have demonstrated that temperature increases in the skin overlying localized areas of heat production within muscle may be obviated if the venous channels between the deeper tissues and the skin are interrupted. This attests to the importance of the veins in the heat transfer process as well as to the efficiency of fat as an insulator. In areas of the body where adipose tissue is attenuated or absent, changes in surface temperatures may well result from conduction of heat from the deeper tissues. However, when a well-developed adipose layer exists, relatively large temperature differences are required to produce a recognizable surface change by conduction. In the presence of fat, it would seem that the process of vascular convection becomes the major transport mechanism.

The above principles are well illustrated in the breast, where the adipose capsule is usually well developed, averaging 0.5 to 2 cm. in the majority of subjects. The venous system of the breast is also well suited for this purpose. Both deep and superficial systems exist, with free communication between the 2. The superficial system is virtually incorporated within the skin, providing for ready conduction of heat from the venous channels to the surface (Fig. 1). It is believed that the heat produced by a cancer or some other biologically active process is the result of accelerated metabolism as compared to the surrounding host tissues. In the past, primarily as the result of poor spatial resolution in the scanning devices, it was assumed that the heat reached the surface by conduction through the intervening tissues, resulting in a "hot spot" over the abnormal area. In fact, this concept made little sense. Not only do the structural characteristics of the breast mitigate against conduction as noted, but, in addition, the breast, as a globular structure, should show a relatively uniform radiation of heat from a centrally located mass rather than an isolated thermal response in one portion of its periphery. Lawson and Gaston (1964) have demonstrated that the temperature of mammary tumors exceeds that of the local arterial and venous blood. The venous blood is warmer than the arterial blood, indicating that the latter serves as a coolant and that the transfer of heat to the other parts of the breast occurs by a process of venous convection. Because the superficial and deep venous systems unite in the plexus of Haller immediately behind the areola, it is possible that blood draining the tumor area may be shunted to any part of the breast. For these reasons, a positive breast thermogram may consist of exaggeration of all or part of the superficial venous system or isolated warming of the areola (Fig.

FIG. 1.—Normal thermographic patterns of the breast. *A*, the superficial venous plexus is well visualized in both breasts. *B*, avascular breasts. The lack of vascularity is a reflection of the metabolic status of the breasts rather than the depth of the venous system. Multiple variations on these patterns may be encountered, but symmetry is the key finding. (Courtesy of Dodd, Zermeno, Wallace, and Marsh, 1973.)

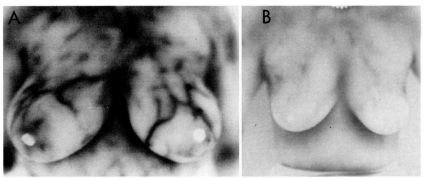

2). Since the surface manifestations of the heat exchange are dependent upon the tissue depth of the veins as well as the temperature of the blood circulating within them, disparities between the location of the abnormal signal and tumor may also occur on this basis.

With the above in mind, some of the problems of thermography become apparent. Since heat is a nonspecific physical parameter, we are searching for a marker which may be common to both benign and malignant processes, an abnormality which may have no spatial relationship to the site of origin and one which is variable in its constancy as a result of the level of biologic activity of the specific abnormality. These drawbacks are reflected in the statistical results that are gradually accumulating in the literature.

FIG. 2.—Abnormal thermograms. *A*, carcinoma of the right breast. The dominant finding is asymmetry of the superficial venous plexus. *B*, carcinoma of the left breast. The dominant finding is notable heat emission about the areola. There is an absence of fat in this area with a rich subcutaneous venous plexus. *C*, carcinoma of the right breast. There is venous channel asymmetry, prominence of the areola, and a significant capillary blush indicating probable involvement of the skin. All of the above findings also may be present with benign processes. There is no difference in the morphological appearance of abnormal thermograms resulting from benign and malignant disease. (Courtesy of Dodd, Zermeno, Wallace, and Marsh, 1973.)

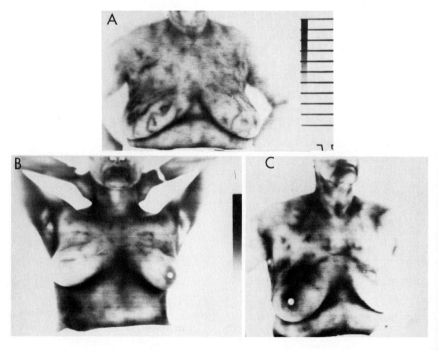

Results

Davey, Greening, and McKinna (1970) have reported a series of 1,768 women screened for breast and cervical cancer over a 1-year period; 11 per cent of the thermographic examinations were reported as suspicious, and 11 (73 per cent) of the 15 cancers detected by thermography, mammography, and clinical examination were in the thermographically suspicious group.

Isard and his associates (Isard, Ostrum, and Shilo, 1969) have reported on a study of 2,696 patients in which 31 per cent of the examinations were classed as suspicious. Of the 55 cancers included in this group, 72 per cent had suspicious thermograms.

Stark and Way (1970) have reported on a series of 5,234 patients who received both thermographic and physical examinations. Mammography was additionally performed on 500 of these women. Of particular interest was the discovery of 9 clinically unsuspected cancers, all nonpalpable and all less than 1 cm. in diameter.

Ohkashi (1970) has reported on a study of 188 cases in which a 0.5°C. increase in temperature was used as a criterion of suspicion. Based on this temperature differential, he reported that 71 per cent of the cancers were correctly classified as suspicious.

Isard, Becker, Shilo, and Ostrum (1972) have also reported on a 4-year study involving 10,000 patients, including 306 instances of malignant disease. Seventy-one per cent of the confirmed cancers produced positive thermograms. Again, it is of interest to note that 22 (61 per cent) of the 36 patients with occult cancers had positive studies.

Dowdy and his associates (1970) performed 1,950 examinations in a screening program. He found that he correctly classified as suspicious 73 per cent of the thermograms of patients with subsequently proven cancers; 17 per cent of all thermograms were reported as suspicious in the process of achieving this true-positive rate.

Tricoire and his associates (1970) utilizing the liquid crystal technique, have reported a true-positive rate for carcinoma of the female breast of about 93 per cent.

Finally, Furnival *et al.* (1970) have reported on a study of 891 patients, 414 of whom had clinical symptoms referable to the breast. In the 77 patients with subsequently proven cancer, the thermographic interpretation was classed as suspicious in only 50 per cent of examinations. The thermograms were read independently by 3 radiologists and the authors note that there was a significant disagreement among the 3 readers.

These results indicate that the thermographic examination may be expected to detect at least 3 of every 4 cases of malignant disease of the breast. In our experience, the accuracy has been higher, with the average in several series of patients being 85 per cent. However, the so-called false-positive rate has increased with greater rapidity than the true-positive rate in order to attain this level. The possible reasons for this distribution of results will be discussed below.

Discussion

Various investigators have attempted to increase the accuracy of thermography by quantifying the heat differential between the "hot spot" and the surrounding normal tissue or the corresponding area of the opposite breast. Since the temperature differences in cancer of the breast may be quite significant, an arbitrary dividing line of 1.5°C. has been suggested, *i.e.*, differences of less than 1.5° tend to indicate benign processes while those above 1.5° are more apt to represent cancer. In our experience, this approach has no basis in fact. Not only do individual tumors differ in their biologic potential and therefore their heat production, but they also are subject to an independent biologic rhythm which may be profoundly out of phase with the normal circadian rhythms of the body. Studies in our laboratory employing continuous telemetric monitoring of breast temperatures indicate that the cyclic fluctuations in tumor temperatures are related to mitosis; the more orderly a mitotic pattern, the more irregular the thermal pattern. As a result, the temperature differential between the cancer and the control area may, at different times, vary from 6° or 7°F. to as little as 0.2° or 0.3°F. Except for general reference purposes, these fluctuations vitiate the utility of a temperature for reference scale or densitometric measurements for more precise quantitation of temperature differences.

While it has been suggested that only very large tumors will generate sufficient heat to produce positive thermograms, this has not proven to be the case in our experience. In our series of patients, more false-negative thermograms occurred with cancers in excess of 1 cm. in diameter than in small nonpalpable tumors. It is difficult to explain how a 3- to 4-cm. carcinoma can show no significant heat production while a cancer 1 cm. or less in size may cause a grossly abnormal thermogram. Certainly, the difference cannot be explained by the bulk of tissue involved. Presumably the biologic activity of a given tumor is the determining factor, but it is our belief that the tumor-host interaction plays a significant part in the production of the abnormal signal. While this concept requires further investigation, it is clear that both very large and very small tumors may not be detectable by thermographic procedures. The latter errors are particularly disturbing, but it is possible that these metabolically inactive tumors would not have become clinical cancers. In any event, the over-all efficacy of thermography can be increased by combining the procedure with physical examination. The potential of the dual approach is indicated by the results of a series of 565 patients surveyed in our institution. In this group, there were 69 proven cancers, 85 per cent of which were considered suspicious by thermography. Of the 9 cancers missed, 5 were readily palpable, *i.e.*, 65 of 69 cancers (94 per cent) were diagnosed by a combination of thermography and physical examination.

While false-negative rates are of concern, false-positive rates have proven to be a greater problem. The procedure is nonspecific, and positive scans may be produced by a variety of benign dieases. Thermography, therefore, may be considered highly sensitive to abnormalities in the breast, but it does not distinguish between active benign and malignant disease. In this respect, it should be noted that the false-positive rate will vary with the types of patients examined. Screening procedures utilizing a nonselected group of asymptomatic patients over age 35 will usually result in an over-all false-positive rate of approximately 15 per cent. If only symptomatic patients are examined, the false-positive rate will increase to 40 per cent or more. This emphasizes the sensitivity of the technique insofar as breast abnormalities are concerned but also underscores its lack of specificity.

It also should be noted that so-called false-positive rates of less than 15 per cent are usually associated with a decline in the true-positive rate. In our experience, a false-positive rate of between 15 and 20 per cent is necessary to achieve a true-positive rate of 85 per cent or better.

Since the basis of thermographic interpretation is the comparison of symmetrical parts, problems are encountered in the examination of the residual breast in the postmastectomized patients. Previous thermograms are of great assistance; in their absence, the interpreter must rely upon his experience, and we have found this to be of dubious value.

Somewhat similar problems are encountered with bilateral carcinoma. Usually only 1 of the cancers is detected, since the thermographic findings are frequently dominant in 1 breast. There is a tendency on the part of the interpreter to regard the least obvious change as within normal limits (Fig. 3).

It would seem that the greatest potential of breast thermography

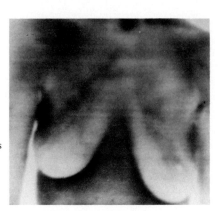

FIG. 3.—Bilateral noninvasive intraductal carcinoma of the breast. The right breast may be considered positive; the left, by comparison, appears normal. (Courtesy of Dodd, Zermeno, Wallace, and Marsh, 1973.)

lies in its use as an initial screening procedure for mammography in clinically normal patients. Although the accuracy of the 2 methods is approximately the same, not all malignant lesions are detectable by both; the procedures seem to be complementary rather than competitive and, indeed, the best case finding figures result from the simultaneous use of the physical examination, thermography, and mammography. Nevertheless, even though screening is most effective when all methodologies are used, the relative simplicity and inexpensiveness of thermography suggest that it might serve to reduce the number of mammograms required to manageable numbers. In our opinion, false-positive rates of up to 20 per cent would be acceptable, provided between 85 and 90 per cent of all cancers were detected by physical examination and thermography.

Of particular interest in evaluating the utility of thermography are those patients with positive thermograms but no other evidence of breast disease. As indicated, because of the dominance of the superficial circulatory pattern in the composition of the abnormal thermogram, there is frequently no spatial relationship between the underlying abnormality and the surface signal (Fig. 4). For this reason, a biopsy cannot be performed on the basis of the majority of positive thermograms. If the physical examination and mammogram are non-contributory, a substantial dilemma is imposed. At present, we must consider these patients to be at risk and follow with serial thermograms at intervals of no less than 3 months. If the thermographic examination continues to be abnormal, a mammogram should be performed at least every 6 months until cancer can be excluded or the thermogram reverts to normal. The potential of this approach is illustrated by 11 of our patients (18.7 per cent of those originally classi-

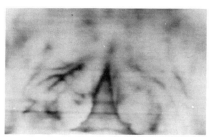

FIG. 4.—Tiny subareolar carcinoma of the right breast. Note that the major thermal changes are in the upper middle and middle quadrants. Biopsy in these areas would not be productive. (Courtesy of Dodd, Zermeno, Wallace, and Marsh, 1973.)

fied as false-positive examinations). All subsequently developed cancer in the breast, initially incriminated by thermography. This would suggest that the procedure may well be a more sensitive case finding method than is currently appreciated.

Future Developments in Thermography

There is still room for improvement in thermographic equipment. The ability of a thermograph to produce a complete scan at conventional television frame rates would be most desirable since it would permit immediate evaluation, avoid technician error, and open up the possibility of convenient storage of all information on computer tape. This development is possible through the use of detector arrays and undoubtedly will supplant other techniques.

Subtraction techniques employing simultaneous infrared photographs and infrared scans may increase accuracy; however this development is presently in the laboratory stage.

Although technical advances are desirable, nonspecificity remains the great weakness of the technique and does not generally appear subject to instrumental manipulation. If a means could be devised to eliminate the need for mammography in those patients with positive thermograms produced by benign processes, then the possibility of surveying the entire female population over age 40 becomes feasible. Admittedly this is a tenuous goal. However, Chiricuta and co-workers (1971) suggests a method by which false-positive rates might be reduced. Using the known difference in the utilization of glucose by benign and malignant neoplasms, he has reported on a study of 115 patients, including 22 controls, 15 with benign tumors and 78 with malignant tumors. In each, a 50-ml. solution of 10 per cent glucose was slowly infused over a period of 30 minutes. Approximately

1½ hours after the completion of the infusion, the patients were found to display the following thermal characteristics in the breast:

1. None of the controls or benign tumors showed any increase in breast temperature.

2. Of those with carcinoma, 96.3 per cent had an increase in the temperature of the suspect breast. The absolute increase in response to glucose was inversely proportional to the base line temperature differential.

We have not been able to confirm Chiricuta's observations in a small series of cases. Nevertheless, the idea of chemically influencing the tumor as a means of differential diagnosis is intriguing.

Obviously, such exogenous substances as alcohol and nicotine have a profound effect upon the thermal patterns of normal people. Whether these or other substances would similarly affect vessels draining benign and malignant tumors remains unknown. It would appear that the field of thermopharmacology offers a promising adjunct to thermal imaging.

Summary

The recorded accuracy of breast thermography varies between 75 and 85 per cent. While the latter figure is an acceptable true-positive rate, false-positive rates as high as 40 per cent may be encountered, depending upon the nature of the population examined and the degree of suspicion of the interpreter. It is the false-positive rate which is the greatest drawback to thermography and one for which no solution has as yet been offered.

When combined with physical examination, a 90 per cent true-positive rate is feasible. Both large and small tumors may be missed by thermography. The explanation for these failures appears to lie in the biologic potential of tumors rather than the sensitivity of the method; most very large and very small tumors are readily detected.

There is no spatial relationship between the location of the thermographic signal and the cancer. This is because of the vascular convection of heat which, in our opinion, is the primary method by which the abnormal thermal gradient reaches the skin surface. For this reason, biopsy on the basis of a positive thermogram is not warranted: Clinical or mammographic evidence is necessary for confirmatory and localization purposes.

Equipment improvements are continuing and pending developments appear entirely adequate to clinical needs. If a means can be devised to stabilize or lower the number of false-positive examinations in thermography, it may well meet the need for a rapid, inexpensive screening technique. In any event, since cancers which are subclinical and subroentgen in character may produce a positive thermogram, the individual with a positive examination is considered at risk until the thermogram reverts to normal or sufficient time elapses to rule out the diagnosis of breast cancer.

REFERENCES

Chiricuta, I., Bucur, M., Opris, I., and Bologna, O.: The correlative value of thermometry and the glucose tolerance test in cancer of the breast. *Romanian Medical Review*, 15:73–77, 1971.

Cooper, T., Randall, W. C., and Hertzman, A. B.: Vascular convection of heat from active muscle to overlying skin. *Journal of Applied Physiology*, 14: 207–211, March 1959.

Davey, J. B., Greening, W. P., and McKinna, J. A.: Is screening for cancer worthwhile? Results from a well-woman clinic for cancer detection. *British Medical Journal*, 3:696–699, September 19, 1970.

Dodd, G. D., Zermeno, A., Wallace, J. D., and Marsh, L. M.: Breast Thermography: The state of the art. In R. D. Moseley, Ed.: *Current Problems in Radiology*. Chicago, Illinois, Year Book Medical Publishers, Inc., 1973, 47 pp.

Dowdy, A. H., Lagasse, L. D., Sperling, L., Barker, W. F., Zeldis, L. J., Longmire, W. P., and Cooper, P. H.: A combined screening program for the detection of carcinoma of the cervix and carcinoma of the breast. *Surgery, Gynecology and Obstetrics*, 131:93–98, July 1970.

Furnival, I. G., Stewart, H. J., Weddel, J. M., Davey P., Gravelle, I. H., Evans, K. T., and Forest, A. P. M.: Accuracy of screening methods for the diagnosis of breast disease. *British Medical Journal*, 4:461–463, November 21, 1970.

Isard, H. J., Becker, W., Shilo, R., and Ostrum, B. J.: Breast thermography after four years and 10,000 studies. *The American Journal of Roentgenology, Radium Therapy and Nuclear Medicine*, 115:811–821, August 1972.

Isard, H. J., Ostrum, B. J., and Shilo, R.: Thermography in breast carcinoma. *Surgery, Gynecology and Obstetrics*, 128:1289–1293, June 1969.

Lawson, R. N.: Implications of surface temperatures in the diagnosis of breast cancer. *Canadian Medical Association Journal*, 75:309–310, August 15, 1956.

Lawson, R. N., and Gaston, J. P.: Temperature measurements in localized pathologic processes, thermography and its clinical applications. *Annals of the New York Academy of Sciences*, 121:90–98, October 9, 1964.

Lloyd Williams, K.: Infrared thermometry as a tool in medical research, thermography and its clinical applications. *Annals of the New York Academy of Sciences*, 121:99–122, October 9, 1964.

Lloyd Williams, K., Lloyd Williams, F. J., and Handley, R. S.: Infrared thermometry in the diagnosis of breast disease. *The Lancet*, 2:1378–1381, December 23, 1961.

Ohkashi, Y.: On the diagnosis of breast cancer by thermography. *Cancer Institute Hospital Journal*, Tokyo, Japan, 1970.

Samuel, E.: Thermography. In *Modern Trends in Diagnostic Radiology.* New York, New York, Appleton-Century-Crofts, 1970.

Stark, A. M., and Way, S.: Screening for breast cancer. *The Lancet*, 2:407–409, August 22, 1970.

Tricoire, J., Mariel, L., Amiel, J. P., Poirot, G., Lacour, J., and Fajbisowicz, S.: Thermography en plaque de 300 malades atteintes d'affections variees du sein. *La Presse Medicale*, 55:2483–2668, December 26, 1970.

The Detection of Breast Tumors by Ultrasonic Methods

GILBERT BAUM, M.D.
Ultrasound Laboratory, Albert Einstein College of
Medicine, Bronx, New York

THE ABSENCE OF A FIXED, rigid anatomy makes the breast one of the most difficult organs of the body to examine ultrasonographically, so that special ultrasonographic equipment and techniques are required.

For coherence, I shall discuss these requirements first and then go on the application of these to the breast.

Classical ultrasonographic diagnosis is based upon the anatomic distortion produced by a disease. A simple black and white silhouette is all that is needed to display such anatomical distortions, so most commercial ultrasonographic equipment produces a silhouette type of image.

The limitations of silhouette imagery are demonstrated by a silhouette of a male and female both of whom wear long hair (Fig. 1). In the anterior-posterior position, it is essentially impossible to distinguish male from female. However, in the lateral position, it is fairly simple to do so because of the girl's breasts.

Similarly, in organs possessing a rigid anatomy, such as is the case with the eye, the anatomy is clear-cut and the vitreous space is normally clear (Fig. 2). A retinal detachment has a classical location and shape so that a simple silhouette ultrasonogram is diagnostic (Fig. 3).

The lack of a definitive anatomy makes the interpretation of a silhouette ultrasonogram of the breast virtually impossible (Fig. 4).

Optically, the solution to the limitations inherent in silhouette

405

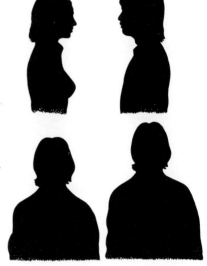

FIG. 1.—Silhouette of a boy and a girl, both of whom wear their hair long. In the anterior-posterior position, it is impossible to distinguish male from female. In the lateral position, it is possible to do so because of the girl's breasts.

imagery is the use of a gray scale, *i.e.* a simple snapshot. When gray scale or a snapshot (Fig. 5) is used, it is very simple to distinguish male from female because, rather than being limited to an outline of the breasts, a number of characteristics may be used for differentiation.

Although snapshots provide more information than a simple sil-

FIG. 2 *(left).*—A compound-scan ultrasonogram of a human eye. Note the similarity to an anatomical cross-section.

FIG. 3 *(right).*—An ultrasonogram of an eye with a retinal detachment. The classical shape of a retinal detachment on an ultrasonogram and the connection of the retina to the optic disc is diagnostic.

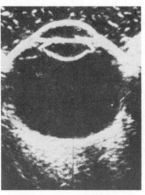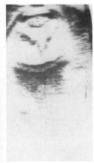

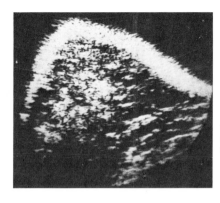

FIG. 4.—A silhouette ultrasonogram of the breast. Because of the lack of a definitive anatomy, interpretation is virtually impossible.

houette, the gray scale limitations of cathode ray tube display systems result in such minimal changes in gray scale that we have used color-coded isodensitometry to make these small changes in gray scale visible to the naked eye. This facility is demonstrated in the next 2 figures.

The first, Figure 6, is a black and white ultrasonogram of the remaining breast of a patient who had had the opposite breast removed because of breast cancer. A color-coded isodensitometric printout of Figure 6 demonstrates the ability of the eye to pick out a minute area of amplitude discontinuity when a color system is substituted for the gray scale (Fig. 7, arrow).

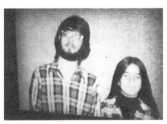

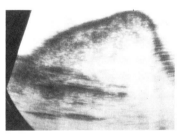

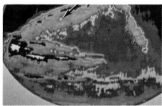

FIG. 5 *(above left)*.—A snapshot of a boy and girl with long hair. The addition of gray scale makes it possible to distinguish male from female even in the anterior-posterior position, although the image has deliberately been defocused.

FIG. 6 *(above)*.—A black and white gray scale ultrasonogram of a breast.

FIG. 7 *(left)*.—A color-coded isodensitometric printout of the previous figure illustrates a minute gap of amplitude discontinuity which may be distinguished when color is substituted for gray scale (arrow).

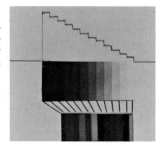

FIG. 8.—An explanation of color-coded isodensi-tometry. The upper portion of the figure shows the A-mode pattern. The central portion shows the gray scale produced in B-mode, and the lower portion shows the substitution of color for each shade of gray. Each shade of gray corresponds to an echo of known amplitude. The use of a fixed, reproducible color code assists the physician in pattern recognition just as staining does in histopathology.

I must emphasize that color coding is only of assistance if it is re-producible. The repeated use of a reproducible color code enables the physician to learn how to interpret the amplitude data, just as staining of histological tissue enables the physician to learn how to interpret histological slides.

Randomized coloring is more confusing and difficult to interpret than the black and white ultrasonogram. Reproducibility is achieved by assigning a specific color code to each shade of gray (Fig. 8). Each gray density in turn corresponds to an echo of known amplitude. This color code is never altered. By the use of such equipment, we have been able to discern 4 basic types of normal anatomical variants as well as ultrasonographic patterns characteristic of the major types of breast disease. A system possessing these characteristics is essen-tial for ultrasound mammography (Table).

Clinical Application

The breast is examined with the patient in a sitting position. The breasts are suspended in a special examining tank filled with water at 37°C. Serial horizontal scans at 3-mm. vertical steps are taken from the top to the bottom of the breast. Only sector scanning can be used with our present scanner, but a scanner presently under construction will be capable of carrying out arc, linear, and compound scanning as well.

Table
Equipment and Operational Characteristics

1% amplitude stability
Dynamic range greater than 2 density units
Constant velocity electromechanical scanner
Standardized operation
Corrections for absorption and viewing angle

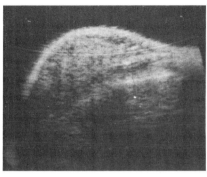 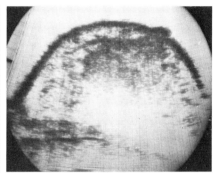

FIG. 9 *(left).* – A gray scale ultrasonogram of the young, normal breast. (Courtesy of Baum, 1974.)

FIG. 10 *(right).* – An ultrasonogram of a 64-year-old female, which demonstrates a dense, fibrous pattern. (Courtesy of Baum, 1974.)

The Normal Breast Patterns

The 4 types of normal anatomical breast patterns that we have been distinguishing are the young, mixed, fibrous, and atrophic patterns. Figure 9 is a black and white ultrasonogram of a 25-year-old female with an essentially normal breast pattern. Figure 10 is a black and white ultrasonogram of a 64-year-old female with a dense fibrous breast pattern. Although there are differences on the black and white ultrasonograms, it is virtually impossible for the eye to define the differences in the amplitude patterns.

Figure 11 is the color-coded isodensitometric printout of the normal young breast shown in Figure 9. On the color-coded printout,

FIG. 11 *(left).* – A color-coded isodensitometric printout of the ultrasonogram of the normal, young breast shown in Figure 9. (Courtesy of Baum, 1974.)

FIG. 12 *(right).* – A color-coded isodensitometric printout of the fibrous breast shown in Figure 10. Note the differences in amplitude distribution displayed on the isodensitometric printout. (Courtesy of Baum, 1974.)

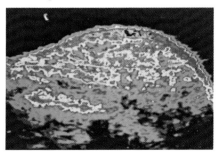 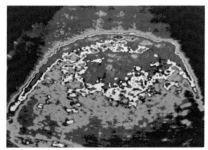

one can ascertain that there is a fairly uniform distribution of loud echo-producing structure throughout this breast. The color-coded isodensitometric printout of the fibrous breast shows that the loud echo-producing remnants of parenchymal structures are concentrated into a continuous centrally located mass (Fig. 12.)

In the mixed pattern, the loud echoes which arise in the parenchymal structures of the breast come to lie in the center of the breast and are surrounded on both sides by an intervening layer which consists primarily of fatty tissue (Fig. 13).

In the atrophic breast, virtually all of the parenchymal tissue is replaced by fat, giving rise to the loose, lacelike pattern shown in Figure 14. An isodensitometric analysis of this figure confirms the

FIG. 13 *(top left)*.—An ultrasonogram of the mixed pattern observed in the normal breast. (Courtesy of Baum, 1974.)

FIG. 14 *(top right)*.—The ultrasonographic pattern observed in an atrophic breast. (Courtesy of Baum, 1974.)

FIG. 15 *(bottom left)*.—A color-coded isodensitometric printout of Figure 14 confirms the replacement of the parenchymal tissue echoes by fat, giving rise to a loose, lacelike pattern. (Courtesy of Baum, 1974.)

FIG. 16 *(bottom right)*.—An echo-free zone, which frequently is observed in the nipple of some patients.

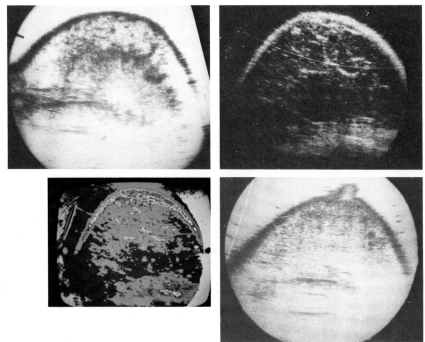

impression of very few echoes of high amplitude (Fig. 15). The echo-free zone which corresponds to the passages of the ducts through the nipple is shown in Figure 16.

Breast Diseases

Ultrasound mammography is the diagnostic method of choice for determining the size, position, and location of cysts of the breasts. In this instance, simple black and white ultrasonograms may suffice because of the major anatomical and acoustic changes produced by these cysts.

Figure 17 is an X-ray mammogram of a patient with a large cyst of the breast. The ultrasonogram through the same breast shows the unmistakable lesion on the black and white ultrasonogram (Fig. 18). The characteristic ultrasonographic features of a breast cyst are the improved transmission through the cyst resulting in a tail and the smooth, complete posterior wall. Multiloculated cysts may also be

FIG. 17 *(top)*. — An X-ray mammogram of a breast containing a huge cyst.

FIG. 18 *(bottom left)*. — An ultrasonogram of the same breast clearly demonstrates a huge cyst within this breast. Ultrasonographically, a cyst is characterized by an acoustic tail and a smooth, complete posterior wall. The acoustic tail is the result of improved transmission through the cyst resulting in increased echo amplitudes behind the cyst.

FIG. 19 *(bottom right)*. — A multiloculated cyst of the breast.

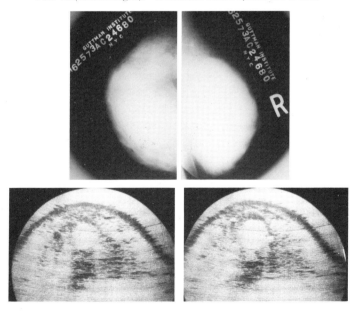

identified (Fig. 19). Fibroadenomas may show a similar pattern but lack a tail of tissue (Fig. 20).

In contrast, in cases of breast carcinoma, the echoes arising from within the leading portions of the scirrhous carcinoma are of medium amplitude (yellow) and are of high absorption causing the acoustic shadow behind the lesion (Fig. 21).

At present, there is no one ultrasonographic sign which conclusively demonstrates the malignancy or nonmalignancy of a lesion. Rather, it is a combination of ultrasonographic findings which leads to the diagnosis of malignant change within the breast.

The outstanding feature of malignant change of breast tissue is a replacement of a portion of one of the normal breast patterns described previously by tissues that produce very weak echoes but have an extremely high coefficient of absorption so that a pronounced shadow is observed behind such a lesion. Thus, it is the combination of distorted, replaced breast parenchyma plus shadow which is diagnostically significant and not each feature by itself.

Cysts however usually produce only weak echoes or no echoes from their centers but have excellent transmission characteristics, so that there is better visualization of the structure behind the cyst. It is imperative that cysts be in front of an area of improved transmission because a pseudo-tail or tail does appear lateral to the shadows cast

FIG. 20 *(left).* — An ultrasonogram of a fibroadenoma of the breast. Fibroadenomas also show weak central echoes because they contain fewer acoustic interfaces than normal tissues. Their absorption equals or slightly exceeds that of an equivalent volume of normal tissue.

FIG. 21 *(right).* — An ultrasonogram of a carcinoma of the breast. The echoes arising from the leading portions of the scirrhous carcinoma are of medium amplitude (characterized by yellow) and are of high absorption, causing an acoustic shadow behind the lesion. Also note the major changes in the ultrasonographic anatomy of the affected portions of the breast.

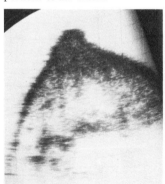 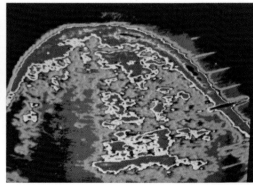

by a malignant lesion. These tails consist of normal tissue echoes and the sides of the acoustic shadow.

Fibroadenomas are echo-producing tissues whose absorption characteristics lie between those of scirrhous carcinomas and cysts of the breast; hence, the internal echoes are weaker and the shadowing effect is less.

Scirrhous carcinomas may also display a unique pattern when viewed with a low-contrast gray scale gradient. Another pattern frequently observed in breast carcinoma is demonstrated in the next series of figures. The first is the X-ray mammogram of a scirrhous carcinoma (Fig. 22). The ultrasonogram of this lesion (Fig. 23) shows the tumor mass surrounded by a dense band of echoes which give the impression of the tissue being compressed and distorted by the advancing lesion. Behind this dense, leading edge there is a virtually echo-free zone or a zone producing only a minimal intensity, somewhat suggestive of a moat about a castle. Regular, finger-like projections extend from the clear zone in the surrounding tissue. In the

FIG. 22 *(top left).*—An X-ray mammogram of a scirrhous carcinoma of the breast.

FIG. 23 *(right).*—An ultrasonogram of the preceding-figure shows that the tumor mass is surrounded by a dense band of echoes which gives the impression of the tissue being compressed and distorted by the advancing lesion. Behind this dense leading edge there is a virtually echo-free zone or a zone producing only a minimal intensity, somewhat suggestive of a moat about a castle. Regular, finger-like projections extend from the clear zone into the surrounding tissue. In the center of this zone, there are irregular clumps of variable size and intensity. These may also show finger-like projections into the surrounding tissue.

FIG. 24 *(bottom left).*—A data-processed ultrasonogram to simplify the identification of malignant lesions of the breast. (Courtesy of Baum, 1974.)

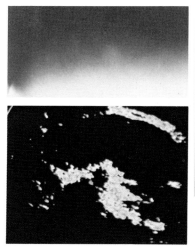

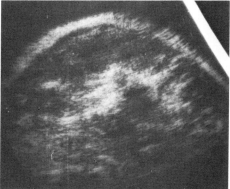

center of this zone, there are large, irregular clumps of variable size and echo intensities. These may also show finger-like projections. The echoes from these areas are significantly weaker than those produced by normal, adjacent tissues.

Figure 24 illustrates what we expect to achieve by our photodensitometric technique; namely, a simple way of outlining and demonstrating these tumors for survey purposes.

In summary, ultrasound mammography requires a diagnostic system which simultaneously displays the undistorted anatomical and acoustic characteristics of the breast. Such a system enables one to determine the range of normal anatomical patterns which the breast displays. Fibroadenomas, fibrocystic disease, and breast cancer have been visualized. The ability of ultrasound mammography to visualize large carcinomas of the breast is unequivocal. The task which remains is that of finding the acoustic characteristics which identify the earliest ultrasonographic signs of malignant change in the breast. This may be accomplished by means of refinements in instrumentation and techniques.

Acknowledgments

This work was made possible by Grant C-127 from the American Cancer Society and by Contract NIH NCI-G72-3872 from the Breast Cancer Task Force of the National Insitutes of Health, U. S. Public Health Service.

REFERENCES

Baum, Gilbert: *Fundamentals of Medical Ultrasonography*. New York, New York, G. P. Putnam's Sons, 1974, pp. 376–386.

Electronic Mammography in the Diagnosis of Early Breast Cancer

DONALD SASHIN, Ph.D. and CLIVE W. MORRIS,
M.B.B.S., F.R.A.C.S., F.F.R.
Department of Radiology, School of Medicine,
University of Pittsburgh, Pittsburgh, Pennsylvania

DESPITE ALL EFFORTS, the treatment for breast cancer has not become conspicuously more successful over the years. There is evidence that biological factors, over which we have little control, may be of great importance (Handley, 1969) and that the dissemination of metastases and the ultimate fate of the patient may be more closely related to such factors than to the size of the tumor when first detected (Fisher, Slack, and Bross, 1969).

Nevertheless, there is overwhelming evidence that a small tumor is more likely to be well differentiated and noninfiltrating, less likely to have metastasized, and has a better prognosis than a large one (Kern and Mikkelson, 1971; Payne *et al.*, 1970), and it is generally agreed that hope for more effective treatment lies mainly in earlier diagnosis (Gershon-Cohen, 1970). A method which would regularly and reliably identify small carcinomas, invasive carcinomas less than 5 mm. in diameter, small intralocular carcinomas in situ, and carcinoma confined within the ducts could be expected to improve results (Hutter, 1971).

Meticulous examination of amputated breasts has shown that a diagnostic pattern of calcification is present in a high percentage of small carcinomas (Hassler, 1969; Koehl, Snyder, and Hutter, 1971), and that multiple small carcinomas are common (Hutter and Kim,

1971). Subtle radiographic signs of an early carcinoma, such as an isolated subareolar duct, have been described (Martin and Gallager, 1971). Wolfe has shown in 500 cases of breast cancer that the incidence of malignant calcification was 51 per cent (Wolf, 1973).

Electronic mammography of improved contrasts and resolutions is one of the new hopes we have in identifying small lesions, tiny areas of calcification, and other such signs of breast tumors. Using this method to routinely examine high-risk carcinoma groups (Zippin and Petrakis, 1971), we should be able to make an earlier diagnosis of breast cancer and thus improve the prognosis. Electronic mammography is a method of recording a single television radiographic image on film. This method has become feasible because of electro-optical, radiographic, and phosphor screen discoveries and inventions during the last few years.

Method and Procedure

Electronic mammography is an X-ray recording technique which involves the substitution of the highly efficient photoelectric effect for the relatively inefficient photochemical effect taking place in the ordinary photographic film.

The manner of implementing this method of X-ray imaging may be understood with the aid of the schematic diagram shown in Figure 1. X rays produced in the X-ray tube are incident on the breast and those that penetrate impinge upon an X-ray luminescent phosphor screen which brightens the image (Fig. 2). The image viewed by a television camera focused on the screen is optically focused on the entrance window of the television camera, is intensified in the camera tube, and then is converted to an electrical charge pattern on the target of the camera tube. In effect, the camera tube target represents the analog to the photographic film, storing the pattern representing the spatial distribution of X-rays emerging from the object.

After a short interval, the accumulated charge pattern on the target is converted to an electrical signal inside the camera by a scanning electronic beam moving across the target in the familiar pattern of a television raster.

After suitable amplification, this electrical signal is used to modulate the brightness of a synchronously moving beam of electrons in a television monitor tube, where the original image is thus reconstructed line-by-line; by using a spot stretch technique in the cathode ray tube, we remove the appearance of the lines from the final image (Fig. 3). The electronic mammograph is recorded by photographing

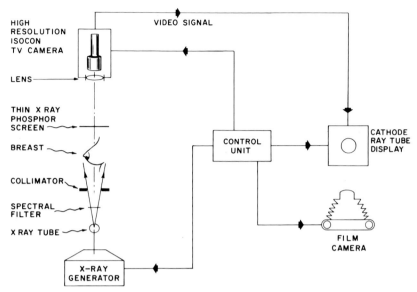

FIG. 1.—Block diagram of the electronic mammographic apparatus.

the screen of the cathode ray tube with a film camera. The entire process is controlled by electronic circuits which pulse the X-ray tube, command the television camera, and advance the film camera (Fig. 4).

Thus, in our system, a permanent mammogram is recorded on photographic film. Hence, the standard radiographic film has been replaced in our system by an X-ray phosphor and photoelectric surface in which nearly every incident X-ray photon can be detected.

The principal advantage of electronic radiographic and mammographic techniques is greater efficiency in utilizing the X-ray quanta, typically 100 to 1,000 times greater than for the best X-ray films, or xerographic recording media available today. In typical electronic imaging systems, this higher efficiency opens up a number of possibilities which may be briefly summarized as follows:

(1) Because of the smaller number of X-ray quanta that must be produced per picture, the X-ray tube current can be reduced. This in turn allows the use of a smaller focal spot, resulting in finer detail in the X-ray image under typical clinical situations.

(2) The radiation dose to the patient is lowered in direct proportion to the reduced number of X-ray quanta registered. Depending upon the amount of detail and contrast as dictated by quantum-noise

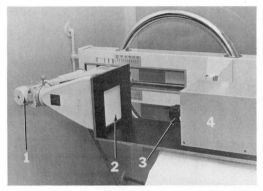
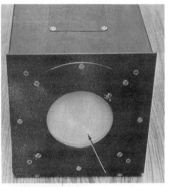

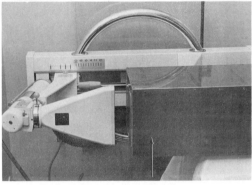

FIG. 2 *(top left).* – This picture of the apparatus with its cover removed shows the relative position of the X-ray tube (1), phosphor screen (2), camera lens (3), and isocon television camera (4).

FIG. 3 *(top right).* – The cathode ray tube (arrow) is viewed by a standard film camera. This component of the apparatus can be located in the X-ray studies darkroom or any other convenient location.

FIG. 4 *(bottom).* – The electronic mammographic apparatus with the cover (arrow) in place.

considerations, the dose can be reduced 100 times in typical clinical situations.

(3) Again, because of the much smaller number of X-ray quanta required per exposure, heavy filtration by a series of specially selected metal filters can be used to eliminate all but the most useful portion of the X-ray spectrum. Recent studies in our laboratory have shown that in this manner, nearly monochromatic X-rays can be produced which have optimum properties in producing image contrast, well beyond that possible with simple aluminum filters.

(4) The high efficiency of such a system as compared to film also allows a reduction in the length of the exposure time, and therefore

reduces the blurring caused by motion. In mammography, with new low-dose film (Dupont, single emulsion and single screen vacuum packed), the dose and therefore exposure time has been lowered by a factor of 2.4 from nonscreen film-medical (Osray-M) (Ostrum, Becker, and Isard, 1973). In our department, the low-dose system reduced the exposure 10–20 times.

(5) As a further consequence of the greater efficiency with which the X-ray quanta are utilized in forming the image, the patient to X-ray focal spot distance can be increased, reducing focal spot blurring.

(6) Since the image is produced in electronic form, various techniques of electronic contrast enhancement can be employed to bring out small density differences by controlling the television camera characteristics. For the same reason, this technique lends itself very simply to computer coupling for a variety of purposes such as computer-aided diagnosis or various forms of image analysis and presentation.

Many of these items have been confirmed in present electronic radiographic systems. In the last 4 years, we have developed high-resolution electronic radiography (Sashin, Rocchio, Matta, and Sternglass, 1969) to eliminate many of the disadvantages in film and fluoroscopic techniques. We have applied electronic radiography clinically to gastrointestinal examination (Sashin, Short, Heinz, and Sternglass, 1973), angiography (Sashin, Porti, Heinz, and Sternglass, 1972), interventional repair of intracranial arteriovenous malformation and aneurysms (Sashin, Goldman, Zanetti, and Heinz, 1972), pelvimetry, and intrauterine transfusion (Sashin, 1972).

The complete electronic mammographic system incorporates the following components and techniques to optimize the image quality:

(1) A small focal spot.

(2) A short exposure time.

(3) Use of a low operating potential for the X-ray tube, resulting in higher contrast between water density tissue and fat and between tissue and calcium.

(4) Thin X-ray phosphor intensifying screen yielding high contrast at low exposure factors.

(5) An isocon television tube with a spectral response matching the emission spectra of the X-ray intensifying screen, giving a high sensitivity, large dynamic range, and high contrast.

(6) A television camera possessing a wide band width and low noise characteristics.

(7) Use of electronic contrast enhancement in the television camera.

Conclusion

An electronic mammographic system is being developed which is specifically designed to permit mass screening for the early detection of breast tumors by increasing the ability to visualize soft-tissue detail and contrast while at the same time reducing the radiation dose required in present mammographic techniques.

This method involves the substitution of image intensification and television techniques for X-ray film, thereby greatly increasing the efficiency with which X rays can be recorded and permitting reductions in the required number of X-ray quanta that must pass through the breast and reach the phosphor intensifying screen. This efficiency allows the use of various techniques to enhance the inherent contrast and detail recorded in the X-ray image. These include the use of lower X-ray tube voltages which at present cannot be applied in mammography because of severe heat-loading limitations in X-ray tubes.

The improvement in the quality of mammography is a consequence of the recent developments of electronic radiographic imaging, high sensitivity, intensifying screens, and the very efficient, high dynamic range, and low noise isocon television cameras.

Electronic mammography for mass screening of the population at risk should result in better diagnosis in shorter examination times with lower radiation exposure; therefore, this technique may reduce the mortality and morbidity of breast cancer.

Acknowledgment

This work is supported by a contract from the National Institutes of Health, National Cancer Institute, Grant No. 1-CB-33904.

REFERENCES

Fisher, B., Slack, N. H., and Bross, I. D. J.: Cancer of the breast: Size of neoplasm and prognosis. *Cancer*, 24:1071–1080, November 1969.

Gershon-Cohen, J.: *Atlas of Mammography*. New York, New York, Springer-Verlag, 1970, 264 pp.

Handley, R. S.: A surgeon's view of the spread of breast cancer. *Cancer*, 24: 1231–1234, December 1969.

Hassler, O.: Microradiographic investigations of calcifications of the female breast. *Cancer*, 23:1103–1109, May 1969.

Hutter, R. V. P.: The pathologist's role in minimal breast cancer. *Cancer*, 28: 1527–1536, December 1971.

Hutter, R. V. P., and Kim, D. U.: The problem of multiple lesions of the breast. *Cancer*, 28:1591–1607, December 1971.

Kern, W. H., and Mikkelsen, W. P.: Small carcinomas of the breast. *Cancer*, 28:948–955, October 1971.

Koehl, R. H., Snyder, R. E., and Hutter, R. V. P.: Use of specimen roentgenography to detect small carcinomas not found by routine pathological examinations. *CA: A Cancer Journal for Clinicians*, 21:2–10, January–February 1971.

Martin, J. E., and Gallager, H. S.: Mammographic diagnosis of minimal breast cancer. *Cancer*, 28:1519–1526, December 1971.

Ostrum, B. J., Becker, W., and Isard, H. J.: Low-dose mammography. *Radiology*, 109:323–326, November 1973.

Payne, W. S., Taylor, W. F., Khonsari, S., Snider, J. H., Harrison, E. G., Jr., Golenzer, H., and Clagett, O. T.: Surgical treatment of breast cancer. *Archives of Surgery*, 101:105–113, August 1970.

Sashin, D.: Dose reduction in diagnostic radiology by electronic image storage techniques. In *Reduction of Radiation Dose in Diagnostic X-ray Procedures*. Bethesda, Maryland, Department of Health, Education and Welfare, 1972, pp. 179–210.

Sashin, D., Goldman, R. L., Zanetti, P., and Heinz, E. R.: Electronic radiology in stereotaxic thrombosis of intracranial aneurysms and catheter embolization of cerebral arteriovenous malformations. *Radiology*, 105:359, November 1972.

Sashin, D., Porti, A., Heinz, E. R., and Sternglass, E. J.: Video techniques in diagnostic radiology. In *Application of Optical Instrumentation in Medicine*. Society of Photo-Optical Instrumentation Engineers, 1972.

Sashin, D., Rocchio, R., Matta, R. K., and Sternglass, E. J.: Resolution contrast and dose reduction performance of electronic radiographic systems. (Abstract) *Second International Conference on Medical Physics*, 2:7, 1969.

Sashin, D., Short, W., Heinz, E. R., and Sternglass, E. J.: Electronic radiology for spot-filming in gastrointestinal fluoroscopy. *Radiology*, 106:551–553, March 1973.

Wolfe, J. N.: Analysis of the radiographic and related features of breast carcinoma. (Abstract) *American Roentgen Ray Society*, 1973, p. 146.

Zippin, C., and Petrakis, N. L.: Identification of high risk groups in breast cancer. *Cancer*, 28:1381–1387, December 1971.

Specimen Radiography

H. STEPHEN GALLAGER, M.D.
Department of Pathology, The University of Texas
System Cancer Center M. D. Anderson Hospital and
Tumor Institute, Houston, Texas

THE RADIOGRAPHY OF SPECIMENS as an adjunct to pathologic examination has, until recently, received little attention. To be sure, postmortem coronary angiography has been an accepted research method for many years (Rissanen, 1970), but other systematic applications of radiography in pathology have been few. The wide acceptance of soft tissue mammography in the diagnosis of breast cancer and the resulting need for an effective means of localizing nonpalpable lesions in breast specimens have made the rapid development of specimen radiography obligatory. It is the intent of this paper to review the indications for and techniques of specimen radiography in the diagnosis of mammary carcinoma, and also to discuss applications of the technique in other areas of surgical pathology.

Specimen Radiography in Breast Cancer

Since its reintroduction as a diagnostic technique in breast cancer (Egan, 1960), mammography has become widely accepted. Early experience indicated that mammography is capable not only of confirming the findings of palpation but also of discovering carcinomas which are not palpable (Egan, 1962). Some of these occult tumors are fully invasive mass lesions, simply obscured by large breasts or by excessive density and nodularity of mammary tissue. Many neoplasms, however, are of microscopic size, noninvasive, and invisible in specimens and represented only by the presence of a cluster of

423

characteristic calcifications or a distortion of architecture on a mammogram (Martin and Gallager, 1971). Such circumstances present a problem for both surgeon and pathologist. The surgeon finds himself asked to excise a lesion he cannot feel or localize by physical examination and the pathologist is asked to find and make sections from a lesion which is neither visibly nor palpably different from the adjacent tissue. Specimen radiography as a solution to this dilemma was first proposed by Patton, Poznanski, and Zylak in 1966 and rapidly adopted in other institutions (Sherman, Brasfield, Snyder, and Hutter, 1967). Currently, it is generally agreed that facilities for specimen radiography are indispensable in any pathology laboratory where breast specimens are examined (Bauermeister and Hall, 1973; Pathology Working Group, Breast Cancer Task Force, 1973).

The objectives of specimen radiography in this situation are twofold (Gallager, 1972). First, it is necessary in order to ascertain that the mammographically demonstrated lesion is within the biopsy specimen. Second, the specific part of the specimen from which sections are to be made must be localized. To accomplish these ends, the following procedure has been adopted in many laboratories, including our own.

Using the mammogram for guidance, a sizable segment of mammary tissue, usually an entire quadrant, is resected. This specimen is first examined grossly. If no palpable mass is present, the intact specimen is radiographed. A self-contained, integrally shielded radiographic unit (Fingerhut, 1968) has been installed in the Frozen Section Laboratory for this purpose (Fig. 1). The film used is relatively slow, fine-grained, machine-processable, and capable of high resolution. Exposure time is 3 minutes at 3 Ma.S. and a kvp. between 15 to 25, depending on the thickness of the specimen. The film is immediately processed and compared with the mammogram. Should the mammographically demonstrated lesion not be present, surgeon and pathologist confer and additional biopsy material is removed. The radiographic procedure is repeated until changes corresponding to those in the mammogram are identified (Fig. 2).

Once it has been established that the lesion is present in the specimen, it becomes necessary to localize a specific focus from which to prepare microscopic sections. The specimen is sliced at intervals of 2 to 3 mm. and the slices are arrayed on a sheet of radiolucent plastic. A second radiograph is prepared from this assembly and suspect areas are marked on the film (Fig. 3). Tissue blocks are cut from corresponding areas of the specimen slices and are processed either by frozen section technique or by paraffin embedding and sectioning.

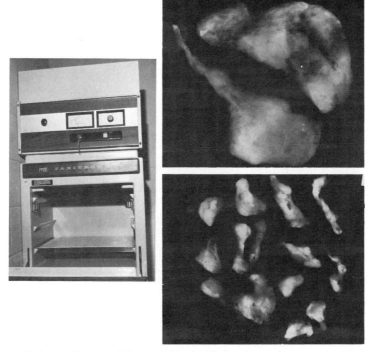

FIG. 1 *(left).*—Self-contained, integrally shielded radiographic unit suitable for use in surgical pathology laboratories.

FIG. 2 *(top right).*—Radiograph of a large breast biopsy specimen. The cluster of calcifications sought can be seen in the lower right corner of the upper half of the specimen.

FIG. 3 *(bottom right).* — Radiograph of a breast biopsy specimen sliced for selection of tissue blocks. Suspicious calcifications are present in several fragments. Pencil markings visible in the photograph are symbols identifying specific tissue blocks.

The locations of selected blocks are numbered on the specimen film to correspond to the tissue blocks. It is important, particularly when searching for lesions represented only by calcifications, that sufficient sections be cut from each block to be sure that the suspect area is represented in sections. Occasional lesions are so small that they may escape detection if only a single random section is made.

Since this procedure may be time-consuming, and since the subtle changes of minimal breast cancer are best appreciated in paraffin sections, it is often preferable to terminate the operative procedure once the presence of the lesion in the biopsy specimen has been established. Definitive surgery can, if necessary, be scheduled 2 or 3 days later. There is no evidence to indicate that a delay of this length is in any way harmful.

Radiography of Mastectomy Specimens

To maintain orientation while dissecting an amputated breast is difficult. Even if excision biopsy has not been done, the inherent flaccidity of the structure interferes with accurate localization of lesions and understanding of their relationships. As a result, data important to subsequent treatment planning may be lost when mastectomy specimens are examined by conventional techniques. For example, it has been well established by whole organ studies that multiple invasive nodules are present in many cancer-containing breasts (Gallager and Martin, 1969), but it is unusual for this phenomenon to be reported in routinely studied surgical specimens. To solve this problem, the following technique, a modification of that proposed by Egan, Ellis, and Powell (1969), has been adopted.

The specimen is oriented in anatomic position, and the axilla is removed in 3 segments (proximal, middle, and distal) and the pectoral muscles are dissected free. The nipple, areola, and subareolar tissues are excised and processed separately. The remaining breast is then divided into 4 quadrants by cutting on the vertical and horizontal axes. Each quadrant is sliced tangentially at about 1-cm. intervals using a long knife (Fig. 4). The slices of each quadrant are arranged in order on a plastic plate and specimen radiographs are prepared (Fig. 5). The processed films are examined and any abnormality in structure is marked. Blocks for paraffin sectioning are selected on the basis of the specimen radiograph. Palpable abnormalities in the

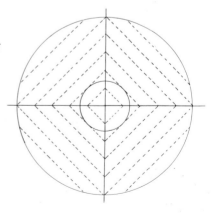

FIG. 4. – Diagram showing placing of cuts for slicing a mastectomy specimen preparatory to specimen radiography.

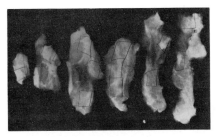

Fig. 5.—Radiograph of one quadrant of a mastectomy specimen prepared as described in the text. Pencil markings indicate areas chosen for histologic examination.

specimen which are not visible on the films are also marked as the gross examination proceeds. The site of each block is numbered on the film to correspond to the slide which will ultimately represent it. Slides and films are studied concomitantly, and thus any lesion found in the sections can be specifically identified and related to other structures present in the breast.

This technique not only makes possible a measure of accuracy in interpretation not otherwise obtainable, but also aids in the identification of the nonpalpable lesions which frequently accompany carcinoma and are of diagnostic and prognostic significance. The specimen radiograph serves as a bridge between the preoperative mammogram and the histologic preparations. Nonspecific mammographic densities may, by the use of this intermediate, be specifically related to histologic abnormalities.

Other Applications

VISUALIZATION OF LYMPH NODES

Normal and neoplastic lymph nodes are sufficiently different in radiographic density from adipose tissue that they can be readily identified in radiographs (Fig. 6). The procedure is useful in the study of specimens from cervical, axillary, inguinal, and retroperitoneal node dissections. Specimen radiography makes it possible to enumerate the nodes present in the specimen and to identify their locations. Since small or fatty lymph nodes can be missed by this technique, careful gross examination also is necessary. The specimen radiograph does not differentiate between nodes involved by tumor and normal nodes, but provides a means by which a maximum number of nodes may be recovered for histologic examination. It is necessary to remove from the specimen all extraneous tissue, such as mus-

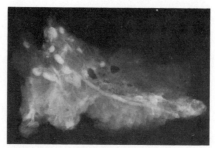

FIG. 6. — Radiograph of a surgical specimen from a radical axillary dissection demonstrating visualization of lymph nodes in adipose tissue.

cle, large arteries and bone, for optimal visualization of soft tissue structures.

LYMPH NODES AFTER LYMPHANGIOGRAPHY

Certain patients with carcinoma of the uterine cervix as well as patients with nonseminomatous germ cell neoplasms of the testis are routinely subjected to selective retroperitoneal node dissection for the purpose of planning radiation therapy. It is important that the locations of positive nodes be identified and plotted with exactitude. The following technique takes advantage of the fact that radiopaque dye is retained in lymph nodes for a relatively prolonged period to obtain the desired precision in localization.

Prior to the operative procedure, a pedal lymphangiogram is performed. Lymphangiography is capable of identifying distortions in lymph, vascular, and nodal patterns which indicate the presence of metastatic neoplasm. Small metastatic nodules, however, are below the limit of resolution of the technique, and nodes completely replaced by tumor may fail to be opacified.

At the time of node dissection, each group of nodes as it is removed is placed on a plastic plate in which fine wires have been embedded to form an outline of the lower abdominal great vessels. The nodes are placed on this template as nearly as possible in the position which they occupied in the body. In the laboratory, the plate, with lymph nodes in place, is radiographed (Fig. 7). Each node is individually marked on the film and numbered to correspond to slide numbers. In this way, each node can be related to a specific image in the specimen radiograph. By comparison with the preoperative lymphangiogram, the precise localization of positive nodes can be obtained. Nonopacified nodes discovered by gross examination are also marked on the specimen film and can be readily related to

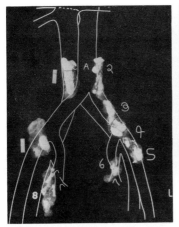 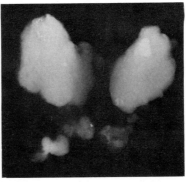

FIG. 7 *(left).* — Opacified lymph nodes from a selective abdominal dissection arrayed on a template as described in the text. Markers indicate specific lymph node groups.

FIG. 8 *(right).* — Radiograph of a radical thyroidectomy specimen. The coarse calcifications in both right and left lobes indicate multiple foci of mixed papillary and follicular carcinoma. Similar calcifications can be seen in 1 pretracheal lymph node, indicating a site of metastasis.

the preoperative lymphangiogram by reference to adjacent opacified structures. Data from this procedure are of value in planning the fields for radiation therapy.

THYROID CARCINOMA

Papillary or mixed papillary and follicular carcinomas of the thyroid gland often contain considerable calcium, which typically appears as sharply circumscribed groups of coarse, angular particles. Specimen radiographs of lobectomy or thyroidectomy specimens readily localize such neoplastic foci (Fig. 8). Lymph nodes containing metastases from thyroid carcinomas may contain similar calcific deposits which can be recognized radiographically. The technique is useful in identifying locations from which blocks for histologic study are to be taken. It also serves as a partial substitute for whole-organ sectioning in situations where the requisite delay for the more extensive procedure would be undesirable.

GERM CELL TUMORS OF THE OVARY

Gonadoblastoma, a neoplasm of dysgenetic gonads found in phenotypic females, has a characteristic pattern of coarse calcification. Since these tumors are frequently overgrown by other forms of germ

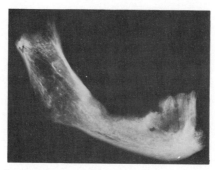

FIG. 9.—Radiograph of the specimen from a hemimandibulectomy for squamous carcinoma of the gingiva. The ragged defect in the cortex indicates the site of invasion of bone by the neoplasm.

cell tumors, notably dysgerminoma, it is easy to miss an underlying neoplasm. The identification of gonadoblastoma is clinically important because its presence makes contralateral gonadectomy mandatory, whereas when dysgerminoma is not associated with gonadoblastoma, conservation of normal ovarian tissue is desirable. Specimen radiography is a rapid and convenient means of localizing foci in which histologic discovery of gonadoblastoma is likely. Additionally, in teratomatous tumors, specimen radiography can be used to identify organoid bone or dental structures not readily subject to histologic sectioning. The occurrence of such structures is definite evidence of the teratomatous nature of the tumor, even when the bulk of the neoplasm may be of some other pattern.

BONE SPECIMENS

In both primary and secondary neoplasms of bone, specimen radiography has particular usefulness(Fig. 9). By showing in detail the trabecular structure of cancellous bone, the extent of a neoplastic lesion within the medullary cavity can be accurately mapped. Cortical defects in bones adjacent to neoplastic soft tissue masses indicate the probability of osseous involvement.

Summary and Conclusions

Specimen radiography in only a few years has become an indispensable tool in the management of biopsy specimens of breast lesions demonstrable by mammography only. Failure to utilize specimen radiography under these circumstances can result in overlooking a microscopic carcinoma of the breast and thereby missing the opportunity of managing it at a stage when the probability of cure is high. It seems inevitable, therefore, that as the utilization of mammography increases the availability of facilities for specimen radiography will also increase rapidly. Ability to interpret radiographs of specimens promises to become one of the standard skills expected of pathologists. Our own experience indicates that the technique has many other uses, not only in the study of breast carcinoma, but also in the management of specimens from a diversity of anatomic sites.

REFERENCES

Bauermeister, D. E., and Hall, M. H.: Specimen radiography—a mandatory adjunct to mammography. *American Journal of Clinical Pathology*, 59: 782–789, June 1973.

Egan, R. L.: Experience with mammography in a tumor institution. Evaluation of 1000 studies. *Radiology*, 75:894–900, December 1960.

————: Mammography, an aid to diagnosis of breast carcinoma. *The Journal of the American Medical Association*, 182:839–843, Nov. 24, 1962.

Egan, R. L., Ellis, J. T., and Powell, R. W.: Team approach to the study of diseases of the breast. *Cancer*, 23:847–854, April 1969.

Fingerhut, A. G.: A self-contained radiographic unit. *Radiology*, 90:1030, May 1968.

Gallager, H. S.: The pathologist and modern breast cancer management. In Sommers, S. C., Ed.: *Pathology Annual 1972.* New York, New York, Appleton-Century-Crofts, 1972, pp. 231–250.

Gallager, H. S., and Martin, J. E.: The study of mammary carcinoma by mammography and whole organ sectioning. Early observations. *Cancer*, 23:855–873, April 1969.

Martin, J. E., and Gallager, H. S.: The mammographic diagnosis of minimal breast cancer. *Cancer*, 28:1519–1526, December 1971.

Pathology Working Group, Breast Cancer Task Force: Standardized management of breast specimens. *American Journal of Clinical Pathology*, 60: 789–798, December 1973.

Patton, R. B., Poznanski, A. K., and Zylak, C. J.: Pathologic examination of specimens containing nonpalpable breast cancers discovered by radiography. *American Journal of Clinical Pathology*, 46:330–334, September 1966.

Rissanen, V. T.: Double contrast technique for postmortem coronary angiography. *Laboratory Investigation*, 23:517–520, November 1970.

Sherman, R. S., Brasfield, R. D., Snyder, R. E., and Hutter, R. V. P.: The pursuit of the occult cancer of the breast. (Letter to the editor) *The Journal of the American Medical Association*, 201:782–783, Sept. 4, 1967.

Indications for Lymph Node Scanning Utilizing Colloidal Gold - 198

JOHN R. GLASSBURN, M.D., LUTHER W. BRADY, M.D.,
HARRY LESSIG, M.D., and
MILLARD N. CROLL, M.D.
*Department of Radiation Therapy and Nuclear
Medicine, Hahnemann Medical College and Hospital,
Philadelphia, Pennsylvania*

ONE OF THE GREATEST DIFFICULTIES facing the clinician is the early detection of neoplastic involvement of inaccessible lymph nodes in patients with malignant disease. As discussed in the preceeding papers, Ethiodol lymphangiography as first described by Kinmonth (1952) has gained wide acceptance, and is extremely useful in determining pelvic and retroperitoneal lymph node involvement. However, this procedure is tedious and time-consuming and its accuracy varies widely from institution to institution depending upon the skill and interest of the diagnostic radiologist (Wiljasalo, 1965; Takahasi and Abrams, 1967; Lee, 1968; Piver, Wallace, and Castro, 1971; Lee *et al.*, 1971).

Radioactive colloidal gold-198 has been used for visualization of the pelvic and retroperitoneal lymph nodes for more than 15 years, but its place as a diagnostic study has not been well defined (Lang, 1960; Sherman and Ter-Pogossian, 1965; Zum Winkel and Scheer, 1965; Zum Winkel and Muller, 1965; Grönross, Laakso, Rauramo, and Aalto, 1968; Mortel, Lewis, and Brady, 1972; Littman, Davis, and Lepanto, 1973; Glassburn *et al.*, 1972; Kazem *et al.*, 1968).

Clinical Method

Colloidal gold lymph node scanning is safe and easily performed. In all patients, 100μCi. of gold-198 in a volume of 0.3 ml. to 0.5 ml. is injected subcutaneously in the interdigital webspace between the first and second toe of each foot. The patients are instructed to walk for 1 hour or to undergo massage of the lower extremities to facilitate the transport of the material through the lymphatic channels. The patients are scanned at 24 hours with a rectilinear scanner according to a method that has been described in previous publications (Glassburn *et al.*, 1972, Kazem *et al.* 1968).

Interpretations

Abdominal lymph scans are considered to be positive when 2 or more of the following criteria are met:

1. Failure of the pelvic and the periaortic lymph nodes to be visualized at 24 hours.

2. Asymmetry in configuration in the distribution of the activity within the nodal areas.

FIG. 1 *(left)*.—A normal abdominal lymph scan with symmetrical distribution of activity throughout the abdominal and para-aortic lymph nodes and good liver activity.

FIG. 2 *(right)*.—This patient had an established diagnosis of diffuse lymphocytic lymphoma. The scan demonstrates poor uptake in the liver and para-aortic nodal area, along with ballooning of the distal node groups.

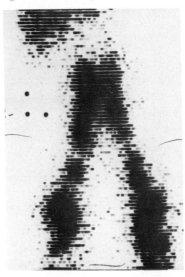 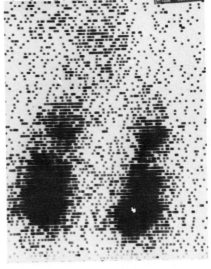

3. Absent or decreased radionuclide localization in the liver.

4. Mottled or patchy appearances of the activity at 1 or more sites.

5. Presence of abnormal collateral channels.

6. Enlargement of the width of a node group.

7. Absence or interruption of activity in the lymph node chain (Figs. 1, 2, 3, 4, and 5).

Edema, stasis, or failure to exercise may cause poor visualization of the node groups examined. Liver visualization is obtained without

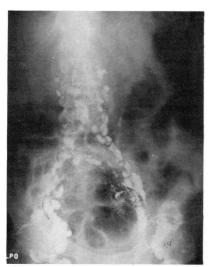
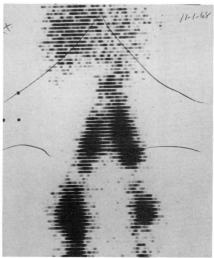
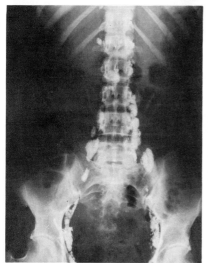

Fig. 3 *(above left).* – The Ethiodol lymphangiogram in the same patient as shown in Figure 2. Diffuse nodal involvement is demonstrated.

Fig. 4 *(above).* – Scan of a patient with Stage IIIA Hodgkin's disease. Asymmetry in configuration of the isotope, poor liver activity, and interruption of activity are demonstrated.

Fig. 5 *(left).* – The Ethiodol lymphangiogram of the same patient as shown in Figure 4, demonstrating obvious lymph node involvement.

visualization of the pelvic and periaortic lymph nodes when the radionuclide is injected intravenously. A repeat study is indicated when this distribution of activity is noted.

Accuracy

A retrospective analysis was made, at our institution, of 871 abdominal lymph scans performed on 757 patients from January 1, 1967, to June 30, 1973. Of this group, 180 patients subsequently underwent lymphangiography. Table 1 is a comparison of the Ethiodol lymphangiography results with those of colloidal gold in lymph scanning. It is evident that the number of patients with negative lymph scans who underwent lymphangiography is quite small. The best correlation between the 2 studies is in the group of patients with lymphomas and Hodgkin's disease, who had positive lymph scans.

More meaningful, however, is Table 2, in which colloidal gold-198 lymph node scanning is compared to the results of lymph node biopsies obtained from 1 or more visualized areas. Again, it is quite evident that the number of patients with negative lymph scans who underwent biopsy procedures is quite small. Good correlation is seen in the group of patients with lymphoma and Hodgkin's disease who had positive lymph scans, with an accuracy rate of 88 per cent. Very poor correlation is seen in the group of patients with the established diagnosis of carcinoma of the cervix, between the positive lymph scan and the biopsy results. This is believed to be because of the large number of these patients who have inflammatory or hyper-

Table 1
Lymph Scan vs. Lymphangiogram

	Lymphoma	Cervix	Other	Total
Positive lymph scan Positive lymphangiogram	65	18	28	111
Positive lymph scan Negative lymphangiogram	16	10	14	40
% agreement with positive scans	80%	64%	66%	74%
Negative lymph scan Negative lymphangiogram	11	5	4	20
Negative lymph scan Positive lymphangiogram	6	0	3	9
% agreement with negative scans	64%	100%	57%	68%
Total patients	98	33	49	180

Table 2
Lymph Scan vs. Lymph Node Biopsy

	Lymphoma	Cervix	Others	Total
Positive lymph scan Positive biopsy	57	23	43	123
Positive lymph scan Negative biopsy	8	25	16	49
% agreement with positive scan	88%	48%	73%	72%
Negative scan Negative biopsy	4	10	7	21
Negative scan Positive biopsy	3	1	3	7
% agreement with negative scans	57%	91%	70%	85%
Total patients	72	59	69	200

plastic changes in the regional lymph node groups. In the heterogeneous group designated as "other," there is 73 per cent accuracy in the positive scan group, and 70 per cent accuracy if the scan is negative.

Indications for Abdominal Lymph Scanning

Colloidal gold-198 lymph scanning is not as accurate as Ethiodol lymphangiography. Furthermore, information concerning the size and morphology of the lymph nodes is not obtained with the isotopic study. This information is necessary when defining a radiation field or when contemplating a lymph node dissection. We have found the isotopic study quite useful in patients with lymphoma and Hodgkin's disease as an aid in interpreting the all-too-frequent equivocal lymphangiogram. A suspicious area on the Ethiodol study may show as a very notable obstruction with the gold-198 study. A gold-198 lymph node scan must be performed prior to Ethiodol lymphangiography, since reactive changes in the nodes from the Ethiodol lymphangiogram are sufficient to cause a positive isotopic study. Repeat lymph scans are also useful in following patients with lymphoma or Hodgkin's disease after radiation because the study can be repeated without difficulty.

In patients with other malignant diseases in whom Ethiodol lymphangiography is contraindicated because of sensitivity to iodine or marked pulmonary disease, useful information can be obtained with the gold-198 lymph scan. We have also found this study to be quite reproducible, and changes from a baseline study invariably signify progressive disease.

Conclusions

Our original enthusiasm for colloidal gold-198 lymph scanning has been tempered with time. It is a useful adjunct to lymphangiography in patients with lymphoma and Hodgkin's disease, and is a useful study in patients who have contraindications to lymphangiography. However, at this time, Ethiodol lymphangiography remains the best method of determining the presence or absence of malignant disease in pelvic or periaortic lymph nodes.

Acknowledgments

This work was supported by PHS Training Grant No. T01-CA05185, PHS Research Grant No. 1-R10-CA12252, and PHS Research Grant No. 5-R01-CA12478, all from the National Cancer Institute; by the Alperin Foundation; and by the Friends of the Radiation Therapy Center.

REFERENCES

Glassburn, J. R., Prasasvinichai, S., Nuss, R. C., Croll, M. N., and Brady, L. W.: Correlation of [198]Au abdominal lymph scans with lymphangiograms and lymph node biopsies. *Radiology*, 105:93–96, October 1972.

Grönross, M., Laakso, L., Rauramo, L., and Aalto, T.: Value of lymphoscintigraphy in evaluation extent of malignant tumors in female pelvis. *Acta Obstetrica et Gynecologica Scandinavica*, 47:501–516, 1968.

Kazen, I., Antoniades, J., Brady, L. W., Faust, D. S., Croll, M. N., and Lightfoot, D.: Clinical evaluation of lymph node scanning utilizing colloidal gold[198]. *Radiology*, 90:905–911, May 1968.

Kinmonth, J. B.: Lymphangiography in man; method of outlining lymphatic trunks at operation. *Clinical Sciences*, 11:13–20, February 1952.

Lang, E. K.: Demonstration of blockage and involvement of the pelvic lymphatic system by tumor with lymphangiography and scintiscanograms. *Radiology*, 74:71–73, January 1960.

Lee, B. J.: Correlation between lymphangiography and clinical status of patients with lymphoma. *Cancer Chemotherapy Reports*, 52:205–211, January 1968.

Lee, K. F., Greening, R., Kramer, S., Hahn, G. A., Kruoda, K., Lin, S.-R., and Koslow, W. W.: The value of pelvic venography and lymphography in the clinical staging of carcinoma of the uterine cervix: Analysis of 105 proven cases by surgery. *The American Journal of Roentgenology, Radium Therapy and Nuclear Medicine*, 111:284–296, February 1971.

Littman, P., Davis, L. W., and Lepanto, P.: Evaluation of nodal metastasis in patients with cervical carcinoma. *Cancer*, 31:1307–1311, June 1973.

Mortel, R., Lewis, G. C., and Brady, L. W.: Evaluation of abdominal lymph scanning in gynecologic cancer. *Gynecologic Oncology*, 1:36–43, November 1972.

Piver, M. S., Wallace, S., and Castro, J. R.: The accuracy of lymphangio-graphy in carcinoma of the uterine cervix. *The American Journal of Roent-genology, Radium Therapy and Nuclear Medicine,* 111:278–283, Febru-ary 1971.

Sherman, A. I., and Ter-Pogossian, M.: Lymph-node concentration of ra-dioactive colloidal gold following interstitial injection. *Cancer,* 6:1238–1240, November 1953.

Takahasi, M., and Abrams, H. L.: The accuracy of lymphangiographic diag-nosis in malignant lymphoma. *Radiology,* 89:448–460, September 1967.

Wiljasalo, M.: Lymphographic differential diagnosis of neoplastic diseases. *Acta Radiologica Supplement,* 247:1–143, 1965.

Zum Winkel, K., and Muller, H.: Technique, evaluation and roentgenologic control of abdominal isotope lymphography. *Der Radiologe,* 5:381–393, October 1965.

Zum Winkel, K., and Scheer, K. E.: Scintigraphic and dynamic studies of the lymphatic system with radio-colloids. *Minerva Nucleare,* 9:390–398, No-vember–December 1965.

CLINICOPATHOLOGICAL PANEL DISCUSSION —

Problems in Tumor Diagnosis: Interaction of Pathology with Radiology and Other Biophysical Methods*

MODERATORS: WILLIAM O. RUSSELL, M.D.†, and DOROTHY PATRAS, M.D.‡

†Head, Department of Pathology, The University of Texas System Cancer Center M. D. Anderson Hospital and Tumor Institute; ‡President, Texas Society of Pathologists

THE FINAL SESSION of the M. D. Anderson Hospital Eighteenth Annual Clinical Conference was the Sixth Annual Special Pathology Program. The panel included the following staff members of The University of Texas System Cancer Center M. D. Anderson Hospital and Tumor Institute in addition to Drs. Russell and Patras: A. G. Ayala, J. J. Butler, H. S. Gallager, T. P. Haynie, D. E. Johnson, B. Mackay, J. A. Murray, R. S. Nelson, S. Wallace, J. T. Wharton, and E. C. White. Traditionally, these informal panel discussions are made up of a series of case presentations illustrating the clinicopathologic

---

*Arranged by the Department of Pathology of The University of Texas System Cancer Center M. D. Anderson Hospital and Tumor Institute and Co-sponsored by Texas Society of Pathologists.

aspects of subjects covered by speakers during the previous sessions of the Annual Clinical Conference. Therefore, in keeping with the topic of the conference, Radiologic and Other Biophysical Methods in Tumor Diagnosis, 8 case histories were selected to illustrate, in addition to conventional histopathologic techniques, procedures such as organ scans, radiography, organ perfusion, fiberoptic endoscopy, specimen radiography, angiography, and electron microscopy, as well as advances in surgical techniques, including bone transplantation.

As in previous special pathology programs, the emphasis in the panel discussions was on the multidisciplinary team approach to the management of patients with cancers of all sites. The 8 case discussions included patients with tumors of bone, liver, stomach, prostate, testis, cervix and breast.

CASE 1.—*Giant Cell Tumor of the Tibia Illustrating Diagnostic Procedures and Advances in Surgical Management.* This 55-year-old migrant farm worker had been experiencing pain, weakness, and swelling of the right knee for approximately 1 year before he was admitted to M. D. Anderson Hospital in March 1973. Initial physical examination showed a warm, pulsatile mass measuring 8 × 5.5 cm. palpable over the medial aspect of the upper end of the right tibia. However, no limitation of motion was observed and all other physical findings were negative.

DISCUSSION

RADIOLOGY.—Roentgenograms demonstrated a large lytic lesion, the inferior aspect of which was not sharply defined. No reactive changes were associated with the lesion but there was a pathologic fracture in the cortex anteriorly and superiorly. On arteriograms, the lesion appeared to be moderately vascular with some tortuous or coiled vessels throughout. However, no vessel showed the criteria which radiologists consider characteristic of neoplastic invasion or encasement of a vessel by malignant tumor. Although not absolute, 1 of the criteria for malignant invasion of vessels is the appearance of many irregularities, such as small narrowings and dilatations, compared to the somewhat smooth tapering of normal vessels from the take off to the periphery. Another criterion is neovascularity or the pocketing of contrast material. While not conclusive, these radiological features—irregularities in vessels, neovascularity, arterial venous shunting—afford fairly reliable evidence of malignancy. Depending upon the primary tumor, metastatic lesions also may demonstrate vascularity. For example, 65 per cent of renal neoplasms are highly vascular and most of the metastatic disease from those lesions is also highly vascular. This vascularity seen in the secondary lesions frequently mimics vascularity of the primary tumor.

In this particular tumor, the arteriograms demonstrated specific characteristics which have been seen in other giant cell tumors of bone. The number and the tortuosity of vessels was increased. The radiologists concluded that their findings were very compatible with a giant cell tumor, but the age of the patient and the pulsation of the mass introduced a note of doubt, preventing the firm establishment of giant cell tumor as the final diagnosis for the bone lesion.

PATHOLOGY. — Following review of the radiological findings, a biopsy of the lesion was performed. The diagnosis was giant cell tumor of bone. With this diagnosis established, the proximal one third of the tibia was resected. The surgical specimen showed a 9 cm. mass occupying both the metaphysis and epiphysis of the bone. Thinning of the cortex was seen but the tumor had not extended into the soft tissues. The previous biopsy was represented by a white fibrous area. The rest of the specimen evidenced the classical appearance of giant cell tumor of bone with rusty brown discoloration. Microscopically there were multiple benign giant cells and a benign stroma, with occasional mitotic figures.

Several other giant cell tumors of bone were illustrated and discussed to emphasize the classical features previously described. Combined radiographs and gross specimen photographs were shown to illustrate correlation between the 2 diagnostic procedures.

SURGERY. — The preoperative evaluation was primary giant cell tumor of bone. At the present time in this country, most institutions manage these giant cell tumors of bone with curettage and autograft packing. The lowest reported recurrence rates are 35 to 40 per cent, but experience at M. D. Anderson Hospital suggests that studies showing the recurrence rate actually is 60 per cent probably are more correct.

At this institution, the members of the treatment teams associated with the Bone Tumor Clinic favor extraperiosteal resection and allograft transplantation as the treatment of choice for patients with giant cell tumors of bone. Arteriography is an important part of the preoperative diagnostic procedures. While it does not necessarily establish a definitive diagnosis, it does provide the surgeons with important information as to the extent of the procedures which will be required. None of the giant cell tumors have recurred in the more than 30 patients who have been treated by resection and allograft transplants to date. Some extremities have been lost because of graft failure, but the cure rate is better than that recorded for any other known series of patients. Best results have been achieved when surgeons can salvage at least half of the affected joint. The major aim is to achieve intermedullary as well as cross-through stabilization in performing the initial step-cut resection. The only problems encountered to date have been in those patients where good mechanical stability could not be maintained. For the particular patient under discussion, the donor bone was slightly larger than the tibia of the recipient. Nevertheless, good mechanical stability was achieved. Union of the bone was successful despite an episode of wound infection and fistula formation. These difficulties appeared to be attributable to the slight discrepancy in size between the transplant and the recipient bone.

Several of the previous case histories of patients treated by allograft transplantation for giant cell tumors were illustrated and discussed. One patient was a woman who had fallen down the steps who, when told by her physicians that she had a tumor, remained in bed for 2 months refusing to have treatment because she was afraid she had cancer. Nevertheless, at the 5-year follow-up after resection and allograft transplantation at this institution, complete consolidation of the step-cut procedure was observed. The patient had no effusion, no symptoms, maintained 90 degrees of knee motion, and was fully ambulatory. Another patient was a 19-year-old girl who was referred to this institution for consideration of resection following recurrence after treatment by curettage and autograft packing at another institution. The diagnostic polytome illustrated some residual tumor in the graft, but demonstrated that good margins existed and half the joint could be salvaged. At the 4-year postoperative follow-up after allograft transplant, it was discovered that the patient had returned to water skiing (against the advice of her physician). The long-term roentgenographic follow-up studies of these patients emphasized that they all develop rather profound degenerative arthritic changes in the joint involved. In some patients, the degree of arthritis is such that they would be expected to need crutches, but the arthritis does not bother these patients, all of whom have maintained 90 degrees of knee motion and are fully ambulatory. These arthritic changes currently are believed to be attributable to the fact that even in the best fitting transplants, significant incongruity of the joint surface remains. Nevertheless, when the grafts survive, the patients regain full weight-bearing, full range of motion, and continue to be fully ambulatory despite the degenerative arthritic changes which are observed within 4 to 5 years.

FOLLOW-UP

This patient was last seen shortly before the discussion of this case. He was 6 months postoperative and the fistulas were healing. He was ambulatory on crutches and had no evidence of residual or recurrent neoplasm.

CASE 2.—*Carcinoma of the Prostate with Metastasis to Rib, Emphasizing the Importance of a Multidisciplinary Approach to Management of Patients with Prostatic Carcinoma.* In July 1973, a 68-year-old retired oil field worker began experiencing difficulty in voiding as well as other signs of lower urinary tract obstruction. After several months, he consulted a urologist who performed a transurethral biopsy of the prostate. The patient was then referred to M. D. Anderson Hospital for further care. At the time of admission in October 1973, rectal examination showed the prostate gland to be stony hard and apparently entirely involved by tumor. It was fixed to the left pelvic wall. Laboratory studies showed the acid phosphatase levels were within normal limits.

DISCUSSION

PATHOLOGY.—Histologic sections from the transurethral biopsy demonstrated the classical picture of prostatic carcinoma—multiple small glands with practically no intervening stroma and perineural space invasion. With this diagnosis, the patient was referred for a complete skeletal survey as a routine procedure for staging purposes.

RADIOLOGY.—The pyelogram showed the kidneys to be normal in size; no abnormalities were observed in the ureters although they curved slightly inward at the ureterovesical junction. Some thickening of the bladder wall was observed as was early trabeculation which usually accompanies a lesion obstructing the outlet. Benign or malignant prostatic lesions can produce such features. In routine X-ray studies, there was some discussion as to whether the fourth rib was normal or abnormal, but the final reading of the film was that the changes were not significant. Slight expansion of the rib was seen at 1 point; the cortex was fairly well outlined and appeared a little thin, although there was some question of a slight increase in density in 1 area. Differential diagnoses of such features could include: an old fracture which was healed and left some slight expansion, or perhaps a metastatic lesion, inasmuch as carcinoma of the prostate frequently produces osteoblastic metastases. Osteolytic metastases are seen in about 15 per cent of patients. The specific X-ray diagnosis was not established at this point.

A total body scan was performed for this patient using ^{99m}Tc polyphosphate. The procedure entailed injecting 10 millicuries of the medium and scanning the patient 3 hours later using a total body rectilinear scanner with the minification attachment which affords an almost complete scan of the patient. The dual-probe scanner was used to provide simultaneous views of anterior and posterior projections (Fig. 1). Such scans show many areas of normal media concentration. For example, background activity usually is seen in the heart, mediastinum, sternum, and pelvis. Also, the kidneys concentrate the agent and excrete it into the bladder. Such observations cannot be completely eliminated because the agent adheres to the bladder wall. The scan showed an abnormality on the left posterior aspect of the chest which corresponded to the previously questionable abnormality seen on the X-ray films. The gamma camera was em-

FIG. 1 *(left).* — The dual-probe scan provides simultaneous views of anterior and posterior projections.

FIG. 2 *(right).* — The gamma camera showed increased concentration of media on the lateral aspect of the fourth rib.

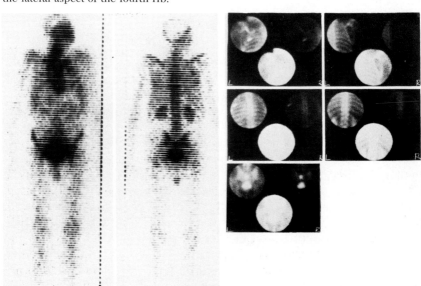

ployed for more detailed resolution of the area in question, and increased concentration of media was seen on the lateral aspect of the fourth rib (Fig. 2). Also, an area of increased concentration was observed in the midsacrum which was thought to be possible evidence of metastatic disease. No evidence of abnormality was found in the skull or the anterior chest. However, final judgments were reserved for assembly of the total clinical picture because abnormal bone scans may be produced by fracture processes which lead to osteoid formation, as well as by many benign conditions such as osteomyelitis, arthritis, and certain infections.

SURGERY. — Discussion of this case emphasized the importance of the multidisciplinary approach to staging carcinoma of the prostate. This patient was asymptomatic for metastatic disease and the skeletal survey was performed as part of routine evaluation. Clinically, the patient was classified as stage C — locally invasive disease with involvement of the seminal vesicles. With no evidence of disseminated disease, 7,000 rads tumor dose would have been recommended, delivered over 7 weeks to the prostate, as an approach to cure. With the indication of metastatic disease in this patient, the initial procedure was excision of 15 cm. of the fourth rib. An obvious metastatic lesion was diagnosed, similar to the lesion in the prostate. Both osteoblastic and osteolytic patterns could be seen. With confirmation and diagnosis of the metastatic lesion, bilateral orchiectomy was then performed. At this institution, the therapeutic approach to patients with carcinoma of the prostate is to recommend bilateral orchiectomy at the time metastatic disease is diagnosed. If the patient relapses, he is placed on estrogen therapy, usually diethylstilbestrol.

This approach recognizes the fact that considerable controversy still remains regarding the use of hormones and orchiectomy for these patients. However, until more conclusive studies are available, or until the institutional experience suggests some other form of therapy, the policy of initial orchiectomy followed by estrogens on relapse will be continued. For the average patient with metastatic disease at the time of initial diagnosis, the 5-year survival rate is approximately 20 per cent.

In an effort to improve this situation, recent emphasis has been placed on the use of chemotherapy for prostatic cancer. This institution is participating in a randomized study evaluating the use of chemotherapeutic agents for these patients. While progress appears to be evident with the use of chemotherapy for prostatic cancer, the results are not yet sufficiently conclusive to develop and apply a protocol.

Discussion also covered the grading of prostatic tumors, and in studies of a group of patients under 50 years of age with carcinoma of the prostate, results showed that degree of anaplasia had no correlation with survival. Furthermore, several years ago, 618 patient histories were reviewed and no correlation could be found between histologic grade and survival or prognosis. In fact, depending upon where the biopsy is taken, most histologic sections will show areas of Grades I, II, and III malignancy. Furthermore, whole organ sections have shown that areas of all 3 histologic grades are intermingled in the tumors; so grading has proved to be of limited value.

FOLLOW-UP

This patient, recently released from the hospital, was approximately 6 weeks postsurgery at the time of this case discussion. The routine follow-up procedures, including the determination of phosphatase levels and radiologic evaluation of the rib area will be repeated at regular intervals in the future. This will continue for 3 years and if this patient remains in good health, the follow-up clinical visits will be scheduled at 6-month intervals. As an indication of possible prognosis, the discussion concluded with mention of 2 male patients who were recently seen in the clinic for follow-up of carcinoma of the prostate with metastasis to ribs. One patient who also had local involvement of the muscle is now 3 years postresection. He had undergone rib resection plus postoperative irradiation because of the extra rib involvement. He is now 3 years without evidence of any other metastatic lesions. The other patient is a little over 1 year postsurgery without evidence of metastatic disease. They are receiving the same follow-up procedures previously described.

CASE 3.—*Mixed Teratoma and Embryonal Carcinoma of Testis, Demonstrating the Application of Lymphangiography and Specimen Radiography.* Right inguinal orchiectomy for mixed teratoma and embryonal carcinoma of the testis had been performed for a 27-year-old Caucasian salesman before he was referred to M. D. Anderson Hospital in December 1972. His physical examination was negative at the time of admission. Intravenous pyelogram showed no abnormalities. A lower extremity lymphangiogram demonstrated metastasis in 1 para-aortic node at the level of L–3. Several other nodes were suspicious.

DISCUSSION

RADIOLOGY.—At this institution, pedal lymphangiography is performed for all patients with malignant neoplasms of the testis.

(Testicular lymphangiography cannot be used because most frequently the testicle has been removed.) This patient also had a pyelogram in which the kidneys and ureters appeared normal. However, in the lymphangiogram, 1 node at the level of L–3 was crescent shaped and contained a defect which was not traversed by lymphatics. A metastasis to a lymph node occludes the marginal sinusoids, and lymphatics cannot permeate through a focus of carcinoma. This is evidence of metastases, with an accuracy of 95 per cent. However, other conditions such as an abscess in the node, tuberculosis, or necrosis of a portion of a node occasionally can produce similar radiologic features.

NUCLEAR MEDICINE. — A gallium-67 citrate scan also was performed on this patient. Approximately 3 millicuries of gallium-67 citrate were injected and the patient scanned 48 hours later. However, this scan was interpreted as negative, probably because the node observed radiographically was too small for detection by the gallium procedure, the lower limit of which is approximately 2 cm.

PATHOLOGY. — The specimen from the orchiectomy showed at least 2 patterns of germ cell tumor. One consisted of cartilage intermixed with some tall columnar mucous epithelium. In addition, foci of poorly differentiated embryonal carcinoma were observed. The histologic diagnosis was mixed malignant teratoma and embryonal carcinoma or, colloquially, teratocarcinoma.

At the time of retroperitonel node dissection, the removed nodes were placed on a template containing an outline of the abdominal great vessels, and a radiograph of the specimen was performed (Fig. 3). This procedure, developed at this institution, helps to identify the lymph nodes which still contain contrast medium from lymphangiography. It also assists in identifying suspicious nodes and in establishing a correlation with the preoperative lymphangiogram. The large lymph node with the filling defect showed a cystic area with obvious necrosis and fibrosis. No actual tumor could be observed, but evidence of necrosis and reaction suggested the previous presence of a metastatic lesion.

RADIOTHERAPY AND SURGERY. — This patient was judged to have Stage II disease because of lymphangiographic evidence of metastatic tumor. Such patients are treated preoperatively with 2,500 rads tumor dose to the ipsilateral inguinal area and retroperitoneal nodes. This is followed within 24 to 72 hours by bilateral retroperitoneal node dissection. During the postoperative period an additional 2,500 rads are administered. The lymphadenectomy is part of the treatment program but is not a completely definitive procedure in itself. The 5-year survival rates have been about 50 per cent for for Stage II pa-

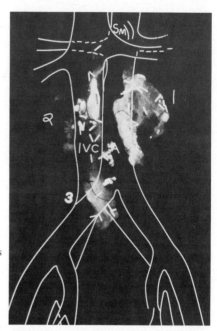

FIG. 3.—Specimen radiography assists in identifying suspicious nodes and establishing correlation with the preoperative lymphangiogram.

tients treated with radiotherapy and surgery including lymphadenectomy. In recent years, patients also have been placed on prophylactic chemotherapy, usually Velban and bleomycin, and survival rates are expected to be significantly improved within the next several years. At surgery, the lymph nodes are not removed en bloc. The left para-aortic chain is removed, then the right para-aortic chain, then the middle chain. Following the surgery and radiotherapy, this patient received multiple courses of Velban and bleomycin.

For Stage I nonseminomatous germ cell tumors in patients with no metastatic lesions, where the tumor is confined to the testis, the treatment program is retroperitoneal lymphadenectomy. It is realized that even with the most detailed surgical procedures, not all of the lymph nodes can be removed. The operation is viewed as a staging procedure, not definitive treatment. About 15 percent of patients with negative lymphangiograms will prove to have metastatic disease in the removed specimens. When lymphangiograms are considered positive, metastatic disease will be present in practically all instances; it has proved to be quite an accurate examination for clinical staging. The 10-year survival rates for patients with Stage I nonseminomatous germ cell tumors with negative lymphadenectomy are slightly over 90 per cent in a series of 76 patients treated at M. D. Anderson Hospital.

The relationship of histologic classification of germ cell tumors to selection of therapy received considerable discussion. It was emphasized that the greatest contribution of the pathologist is separation of pure seminoma from nonseminomatous germ cell tumors. Patients frequently are referred with a diagnosis of seminoma, or embryonal carcinoma and seminoma, or other tumors, when in reality, the picture probably is confused by necrotic tissue and tremendous giant cell reaction. Surgeons and radiologists agreed that it did make an extreme difference, as far as treatment was concerned, whether the patient had pure seminoma or a mixed tumor. Seminomas have proven to be radiosensitive and the prognosis is quite good. Approximately 90 to 95 per cent of patients with Stage I seminoma survive 5 years. For Stage II seminoma, more than 80 to 85 per cent survive 5 years. The treatment is radiotherapy in minimal amounts — 2,500 rads over a 3-week period. The prognosis is not as favorable for patients with nonseminomatous germ cell tumors such as embryonal carcinoma, with or without seminoma, teratoma, or teratocarcinoma. In such cases, the treatment must be much more aggressive, including retroperitoneal lymphadenectomy, more intensive radiation therapy, and chemotherapy. At this institution, differentiated teratomas in adult patients are not considered benign. Approximately 25 per cent of such tumors will metastasize. Nevertheless, elsewhere pathologists and clinicians continue to consider them benign.

FOLLOW-UP

This patient was last seen October 1973, approximately 10 months after treatment and was without evidence of recurrent disease.

CASE 4. — *Metastatic Carcinoid Tumor Masquerading as Primary Carcinoma of the Liver, Demonstrating the Diagnostic Value of Electron Microscopy.* This 50-year-old female was seen at another institution in July 1972 concerning a 6-month history of epigastric discomfort and pain in the right upper quadrant. Initial examination showed her liver to be enlarged and some evidence of a small amount of abdominal fluid. Tests showed the gallbladder to be normal. Peritoneoscopy was performed and a liver biopsy obtained. The biopsy was interpreted as being histologically compatible with primary liver cell carcinoma. The patient then received several courses of various chemotherapeutic agents but showed no significant response. In December 1972, she was referred to M. D. Anderson Hospital for consideration of hepatic artery infusion. At the time, liver scan showed a large cold area in the left and anterior right lobes of the liver. The celiac arteriogram showed a necrotic mass in the right lobe and vascular metastases in the lower portion of the right lobe as well as the lateral segment of the left lobe. On December 18, exploratory laparotomy was performed at M. D. Anderson Hospital. Extensive tumor was found in both lobes of the liver, and another biopsy was obtained. A catheter was inserted in the hepatic artery.

DISCUSSION

PATHOLOGY. — The wedge-shaped biopsy specimen from the surface of the liver measured 2 cm. The hepatic parenchyma was partially replaced by tumor. The tumor cells were relatively uniform in size and no significant pleomorphism was observed. Some small artifactual clefts were observed but no organoid formation of tumor cells could be seen. The histologic evidence favored a metastatic tumor, and carcinoid tumor was considered as one possibility; however, a primary liver cell carcinoma could not be excluded. A Fontana stain showed very fine stippling in the cytoplasm of the tumor cells, reinforcing the possibility of a carcinoid tumor.

Material was processed for electron microscopy and the findings confirmed the suspicion of carcinoid tumor. The cytoplasm of the tumor cells contained many small dense bodies. At higher magnification, the densities were seen to be spherical, membrane-bound, electron-dense aggregates of secretory material (Fig. 4). These granules are found in the cytoplasm of cells of a number of tumors, notably endocrine neoplasms which secrete polypeptide hormones. Their size range often falls within a fairly narrow limit for a particular tumor type, and this can be of some help in determining the primary site. Carcinoid tumor cells tend to have granules approximately 250 millimicrons in diameter, whereas many other tumors, for example pheochromocytoma, will have significantly smaller granules. In contrast, secretory granules in the cytoplasm of cells of exocrine tumors will be significantly larger. The histopathologic diagnosis in the present case was metastatic carcinoid tumor.

Further information was presented regarding the variations in size and appearance of the granules in carcinoid tumor cells. In bronchogenic carcinoid tumors, the granules are smaller than those from carcinoid tumors arising in the gastrointestinal tract. It has been reported that if the primary lesion is in the stomach, the granules are relatively small and uniform, whereas in tumors arising from the ileum

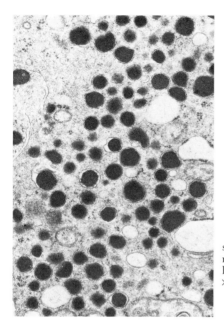

FIG. 4.—Electron micrograph showing a portion of a tumor cell with numerous electron-dense, membrane-limited granules in the cytoplasm. ×60,000.

or appendix, the granules tend to be larger and more pleomorphic. In carcinoid tumors of the rectum, the granules are relatively uniform although somewhat larger than those of the stomach. It was emphasized that these represent preliminary observations which could prove to be very useful in determining the primary site of the carcinoid tumor. Another feature was mentioned regarding carcinoid tumors from the gastrointestinal tract: They frequently contain small aggregates of microvilli identical to those found in normal gastrointestinal epithelial cells. This feature might provide an indication that a metastatic carcinoid tumor was related to a primary lesion within the gastrointestinal tract.

RADIOLOGY.—A celiac arteriogram showed the hepatic artery distribution and a huge mass. Vessels in the right lobe were elongated, stretching over or through the mass. The mass involved most of the right lobe of the liver. The oblique view showed abnormal vasculature in the left lobe in addition to the huge mass. Later phases of the arteriogram showed nodular lesions which varied in size from the huge replaced area to relatively small vascularized areas.

Arteriography can be particularly important in patients with lesions amenable to excision. Very small vascularized lesions also can be detected by this technique. Primary hepatoma was one diagnosis considered by the radiologist. The primary hepatomas may appear as relatively avascular or they may be exceedingly vascular lesions with arteriovenous shunting. Most of them are located in the hypervascular area. Although multiple small nodular lesions rarely are seen in primary hepatoma, they have been observed.

The ultimate conclusion based on the radiological findings was that the changes represented a huge focus of necrotic metastatic tumor.

NUCLEAR MEDICINE. — The preoperative liver scan was performed using technetium-99 sulfur colloid, which localizes in reticuloendothelial cells, Kupffer's cells of the liver, and spleen. Using a gamma camera, the study began with an anterior view, with lead-impregnated rubber strips taped to the costal margin to indicate the relationship of the organ to the external anatomy. The strips were then removed and an anterior view was taken without the costal margin markers. The patient was turned and the right lateral projection was taken; then a posterior projection was done. Finally, a posterior view of the spleen was made. The liver scan for this patient was abnormal, indicating massive replacement by tumor (Fig. 5). Practically no isotope was seen in the left lobe. The right lateral view showed this same replacement in the anterior portion of the right lobe. Following surgery, another liver scan, known as a catheter placement study, was performed by injecting ^{131}I-labeled microaggregated albumin through the catheter which had been placed in the hepatic artery at the time of surgery. The microaggregated albumin particles vary from 30 to 50 microns in diameter, and when injected intraarterially are filtered out in the first available capillary bed. This provided the surgeon with some indication as to the direction of blood flow from the catheter (Fig. 6). This liver scan was performed with a rectilinear scanner. The majority of radioactivity was seen in the periphery of the liver, with large gaps observed in the distribution of blood flow. These were in areas previously identified as being involved with tumor when viewed on the technetium-99 sulphur colloid scan. This indicated that the catheter was well-placed in the hepatic artery.

SURGERY AND CHEMOTHERAPY. — Over the next 4 months, the patient received repeated infusions of 5-fluorouracil at the rate of 500 mg./week. Some subjective improvement was observed and the size of the liver was slightly reduced. However, the follow-up liver scan in July 1973, 4 months after surgery, showed no significant improvement in the appearance of the liver (Fig. 7).

In retrospect, several points from the medical history of this patient were important. She had received excellent diagnostic care, including peritoneoscopy, before she was admitted to M. D. Anderson Hospital. She came with a definite diagnosis of primary liver cell carcinoma. She had received 5-fluorouracil but had not responded. Then Cytoxan had been administered but the patient had continued to lose weight and was becoming edematous and developing ascites. After telephone conversation, she was flown to M. D. Anderson Hospital by air ambulance to have the catheter placed in the liver. Because of the previous diagnostic procedures, a standard laparotomy was performed at this institution. No abnormalities other than those in the liver were found, but a more representative biopsy of that organ was obtained. Subsequent histopathologic study by both light and electron microscopy disclosed the metastatic carcinoid nature of the abnormality previously diagnosed as liver cell carcinoma. What had been interpreted as progressive and rapidly advancing disease was, in fact, the carcinoid syndrome producing diarrhea, hyperpro-

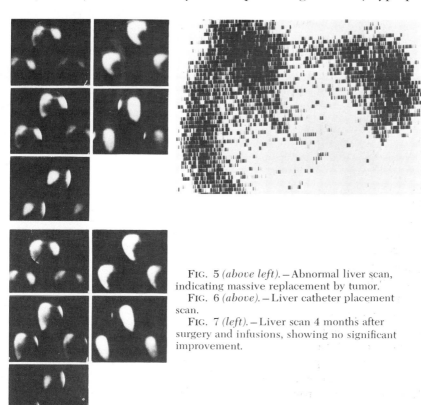

FIG. 5 *(above left)*.—Abnormal liver scan, indicating massive replacement by tumor.

FIG. 6 *(above)*.—Liver catheter placement scan.

FIG. 7 *(left)*.—Liver scan 4 months after surgery and infusions, showing no significant improvement.

teinemia, and edema. The weight loss was not because the patient had become anoretic from tumor. It was merely the result of the fact that she was not eating because this was the only way she could reduce the diarrhea which accompanies the carcinoid syndrome.

FOLLOW-UP

Following repeated infusions of 5-fluorouracil at the rate of approximately 500 mg./week, symptoms of the carcinoid syndrome were partially controlled and a moderate reduction in the size of the liver was observed. However, follow-up liver scans showed little change in the necrotic mass and vascular metastases. It was pointed out that arterial infusion usually does not significantly affect the volume of the tumor; however, it does control the carcinoid syndrome. The patient was last seen at this institution in July 1973, at which time she was returned to her referring physician for further care. The last contact was by letter. She had been off treatment for 4 months and the 5-hydroxyindole-acetic acid levels which previously had been reduced were beginning to rise. It was planned to repeat the courses of arterial infusion. The site of the primary tumor remains unknown. This represented a complicated situation in which it was very difficult to evaluate the results of the chemotherapy. Nevertheless, the institution has had several patients with massive carcinoid tumors of the liver who now have been followed for more than 5 years.

CASE 5. — *Focal Nodular Hyperplasia of the Liver in a Patient Previously Treated for Carcinoma of the Cecum.* This 40-year-old female had a right hemicolectomy for carcinoma of the cecum in May 1972 at another institution. At that time, the lymph nodes were negative but the surgeon noted that the liver appeared nodular. She had an uneventful recovery from surgical procedures and remained asymptomatic for several months. However, in October 1972, she developed epigastric fullness and complained of nausea. Her physician detected an enlarged liver, assumed to be metastatic carcinoma, and the patient was referred to M. D. Anderson Hospital. Physical examination at the time of her admission confirmed apparent enlargement of the liver. Diagnostic procedures included barium enema, which showed no evidence of colonic carcinoma, celiac arteriogram, liver and spleen scans, and liver function tests, which were normal. Exploratory laparotomy was performed and a solitary nodule was removed from the medial segment of the right lobe of the liver.

DISCUSSION

PATHOLOGY.—The resected portion of liver measured 7 cm. in greatest dimension and was firmer than normal liver. The periphery was composed of small aggregates of histologically normal liver tissue. On examination of the gross specimen, some small depressed areas with a radiating, stellate pattern could be observed corresponding to dense bands of fibrous tissue in the middle of the lesion. These were considered to be of diagnostic assistance. The needle biopsies from other areas of the liver confirmed that it was not cirrhotic. Biopsies of abdominal lymph nodes showed no metastatic tumor. Low-magnification light micrographs showed several significant features, including abundant, rather dense connective tissue which radiated through the lesion. In this connective tissue were lymphocytes, plasma cells, and a few eosinophils. At the periphery of the irregular nodules of liver cells were many small proliferating bile ducts (Fig. 8). Some of the vessels appeared thickened with hyperplastic intima and media. This patient had had previous surgical therapy for carcinoma of the cecum but no evidence of metastatic tumor was observed. The hepatocytes were not pleomorphic, indicating a benign lesion. The irregular nodules of hepatocytes were com-

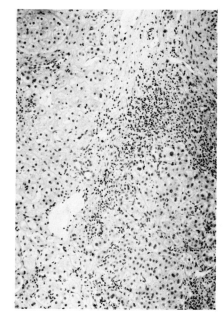

FIG. 8.—Light micrograph showing irregular clumps of hepatocytes exhibiting little pleomorphism. Surrounding the clusters are many inflammatory cells and proliferating small bile ducts. ×150.

posed of uniform, closely packed cells with little evidence of sinus-oid formation. Some of the small bile ducts were intermingled with hepatocytes. All of these features suggested a nonneoplastic entity, frequently solitary, and characteristically occurring in noncirrhotic liver referred to as focal nodular hyperplasia. In summary, the char-acteristic histologic features include (1) abundant connective tissue which radiates from the center of the lesion in a stellate fashion, (2) numerous inflammatory cells in the connective tissue, (3) prolifera-tion of bile ducts, and (4) thickening of vessel walls. The liver cells in the lesion do not exhibit significant pleomorphism and typically are arranged in irregular lobules which may be confluent or separate.

Several other points regarding focal nodular hyperplasia were dis-cussed, including reports of electron microscopic studies contrasting these lesions with hepatic adenoma. The relationship between nodu-lar hyperlasia and von Gierke's disease was mentioned, together with the suggestion that the lesions may in some way be equated with ingestion of estrogens or similar medication for cyclic hormonal treatment. Other theories concerning the etiology of focal nodular hyperplasia included the suggestion that it may be a response to lo-calized trauma to the liver or some form of localized liver cell dam-age. The most widely accepted theory appears to be that it repre-sents some form of vascular malformation. This is supported by vari-ous experimental studies. Also, it was pointed out that liver function tests were normal in this patient and that if she had had a metastatic tumor of this size, it probably would have been reflected by abnor-mal laboratory findings.

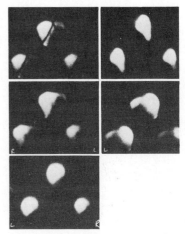

FIG. 9.—Liver scan compatible with diagnosis of focal nodular hyperplasia.

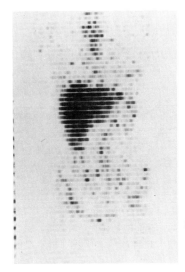

FIG. 10.—Total body scan.

RADIOLOGY.—The celiac arteriogram demonstrated a nodular lesion and suggestion of a few other small densities. The homogeneous vascularity of this lesion was unlike the avascular appearance of metastatic carcinoma. The lesion in this patient did not have a sharp line of demarcation. Similar lesions which have turned out to be adenomas usually have shown clear zones surrounding them. Whether this feature is a consistent angiographic differentiation is not yet established. All of these factors led to the suggestion of focal nodular hyperplasia as the angiographic diagnosis.

NUCLEAR MEDICINE.—The spleen and liver scans were discussed, with emphasis on some of the problems in interpreting the findings. It was pointed out that anatomical variations of the liver are numerous and it is characterized as an individualistic organ. The liver scan did demonstrate a prominent indentation which could have been interpreted as an incisura, a prominent hilus, or a tumor (Fig. 9). Such an observation is compatible with a normal variation and under these circumstances, the tendency is to call the scan normal in order to minimize errors. Therefore, even though the radiologists were aware of the fact that the patient had the tumor, the scan was reported as compatible with normal liver tissue. Likewise, the gallium-67 scan was reported as negative because no abnormal uptake could be observed (Fig. 10). It was pointed out that the reticuloendothelial elements in a lesion, such as focal nodular hyperplasia, may concentrate the isotope and result in a homogenous liver scan.

Follow-up

Following surgery, the patient had some abdominal pain, apparently from an inflamed hiatal hernia. This responded to medical treatment. When last seen in August 1973, 9 months after the operation, the patient was without evidence of disease and had no complaints.

Case 6.—*Pseudolymphoma of the Stomach, Emphasizing the Necessity for Thorough Diagnostic Procedures in Patients with Gastric Lesions.* This 59-year-old housewife was in good health until October 1970, when she had a sudden onset of nausea and hematemesis. The following day she developed pain in the right upper quadrant radiating to the right inguinal region. Persistent melena followed. She was referred to M. D. Anderson Hospital 10 days later. The initial physical examination and laboratory findings were normal. The upper GI series demonstrated a small ulcer on the greater curvature in the midportion of the body of the stomach. A raised, submucosal, ulcerating lesion on the anterior wall near the greater curvature was visualized by fiberoptic gastroscopy. Biopsy from this site showed only ulceration, chronic inflammation, and necrosis. Gastric washings were negative cytologically. The patient was treated medically for 2 months, at which time the GI series and gastroscopy were repeated. The lesion appeared essentially unchanged. Exploratory laparotomy was performed and the lesion was removed by wedge resection.

Discussion

Radiology.—Alterations were seen in roentgenograms of the greater curvature of the stomach. Although they were fairly consistent, they changed from one film to the next suggesting that there was pliability and mobility in this portion of the stomach. Hampton's line, as a thin layer of mucosa that is undermined but normal, was observed. This is a good criterion for a benign ulcer. A tumor mound or edema around an ulcer was observed, together with regular, thickened folds of mucosa. Using the following criteria—Hampton's line, the regular although edematous folds of mucosa, and a mobile portion of the stomach—the radiologic diagnosis was chronic ulcer, benign. Gastroscopy demonstrated that the lesion was raised from the surrounding mucosa making it different from benign peptic ulcer of the stomach. Although inflammatory reactions may be observed surrounding benign ulcers, they are never actually raised. The possibility could not be excluded that this lesion might be a small leiomyoma or some other benign tumor with ulceration. All ulcers observed in the stomach are routinely biopsied, and in more than 100 such cases, only 2 false-negatives have been found. Repeated biopsies taken from the edge of the ulcer showed only chronic inflammation. The radiologist could observe no involvement of the stomach surrounding the localized lesion. Therefore, the surgeon was advised that he could perform a wedge type resection for initial examination.

PATHOLOGY. — Low-power photomicrographs of the initial biopsy showed very little except normal mucosa and an infiltrate which looked lymphocytic but was quite distorted. However, in one small area, typical fibrinous exudate characteristically found at the base of a peptic ulcer was observed. This assured the pathologist that the biopsy had been from the ulcer bed. Low-power cross-sections of the entire resected lesion showed a central area of ulceration with normal mucosa on both sides and very marked lymphoid hyperplasia in the base of the ulcer. Reactive follicles were seen in the underlying tissue extending down to the muscle. This reaction was responsible for the elevation of the lesion observed by gastroscopy. At higher power, the reactive follicles were more evident against a background of lymphoid tissue and normal mucosa. The reactive follicles and lymphoid tissue contained a mixture of mature lymphocytes and histiocytic cells. A small number of plasma cells also were seen. The characteristic mixed cell infiltrate with the reactive follicles is diagnostic of lymphoid hyperplasia of the stomach, also called pseudolymphoma. This is not rare in the base of an ulcer. However, without the reactive follicles, the pathologists may have difficulty in differentiating this type of lesion from malignant lymphoma, but it is very rare to have lymphoma of the stomach composed of small lymphocytes. Most lymphomas of the stomach are diffuse and composed of immature cells in the poorly differentiated lymphocytes or histiocytes. Regarding the initial biopsy, it was observed that obtaining the specimen of any lymphoid lesion with forceps usually distorts the cells to a degree which makes it almost impossible to distinguish the various types.

Further discussion concerned the general problem of lymphomas of the stomach. The opinion was expressed that the older reports in the medical literature concerning very good survivals of patients with lymphomas of the stomach could be accounted for, in part, by the fact that nonmalignant lesions or hyperplastic pseudolymphomas were included in the series. However, some patients with unequivocal lymphoma in the stomach apparently have relatively good prognoses. This was observed to be related to the histologic type of lymphoma. Patients with nodular lymphoma, particularly the poorly differentiated lymphocytic type, apparently have relatively good survival. In contrast, patients with histiocytic lymphoma in a gastric biopsy do not have an equally good prognosis. However, it was emphasized that patients with lymphomatous lesions of the stomach apparently do better than patients with lymphoma occurring in lymph nodes. This was attributed to the fact that the lesions are localized to the stomach. Therefore, the patient has Stage I or at most Stage II disease if regional nodes are involved. Also, it was observed that in any type of lymphoma, particularly the large cell variety, some cases are unpredictable and do not necessarily have the poor prognosis usually associated with this disease.

Lymph node involvement also was discussed in relation to localized lymphoma in the stomach. In such patients, the regional lymph nodes may be very large and hyperplastic but may have no lymphomatous features. It was pointed out that in patients with lymphoma of the gastrointestinal tract accompanied by ulceration, the enlarged nodes probably result from secondary inflammatory reaction. Therefore, it should not be concluded, merely on the basis of size, that the lymph nodes are involved in the disease process. The nodes must be examined histologically in order to determine whether they are involved.

FOLLOW-UP

The patient had an uneventful recovery from surgery and was discharged on the tenth postoperative day. Subsequently, she returned to her home in Tampa, Florida, with instructions for routine postoperative management to be conducted by her family physician. She has remained well according to subsequent reports.

CASE 7.—*Carcinoma of the Cervix, Stage IIIA, Demonstrating the Interaction Between the Various Disciplines Represented on the Treatment Team.* This patient was a 32-year-old female, gravida 5, para 4, abortus 1. She developed a blood-tinged vaginal discharge in September 1971. Her physician treated her for vaginitis for several months without symptomatic improvement. In March 1972, a biopsy of the cervix showed invasive squamous carcinoma. The patient was then referred to M. D. Anderson Hospital. Her cervix was massively enlarged to about 8 cm. in diameter with an ulceration on the posterior lip and palpable induration extending into both right and left parametria. The indurated area was fixed to the left pelvic wall. No evidence of vaginal extension could be seen. The endometrial cavity sounded to a depth of 3 inches. The intravenous pyelogram was normal but pedal lymphangiography showed 2 definite metastatic nodes in the left external iliac region.

The patient was initially treated by supervoltage radiation to a dose of 1,500 rads by transvaginal cone. This was followed by selective retroperitoneal lymphadenectomy. Enlarged tumor-containing nodes were found in both sides of the pelvis and in the left para-aortic region. Following surgery, further radiation therapy was given in the form of radium to a total dose of 6,048 mgh. and external radiation to the pelvic and para-aortic nodes to a total dose of 5,435 rads. At the termination of this treatment, bulky, palpable tumor remained in the central pelvis. Additional vaginal radium was applied. Her recovery was complicated by development of a pelvic cellulitis which responded to antibiotics.

DISCUSSION

PATHOLOGY. — The patient had enlarged, invasive squamous carcinoma. The biopsy presented no diagnostic difficulties. It was classed Stage IIIA by virtue of extension to left and right parametria. The mass measured 8 to 10 cm. in diameter and was fixed to the left pelvic wall.

RADIOLOGY. — The intravenous pyelogram showed the kidneys to be normal. The ureters were interpreted as normal although some variation in ureteric distribution was seen; however, this observation was of small value in reference to possible metastatic disease. Distribution of the nodes presented some concern, in that they were dislocated medially on one side and an impression was seen on the dome of the bladder, probably as a result of an enlarged uterus. The nodal and arterial phases of the lymphangiograms demonstrated a difference in the number of nodes observed as well as abnormal nodes with crescent-shaped defects interpreted as definite evidence of metastatic disease. The hypergastric and extrailiac nodes were positive, and several large inflammatory nodes were observed. One node to the left of the aorta was suspicious. The Planning Lymphangiogram Conference dictated removal of several groups of nodes and careful sampling of others.

The specimen radiograph appeared different than that shown for the patient with testicular tumor (Case 3), because in testicular tumors, the para-aortic nodes are of greatest concern, whereas in cervical cancer, the pelvic nodes are of primary importance. The specimen films are used as a guide, with each node being numbered to correspond to a specific block. Then the block, the film, and the original lymphangiogram can be used to precisely identify the positive nodes. By this technique, nodes having only very small defects can be located even though the metastatic deposits are too minute to be shown by lymphangiography. Occasionally, soft tissue deposits of metastatic tumor adjacent to a node may fail to produce lymphangiographic defects and therefore be overlooked. Based on these findings, the patient had 6,000 mgh. of radium and 5,500 rads of external pelvic radiation. Because of residual tumor, she received additional transvaginal radiation and a boost to a positive node.

GYNECOLOGY. – The history of development of this approach to the management of patients with cancer of cervix was reviewed. In the early 1960's, a group of patients were treated by radiation, and lymphadenectomies subsequently were performed. It was noted that the incidence of positive nodes was about 50 per cent lower than that usually expected, indicating that prior irradiation therapy was effective in controlling cancer in lymph nodes. Examining these data for reasons for failure, 3 points were noted: (1) A certain number of patients had cancer outside the irradiated area, (2) another group had cancer within the irradiated area which was not controlled, and (3) a third group had cancer in both locations.

This led to the present study to determine whether extended-field radiotherapy is effective in controlling metastases from cancer of the cervix. This is a cooperative study between the gynecologists, the diagnostic radiologists, the radiotherapists, and the pathologists. Recent figures show that for Stages I or IIA cancers of the cervix, the recurrence rate is only 1.5 per cent. For patients with Stage IIB cancers, the central recurrence rate is only 5 per cent. Excess tumor volume within the irradiated field is thought to be one cause of failure. Large lesions have anoxic central compartments which are radioresistant and therefore not controlled. The present approach is to perform pre-treatment exploratory laparotomy to reduce the bulk of the tumor and determine its extent and then to plan the radiotherapy fields to encompass all of the potential residual disease. At the time of surgery, nodes are sampled around the great vessels, the vena cava, the common iliac regions, and the pelvis. If the common iliac nodes are positive to the level of L−4, the radiation fields are extended. If the aortic nodes are positive, the radiation field is extended all the way to the diaphragm, fully recognizing the effect of irradiating such large volumes of tissue.

One hundred patients with carcinoma of the cervix have been explored at this institution. On the basis of lymphangiograms, it has been possible to select the nodes which should be removed. Of the 100 patients, 56 had positive nodes. These were patients with locally advanced disease. The larger the volume of tumor, the greater the incidence of extension to regional lymph nodes. Nodal involvement was bilateral in 22 per cent of cases. If surgical dissection is too vigorous, the patient may develop a lymphocyst. Pelvic fibrosis is another problem. Of the 100 patients studied, 13 have died from complications related to extent of radiotherapy and surgical dissection, while 19 patients died of cancer. These were patients who had massive metastases in the common iliac and para-aortic nodes. Another 8 patients are living with known disease. Thus, 60 of the 100 patients are still alive as of July 1973. It should be emphasized that this study concerns only patients who have locally advanced disease.

FOLLOW-UP

This patient was last seen in October 1973. She was without evidence of disease. Recent biopsies of the cervix showed only necrotic material. Vaginal cytology has been consistently negative since the completion of treatment.

CASE 8. — *Carcinoma of the Breast, Illustrating the Importance of Careful Follow-up of Patients with Positive Thermograms and Negative Mammograms.* This 53-year-old social worker was first seen in March 1972, because of a vague mass in the right breast. She had a long history of breast nodularity but believed there had been an increase in the density of the upper outer quadrant of the right breast. On palpation, the breast was diffusely nodular and the mammary tissue was somewhat more dense in the upper half of the right breast. No discrete mass could be detected. A thermogram was interpreted as suspicious. The xeromammogram showed only scattered small calcifications bilaterally. No treatment was given. A year later, thermograms, mammograms, and physical examinations were repeated and considered normal.

In the Fall of 1973, the patient reported she thought the density in the right breast had increased in size. Slight flattening of the right nipple was observed, but no palpable mass could be detected. A xeromammogram in October 1973 was similar to previous studies, but, in addition, a discrete area of increased density and trabecular distortion 1.5 cm. in diameter was detected in the upper outer quadrant on the right. On October 10, this area was resected. By specimen radiography and frozen section, multiple nodules of invasive carcinoma were demonstrated. Radical mastectomy was performed. In the remainder of the breast specimen, several microscopic nodules of invasive carcinoma, as well as diffuse intraductal carcinoma and lobular carcinoma in situ, were detected. The specimen was negative for blood vessel invasion. No axillary lymph nodes were involved.

DISCUSSION

RADIOLOGY. — The initial thermogram performed in 1972 showed the venous heat to be greater in an area crossing the central portion of the right breast, but the mammogram was considered normal. Repeat mammograms in February 1973, demonstrated small, faint calcifications. The vessels of the right breast were fairly prominent. The mammograms of July 1973, again showed prominent vessels in the right breast (Fig.11). When the prominent vessel on the right was compared with a similar vein in the same area on the left, the diameter ratio was greater than 1:4. This, according to recent studies in this institution, strongly suggests the presence of carcinoma. The abnormal calcifications provided some measure of localization of the potential lesion.

PATHOLOGY. — The biopsy performed was essentially a quadrant resection including the site of the calcifications. The breast tissue specimen showed no distinct mass, but one area of thickening was suspicious. Specimen radiography was performed for the purpose of assuring the surgeon that he had removed the proper area and to assist the pathologist in determining where sections should be taken. The suspect region was demonstrated as an irregularly shaped mass with fine calcifications. More detailed examination disclosed not 1 mass, but 3 confluent but discrete invasive masses in a chain going from the periphery down toward the nipple. The largest mass was a small-celled tumor with a single cell infiltrating pattern which is regarded as a classical pattern for infiltrating lobular carcinoma. At higher power, however, 2 cell types could be detected. The small cells tended to be spindle-shaped and very irregular, while in another area of the same mass, the cells were polyhedral with comparatively large amounts of cytoplasm. The nuclei in this area were larger and more variable, and contained less chromatin. At the edge of the mass, a focus of noninvasive intraductal carcinama could be seen leading into the mass and presumably representing the duct from which the tumor invaded. The second mass was composed entirely of duct cell type carcinoma. The third mass appeared to be a mixture of ductal carcinoma and the single cell infiltrating pattern with smaller

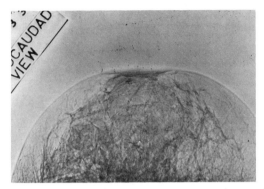

FIG. 11.—Xeromammogram showing prominent vessels in right breast.

cells. Thus, the pathologic findings showed 3 distinct masses, each of which had a different pattern. Specimen radiography was used to study the axillary contents. No positive nodes were found.

SURGERY.—This patient demonstrated 2 points: First, if suspicion is drawn to the breast in a woman 40 or over, follow-up at close intervals is necessary. This patient was followed at 3-month intervals. Second, if clinical changes are present (and there were clinical changes in this patient), another thermogram and xeromammogram should be ordered, regardless of the interval. In this patient, only a few months had passed between a negative study and one with some change in findings. This led to the diagnosis. Also, it was pointed out that the upper outer quadrant lesion was associated with a vague alteration in contour which was protuberant rather than retractive. This provided good orientation as to where to biopsy.

The present trends toward earlier diagnosis and more liberal pathologic interpretation of the material simplify some problems. The surgeon must take out an adequate amount of tissue and wait as long as 10 or 15 minutes for the frozen section diagnosis to tell him whether he had been in the right place. If the specimen is not diagnostic, then the excision must be extended. Again, the specimen must be radiologically examined, and it may prove to be negative. The surgeon may spend an entire morning on a negative case. Nevertheless, it is recommended that these early lesions be approached surgically, because when they are found they can be cured.

FOLLOW-UP

The prognosis for this patient is excellent. The lesion was in the upper outer quadrant, the nodes were negative, and the involved area was small and nonpalpable. The patient will continue to be followed at regular intervals.

Acknowledgment

The narrative summary of this panel discussion was prepared by Mary L. McCrackan, M.Sc., Department of Pathology.

Index